PRAISES FOR HACK YOUR HEALTH HABITS

"*Hack Your Health Habits* is a chock full of useful tips and information for all of us trying to live a more balanced life. Definitely a must-read for anyone looking to get healthy, naturally, inside and out."

— Adria Vasil, best-selling author of the Ecoholic book series

"Dr. Nathalie Beauchamp has dedicated her life to becoming an expert in the field, as well as sharing her health wisdom with others. I don't know many people who are as devoted to helping people live a healthy and happy life as Nathalie. I would highly recommend her new book *Hack Your Health Habits.*"

— Jeffrey Eisen, Life Coach and Author of *Empowered YOUth: A Father and Son's Journey to Conscious Living*

"*Hack Your Health Habits* is a must have for anyone who truly wants to be healthy. It has enough content to be ten books and will prove to be a fantastic investment for all of us. Dr. Nathalie has a wealth of knowledge and clinical experience and walks the reader methodically through the "how to" being healthy. We thoroughly enjoy the humor and real-life stories that are shared in this book. A brilliant insight and interpretation of the current state of health."

— Drs Mike and Celina Spencer B.Sc.,D.C.

"Dr. Beauchamp stepped up to the plate and took a huge swing at writing about the complexities of the human body and breaking them down into manageable sections that are fun and easy to read. So, whether it has been years since your last high school biology class or you are a seasoned clinician, by the time you finished reading this book you will end up saying... *"Huuum, I didn't know that"*... and whenever you learn something new... that's a home run!"

— Dr. Emile Compan B.Sc., N.D.

"Rarely am I excited for "yet another book on health." However, I am thrilled to see *Hack Your Health Habits*. It is relevant, referenced, and asks you to be responsible. This is one book I can totally recommend that asks you to make the decision and take the journey to be healthier and Dr. Nathalie shows you how to do so. I am so looking forward to read the future testimonials of empowered change from those who apply the principles within. I can say, I will be ordering a box of books for gifts to those I care about."

— Dr. Liz Anderson-Peacock BSc., D.C. CEO of Engage In Life Inc.

"This book is a Game Changer! If you apply even half of what you will learn in this book, your body, mind, and soul will be forever grateful. Dr. Nathalie is the real deal; a true warrior for wellness."

— Dr. Brian Wolfs B.Sc., D.C.

"No other industry has as many books as the health industry. Dr. Nathalie has written a incredibly comprehensive manifesto of what TRUE health is all about."

— Dr. Craig Hazel B.Sc., D.C.

"Dr. Nathalie Beauchamp is a leading authority on Health and Wellness. Her new book, *Hack Your Health Habits*, provides a well-structured, no-nonsense, scientific guide to what you need to know to take control of and improve your health. It is a simple approach that covers all the basics including identifying the right foods, using the right vitamins, how to get rid of toxins, how to improve the immune system, how the brain works and the importance of good rest. I highly recommend this book for anyone who wants to understand how the body works and wants to achieve better health and wellness."

— Deborah MacDonald, Author of *Creating Freedom*

"What an amazing book! Wow, it sure got me thinking of the health habits I need to hack. This will definitely become a go-to reference book for me. It covers it all, body, mind and soul. It's great for people like myself who finally decided to do something about their health and how to go about it. The amount of information in this book is incredible, and will definitely become useful knowledge. Thank you Dr. Nathalie!"

— France M. (patient of Dr. Nathalie)

"My new go-to trusted source! Dr. Nathalie has done an awesome job of sifting through all of the literature and presenting it one place. She makes it easier to adopt a healthier lifestyle with her suggestions in terms of different levels of habits. I am hacking away to a healthier me!"

— Ginette T. (patient of Dr. Nathalie)

"I find Dr. Nathalie's new book *Hack Your Health Habits* very enlightening. I can easily relate to several subjects, and reflect on how I do certain things and really how I should be changing them. It has really opened my eyes on how to improve my daily health habits very quickly and easily, in a variety of topics from safe cookware to taking vitamins, even to the brand of makeup I use, and so much more. This book has encouraged me to live a healthier life by making simple changes. It reads very well and I would recommend it to anyone wanting live a healthier, more vibrant life."

— Pierrette L. (patient of Dr. Nathalie)

HACK

YOUR HEALTH HABITS

SIMPLE, ACTION-DRIVEN, NATURAL HEALTH
SOLUTIONS FOR PEOPLE ON THE GO!

Hack Your Health Habits
Simple, Action-Driven, Natural Health Solutions for People On The Go!

Copyright ©2018 by Dr. Nathalie Beauchamp

Published by Rebel Press
Austin, TX
www.RebelPress.com

ISBN: 978-1-68102-810-1

Library of Congress Control Number: 2018944825

Printed in the United States of America

This book is dedicated to the people who are on a quest to be the best versions of themselves.

ix

ACKNOWLEDGMENTS

There are so many people I would like to thank for supporting me in writing this book but the list would truly be too long. From the people who inspired me to publish another book; to the people who read my chapters as I was writing and provided their constructive feedback; and to the people who helped in the publication and promotional process—you know who you are and thank you.

That being said, this book would not be possible without the patience of my husband for the countless hours on my computer researching, writing, editing, editing again and editing yet again. Thank you honey. A special thank you to Parmees Yazdanyar for her invaluable help in writing this book, if it was not for her, I would still be writing, and the book would sure not read the same. Lastly, thank you to my step-daughter and virtual assistant extraordinaire Whitley Languedoc for helping me make sense of my crazy ideas and projects and helping me get organized, execute, and making me shine and share my message and passion.

"Those who keep learning,
will keep rising in life."

— CHARLIE MUNGER

TABLE OF CONTENTS

SECTION 1: GET MOTIVATED, ORGANIZED AND PRODUCTIVE TO TAKE YOUR HEALTH HABITS TO THE NEXT LEVEL

SECTION 2: GET BACK TO BASICS—UNDERSTAND THE FOODS TO CONSUME TO KEEP YOUR BODY PERFORMING AT ITS BEST

SECTION 4: GET RID OF TOXINS—THE KEY TO REAL CELLULAR DETOX FOR OPTIMAL HEALTH

SECTION 6: GET FIT AND STRONG IN LESS TIME

SECTION 7: GET TO KNOW YOUR HORMONES AND FEEL BETTER

SECTION 8: GET YOUR GUT AND IMMUNE SYSTEM PERFORMING OPTIMALLY

SECTION 9: GET YOUR BRAIN TURNED ON TO ITS FULL POWER

SECTION 10: GET REST, RECHARGE AND BE MORE ZEN

SECTION 11: GET IN CONTROL—YOU AND YOUR WELLNESS TEAM

SECTION 12: GET ON PURPOSE—DESIGNING THE LIFE YOU WANT

PREFACE

WE ALL HAVE A STORY

"Owning our story and loving ourselves through that process is the bravest thing that we'll ever do."

— BRENE BROWN

Each person has a unique story. The obstacles and opportunities we have faced have led us to who and where we are today. The amazing thing about our story is that we are in control of it. While we cannot choose every circumstance in our lives, we can choose how we react to each one. We may have had a difficult past or felt that we were dealt an unfair hand, but we can always decide what happens next. We can analyze who we are and where we are in our lives, and then make changes accordingly.

As a preface to this book, I thought it was important to share my own story with you. I want you to know exactly from where my drive and insatiable thirst for knowledge and ideas stem. I hope that you will also take time to reflect on your own story. Understanding who you are and what influences you are important steps when looking to implement healthy lifestyle changes.

MY STORY

I grew up in Montébello, a small town in Québec, Canada, where I was blessed with incredibly supportive and loving parents. I enjoyed school and sports and was always on the go. All was well until the summer of 1983. At 14 years old, my simple life became a heck of a lot more complex. I noticed my body changing. I was very athletic and much more muscular than the other girls in school. I decided that I wanted to be thinner. I started watching what I ate and spent the majority of my summer at the local pool and on the tennis court. When school started in the fall, all my friends told me how great I looked. That's when being thin became an obsession.

At a height of 5'9", I went from being a healthy 128 pounds to a shocking 89 pounds in only a few months. I remember going to a provincial volleyball tournament that fall. Despite being one of the best players on the team, my coach benched me. I was livid. I'm guessing that he was too afraid to play me, and I don't blame him. I looked sickly and weak. I knew I would have to start eating if I wanted to be allowed back on the volleyball court but I could not bring myself to do it. It was like I had lost control of my mind. Food became an enemy. The more people urged me to eat, the less I could. My parents tried helping, but they were at a loss. They brought me to Sainte-Justine Hospital in Montréal, where I stayed for over a month. Though the team there did the best they could, I found it difficult to relate to anyone. What did my 45-year-old bearded psychiatrist know about being a 14-year-old anorexic girl? I felt so alone and did not know how to get out of the dark hole I was in. I was scared.

One day, while taking a bath in the dark—I could not stand the sight or feel of my own body—I had a pivoting moment. I had to do something or I would die. I had to regain control of myself and get better. Nobody else could do it for me. I realized that I was being selfish. My health was impacting not only me, but also my parents and the people who loved me. I realized that I was put on this planet for a reason and I had a purpose to fulfill. Dying at 14 years of age was *not* my purpose. I realized that I had to make health my number one priority if I wanted to live. I realized that I had to take control of my mind and make my own decisions on what was right for me. I could not let classmates, the media, or marketing agencies tell me how to look or how to behave. I had to think for myself.

It became my quest to get better, healthier and stronger, so I read everything I could. I became a student of nutrition, fitness, mindset and anything to do with personal development and performance. I was on a journey to heal myself, to learn and to help others. Around that time, my family started seeing a chiropractor. Interestingly, the chiropractor only spoke English and we only spoke French. I did not understand exactly what he was doing but he was helping my mother with her frozen shoulder, my dad with his anxiety, my uncle with his constipation, and my cousin with her chronic ear infections. I thought to myself, *How cool is this guy's job? He helps people with his hands. No drugs or surgery.* I saw his diplomas on the wall. They were from English schools, and all from the United States. I thought to myself, *Well, there goes that idea. We don't have that kind of money, and I don't speak English.*

I had always been good in school. I liked science and a challenge, so when a friend of mine joined military school, I thought it might be the right fit for me too. That first year in military college was my first encounter with failure. As much as I liked the military experience, I quickly realized that engineering was not for me. I kept joking that if I had to build a bridge, it would collapse! This was an important learning experience for me. My decision to leave was not an easy one, but I knew in my heart that my education and career had to align with my core values and purpose if I wanted to be happy and fulfilled.

Eventually, I entered the French stream of the Human Kinetics program at the University of Ottawa. While in school, I waitressed at a local restaurant; it was a great experience, and I learned a lot about people and their behaviors. I also learned a bit of English. So, when I heard about a chiropractic school in Toronto, I thought, *If I can get by serving people in English at the restaurant, how hard could it be to go to school in English?* As Tony Robbin says, *"It is not about the resources, but about being resourceful."* And resourceful, I was. I barely spoke English and did not have the money but somehow, I found a way. After eight years of postgraduate studies, I became a chiropractor!

Chiropractic school gave me the tools to help people with their physical symptoms: neck pain, back pain, etc. However, it was only after being in practice for a few months that I really started to understand the power of the nervous system on one's overall health and well-being. I started seeing amazing transformations in my patients. I heard reports of no more headaches after twenty years, depression lifting, couples being able to conceive after years of trying, kids having better focus in school, and entire families no longer plagued with recurrent colds and flus.

The power of chiropractic became so obvious to me; I was astonished. I was seeing first-hand how chiropractic was changing people's lives, their relationships, their overall performance, and even their outlook on life. I was now on a quest to be the best doctor I could be for my patients. I wanted to be that resource I did not have when I was 14 years old.

Although I chose to become a chiropractor, the more I think about it, the more I realize that the profession actually chose me. But I have to admit—it has not always been easy. As a chiropractor, you are often challenged and criticized. You are told that you are not a real doctor and that your philosophy is wrong. It can be frustrating, but seeing all these amazing results and being part of a person's health journey makes it all worthwhile.

Chiropractors give their patients the ability to perform and function at their highest potential and live a life of wellness by removing nerve interferences that impact cells, tissue and organs in the body. Ultimately, chiropractors "sell" well-being and optimal function.

Promoting a healthy lifestyle can be difficult in a world where we pay more for a cure than for prevention. Despite this, I know I am meant for more than relieving my patients' aches and pains. My purpose in health is to educate people and provide them with the tools to think critically and create habits that generate a fulfilling life. I want to help people realize the importance of taking control of one's health and well-being because no one else can do it for them. Too often it takes a cancer diagnosis or a brush with death from a heart attack for them to finally take their lifestyle and habits seriously.

I am always searching for ways to spark people's interest in health so they don't have to suffer from illness later on. Just as I invest in myself to be a better doctor, businesswoman and speaker, I believe everyone should invest in themselves physically, emotionally and spiritually in order to design a life they want to lead: a life of meaning. I learned from my own struggles with language barriers, starting a practice from scratch, and dedicating my life to continual growth and personal improvement, that we can *all* design a life that is intentional. Even if we have to start small, it is important to find our passion and help others get to where they want to be by adding value to their lives. In turn, value is added to ours.

Along my journey, I was influenced by many people: educators, authors, speakers and motivators. From attending conferences, taking courses, reading books and doing online programs, I was able to develop into the person I am today. I still continue to learn and grow by feeding my mind with information. Countless people have influenced me through their teaching, experience, guidance, advice and partnership in ways that I cannot explain and that I am so thankful for. They have opened my eyes to the realms of spirituality, business, self-knowledge, purpose, leadership and health. Their influence has helped me create a practice and lifestyle that I am proud of. I truly believe everyone must commit themselves to continuous and ongoing learning.

WHY I WROTE THIS BOOK

If there's one thing I've learned as a natural health practitioner over the past twenty-plus years, it's that a "one-size-fits-all" approach doesn't work for most things. The same goes for this book. Not everything I've written will resonate with everyone who reads it. Some of you will take in the information and adapt the methods to what works for you. Some of you may feel compelled to delve deeper into a certain area that really hits home. I hope that it ignites something in you, or speaks to your intuitive sense in a way that moves you to explore different areas of health in greater depth.

There will be people who will find the more technical sections in some chapters of the book somewhat challenging. If so, I encourage you to bypass it for a bit, move on, and maybe come back to it again later on. This is not to say that I dismiss anything included in the book as extrinsic or dispensable; however, some information may be pertinent only later on for you.

This book isn't a solo diet plan, or an exercise routine, or even a vitamin regimen. The information and ideas are here to make you think about your health, and to provide you with the most relevant, innovative information and processes available today. I want my readers to understand how much control they truly have over their habits and ultimately their realities.

This book is also to make you realize that wellness is subjective; there are countless ways of approaching health and addressing conditions and diseases in ways that are effective and natural, yet you must find the approaches that are right for *you*.

In addition, I also want my readers to realize that true wellness is all-encompassing, multi-faceted, and unique to each individual. I want to shift the one-size-fits-all, diagnosis-based mindset that our society has adopted toward health and direct the attention to getting to the root causes of today's most common health concerns. In other words, get to the "why" of ailments.

THE NEW ERA

There is a new wave of personalized medicine that is developing, which emphasizes the importance of taking each person's unique nature and nurture into account. With this, the future of medicine is shifting toward an approach that includes the various aspects of one's health, such as genetic make-up, biochemistry, physical and mental health in order to help each person reach their own subjective potential.

Now, some of you might be wondering, "Why cram so much into one book?" Most health and wellness authors focus on one thing and one thing only: a certain meal plan, an exercise regime, or a specific health protocol. The thing is, not everyone reading a book needs to become an expert. In fact, knowing a bit about a lot can go a long way when it comes to your health.

The twelve sections in this book are based on the questions and health problems I hear and see in my practice every single day. Each is an important piece in one's overall health and well-being. The "hack your health" concept—which will be discussed in detail in the first chapter—is all about creating action. What good is information if you don't put it into action? Too often in my practice I hear patients say: "I know, I know. I have to exercise and eat better," and yet they never seem able to act on it. I wanted to create something that didn't just get you thinking about health, but encourage you to take action and make positive changes.

My passion in life is optimal health and the expression of our human potential. Helping people help themselves is what I do, and what I love to do. This book is a product of this passion and philosophy. It's a collection of almost everything you need to plan your health goals and begin your journey to greater health and wellness.

So, I want to congratulate you for picking up this book, for making the decision to take control of your health and establish good habits. The work you do while reading this book will contribute to a lifetime of well-being. Congratulations!

> "Don't go through life, grow through life."
>
> — Eric Butterworth

WHO IS THIS BOOK FOR?

No matter where you fall on the health spectrum, I am sure this book will bring you value. Whether you are just starting on your health journey or far down the road, I'm certain that *Hack Your Health Habits* will inspire you to make positive changes. I do realize that everyone is at a different level. If you happen to be a beginner or fall somewhere in the middle, rest assured—you don't have to implement everything in this book right away.

For some, even taking a daily dose of vitamins is a struggle. It's taken me a long time to get to where I am today. Through much research and a commitment to leading a healthy life, I learned how to hack my *own* health habits and create the vibrant life I now live. With a little help from this book, I'm confident that you can do the same. Though some of the health hacks discussed may seem out of reach at present, don't worry. This book isn't meant to overwhelm you with information. In fact, to help you implement new habits, I have designed a *Hack Your Health Habits Worksheet* that you can download and print to follow along as you read through the chapters. This will not only help you internalize the information, but also will assist you in integrating what you learn from this book into your daily life. You can download the worksheet by visiting:

www.hackyourhealthhabits.com/worksheets

You don't have to implement every hack right away; take it from Catherine. Throughout the book, you will notice comments, ideas and questions from our "character reader," Catherine. Catherine's comments are meant to help clarify the concepts discussed in this book. She will talk about her family, friends and personal health struggles. She will also give tips and tricks that can help you on your health and wellness journey. You may notice that Catherine is more eager to try some hacks than others. She realizes that she can't tackle everything at once. Instead, she focuses on key health hacks in order to be successful. I encourage you to take the same kind of approach when hacking your own health.

To differentiate between Catherine's comments and regular text,

 her comments will look like this.

Note that while these comments are meant to help, you can skip over them, if you prefer. Consider them an added bonus!

SO, WHO IS CATHERINE?

 I wouldn't exactly consider myself a "health nut," but I do try my best to keep my family and me healthy. I do make an effort to occasionally buy some organic products, I work out two to three times per week at a local gym, and I do like to stay up to date on

the latest health trends. I am a 42-year-old mother of two girls (aged eleven and thirteen) and own a home with my husband of fifteen years in the suburb of a big city. I have a Bachelor's degree in Business Administration and work full time at a telecommunications company as a Development Manager.

My core values are family, health and personal development. I also value honesty, humor, physical activity, adventure and loyalty. I really believe that taking care of myself allows me to be a better mother, wife, friend and family member. I keep my kids actively involved in sports and want them to grow up as confident, healthy young women. My goals are to keep improving myself and to grow as a person with an informed and open mind. I want to lead a healthy and vibrant life for years to come and know that hacking some of my not-so-great health habits will play a big role in this.

Now that you know Catherine a little better, before we get started, there is one more thing I would like to address.

Health is our most prized asset, but how do we measure our *net worth* in respect to our well-being? When it comes to money, it is easy to measure how rich we are by looking at our bank accounts. How could we possibly give health a similar value? What separates the wealthy from the not-so-wealthy? I wish measuring how health-rich we are was as easy as getting a monthly bank statement but unfortunately, it is not. Even though we can't truly measure our "health worth," I still gave it my best shot and created what I called a *Health Currency Questionnaire*. The questionnaire is a thorough assessment that attempts to measure how health-rich you are when it comes to your health knowledge and the integration of that knowledge in your lifestyle. I recommend you do the quiz before and after you have read and implemented the tips, tools and strategies you will learn in this book. My goal is for you to be "worth" a *lot* more after reading *Hack Your Health Habits!*

To complete the Health Currency Questionnaire, please go to

www.hackyourhealthhabits.com/healthcurrencyquiz

SECTION 1

Get Motivated, Organized and Productive to Take Your Health Habits to The Next Level

Want to know the secret to building lasting habits, managing your energy, staying motivated and getting stuff done? Section 1 introduces you to the *Hack Your Health Habits* process—the ultimate formula for implementing long-lasting healthy habits.

1

HABITS
You Are What You Do—The Key to Unlocking Your Health Habits

THINK IT OVER

- What are some current habits that you would like to change in the coming week/month/year?

- What are some new habits that you would like to implement in the coming week/month/year?

- How will your life benefit from incorporating these habits into your daily routine?

"First we form habits, then they form us."

— JIM ROHN

Habits are the everyday behaviors that shape who we are. We are the sum of what we do; our repeated behaviors ultimately create our identity. As creatures of habit, we develop behaviors—some good and some not so good—to make things easier for ourselves. Essentially, a habit is a behavior we repeat with little conscious effort.

Consider your morning routine: You wake up, make breakfast, take a shower, get dressed and drive to work. You may still be half-asleep when performing these tasks, but you complete them nonetheless; it's like you're running on autopilot. Habits help us save time, effort and energy. Adopting good habits can help propel us to a better state of health and well-being. While motivation is needed to get us started, learning to harness the power of habits can help sustain our motivation so that we can achieve our goals.

Creating good habits is a way of leveraging our brain's capability to create positive change. The more we establish good habits, the less willpower we need to use, and the easier good behaviors become.

"We are what we repeatedly do. Excellence then, is not an act, but a habit." These are sobering words from Aristotle, and an astute reminder that success doesn't always come right away. I am sure you have heard someone described as "an overnight success." Do you really believe that this is the case, or is this person's success the outcome of perseverance and countless hours spent learning their craft?

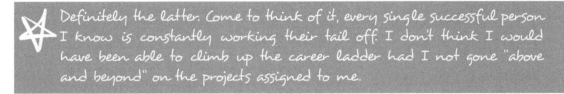

Definitely the latter. Come to think of it, every single successful person I know is constantly working their tail off. I don't think I would have been able to climb up the career ladder had I not gone "above and beyond" on the projects assigned to me.

Remember, we can take control of the development of our habits.

A BRIEF BIOLOGY OVERVIEW

Habits are an efficiency tool for the brain. Our brains are wired for pattern recognition; if they pick up on repetitive behaviors, they will expend less energy to produce that behavior. This ability to change and adapt to our environment is called *neuroplasticity*. As neural connections in the brain create associations between actions and behaviors, new neural pathways are generated, resulting in the development of 'automatic behaviors.'

There are three parts of the brain that are responsible for pattern recognition and the development of neural pathways:

- **The reptilian brain,** the oldest part of the brain, consists of the cerebellum and brainstem and is responsible for autonomic functions, such as body temperature, breathing, heart rate, sweating and even walking. It is also the part of the brain that controls our compulsive primal instincts.

- **The limbic brain**, which consists of the hippocampus, hypothalamus and amygdala. This part of the brain is considered the emotional control center through its ability to develop memories, feel experiences and protect us from risky behaviors.

- **The neocortex,** is the newer portion of the cerebral cortex that serves as the center of higher mental functions for humans. It is responsible for learning, consciousness and abstract thinking.

We are complex, aren't we? To put it simply, these three sections of our brain interplay to recognize patterns. Recognized patterns are neurologically ingrained in order to reduce energy expenditure. In the same way, habits that are not so favorable never fully dissolve, despite our efforts to avoid them.

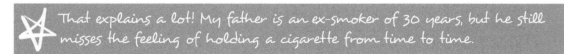

That explains a lot! My father is an ex-smoker of 30 years, but he still misses the feeling of holding a cigarette from time to time.

Once the neural pathways of habits are developed, chances are high they will be continually triggered.

A BRIEF PSYCHOLOGY OVERVIEW

Psychologists Ivan Pavlov and B.F. Skinner were pioneers in the understanding of motivation and habit development. Pavlov developed an experiment demonstrating what is known today as *classical conditioning*. He discovered that repeated exposure to an unconditioned stimulus paired with a neutral stimulus creates a conditioned response. That is, he noticed that with the introduction of food, his test subjects – dogs – began salivating. This was an unconditioned response. However, he discovered that if he rang a bell (a neutral stimulus) before introducing their food several times, the dogs would automatically begin salivating at the sound of the bell. They had been conditioned or developed a habit of associating the sound of a bell with food.

Similarly, B.F. Skinner conducted an experiment with rats that demonstrated the importance of behavior reinforcement through punishment or reward. Skinner showed how rewards work by placing a hungry rat in his "Skinner box." The box contained a lever on the side, and, as the rat moved about the box, it would accidentally knock the lever. Immediately, a food pellet would drop into a container next to the lever. The rats quickly learned to go straight to the lever after a few times of being put in the box. The outcome of receiving food ensured that they would repeat the action again and again. This is known as positive reinforcement, which strengthens a behavior by providing a consequence an individual finds rewarding.

These studies apply to humans: Our minds are programmed for automatic behavior through cues, repeated behaviors and rewards.

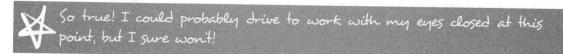

So true! I could probably drive to work with my eyes closed at this point, but I sure won't!

DEVELOPING HEALTHY HABITS

Developing healthy habits requires quite a bit of conscious effort since they take a while to install in our minds. For habits to develop, certain actions and behaviors need to be repeated in a patterned sequence multiple times before they are recognized and hardwired.

The first thing to think about when wanting to develop a habit is to ask yourself *why?* What importance does this action or behavior have to you? What will be the benefits of creating this habit? Does this habit help bring you closer to your personal goals?

We need to have a big enough *why factor* to actually want to commit to changing or creating a behavior. A healthy habit needs to have meaning for us in order for us to implement it; it either helps us become more productive or establishes a positive change in our lives.

Once we have established a strong enough reason to want to change a behavior or develop a new one, we must implement a proper strategy and take action to have it drilled down into our subconscious. This ensures that the behavior does not deplete our limited reservoir of will and discipline.

Following these steps is *key* when adopting a new habit:

- **Prioritizing** – Creating a new habit takes mental and physical energy. Don't overextend yourself with too many new goals. The key is to focus on developing one significant habit at a time while conserving energy. Focusing on individual changes helps minimize distractions and allows you to delve deeper into obtaining that one change. The two components of this step are to determine the new habit and to truly commit to it.

- **Establishing triggers** – These are cues and reminders that generate an autonomic response in the brain. Create an environmental support that will encourage the implementation of your new habit. For example, leave yourself notes or set reminders in your calendar.

- **Setting patterns** – Incorporate actions into your day-to-day activities and develop a routine that your brain will recognize. Focus on the frequency of the behavior and practice it daily so that the psychological and physical patterns develop in your mind.

- **Setting rewards** – Extrinsically motivate your brain to crave a reward the next time you repeat the behavior.

For example, a simple habit to take your shoes off upon arriving home. You probably don't think much about doing it, but you have made it a habit. There is a mental link formed between getting home (the trigger) and your response to that trigger (taking your shoes off). And the reward is not bringing dirt on your floors.

HOW TO DEVELOP HEALTHY HABITS

You will never change your life until you change something you do daily. The secret of your success is found in your daily routine.

- John C. Maxwell

So, how long does it take to develop a habit? Some say twenty-one days; others say six to eight weeks, but how long it takes really depends on the perceived level of difficulty of the habit you want to acquire and how important it is to you. Habits are a process, not an event. Understanding this key aspect of pattern development from the beginning makes it easier to manage expectations and to commit to making incremental changes. When we have a strong desire for the expected outcome, there is a greater inclination to continue the habit.

EXAMPLES OF HEALTHY CONDITIONING

Here are a few examples of triggers, repeated behaviors, and rewards that can be set and maintained in order for a healthy habit to form:

TRIGGER SUGGESTIONS:

- Lay out your workout clothes the night before so that upon waking you are immediately reminded to work out.

> ⭐ *I have even heard of people who sleep in their workout clothes so that they are ready to go in the morning!*

- Leave your daily vitamins beside your car keys to remember to take them.
- Leave a book on your nightstand to remind yourself to read before bed instead of scrolling on your phone or tablet.

REPEATED BEHAVIORS:

- Establish a certain routine at the grocery store that allows you to avoid aisles with unhealthy temptations.

PUNISHMENT:

- Remember how awful it feels to be hungover, to avoid excessive drinking on a night out.

REWARD:

- Remember you may get recognition at work for the extra effort you put in.

A simple way to achieve this is to decide and commit to changing one bad habit and/or adding one new healthy habit each month. Sounds doable, right? This will help you to set manageable and achievable micro-goals. By the end of the year, if you stick with your plan, you will have changed 12 habits!

As mentioned earlier, our habits make us who we are, and we want to remain as congruent with our goals and values as possible. Think to yourself: Who am I? Who do I wish to be? Do my behaviors reflect this? Remember, you are in full control of your actions. I often go as far as asking myself: *How would 'so and so' whom I look up to and admire behave regarding this habit?*

HACK YOUR HEALTH HABITS

My intent with this book is to help you become more aware of your current habits and to discover some new ones that you would like to acquire. The creation of a new habit may seem like a complicated undertaking. To make things easier, I have created a "Habit Hacking Process" that will guide you, step by step, through the phases of habit acquisition. This will help to make the implementation of new habits less intimidating!

Why did I choose the word "hacking?" Well, a "hack" is a clever solution to a programming or computer problem, and "hacking" implies using a novel shortcut or getting around a barrier in a resourceful way. This same concept can be used when wanting to change undesirable habits. The word change elicits negative feedback as, often times, it is associated with effort, with sacrifice, and with stepping out of our comfort zone. Now this 'comfort zone' is not a hypothetical place; it is very well established in our brains. In fact, it is hardwired into our own programming. That's right, our behaviors and habits are quite literally ingrained in our mind through neural connections. You have most likely heard of the saying *neurons that fire together, wire together.* This means that repeated behaviors become programmed in our unconscious minds, making it very difficult to break free.

Fear not, for this is not permanent. This is where our "hacks" come into play. New behavior patterns can be established by creating new neural pathways and thus ingraining new habits. These hacks are small triggers and cues that you can add to your routine to help develop the appropriate habits you are looking to create with maximum change with minimum effort.

As you read through the chapters, note the behaviors and routines that you would like to add to your current lifestyle. If you are struggling to think of changes, don't worry, I provide examples of hacks at the end of each chapter to guide your thinking.

THE THREE HACK-YOUR-HEALTH LEVELS

In my years of experience in the health field, I've found that most health habits fall into three different levels in terms of their complexity and difficulty in execution.

WHAT IS A LEVEL ONE HACK?

It is a simple habit that can be executed quickly and easily and is often a one-time effort.

Examples include:

- replacing your deodorant with a natural deodorant
- replacing your cooking oil with a healthier oil
- replacing your brand of multivitamin with a healthier brand

THE FIVE STEPS TO A LEVEL ONE HACK:

1. **Be aware:** What have you become aware of that you would like to change? What have you learned that you would like to add to your daily routine?

2. **Decide:** Make the decision to make a change. Set a goal and affirm why it is important to you.

3. **Plan:** What are the steps you need to take to implement this habit? What is your overall plan?

4. **Implement:** What do you need to do to follow through with your plan of action? How will you integrate the steps of your plan into your daily life?

5. **Reflect:** What did and did not work, and what could have been done differently to achieve greater results next time? How do you feel when the habit or change has been fully implemented? How does it improve your current lifestyle?

WHAT IS A LEVEL TWO HACK?

A more complex habit that requires the implementation of a routine to be sustainable.

Examples include:

- taking vitamins daily
- working out four times per week
- eating 6–8 servings of vegetables every day

THE SEVEN STEPS OF A LEVEL TWO HACK:

There are two new steps added to the ones from a Level One Hack.

1. **Be aware.**
2. **Decide.**
3. **Plan.**
4. **Implement.**
5. **Repeat:** For a behavior to become a habit, your brain must have repeated exposure to it to develop the neural pathways that create the automatic response. Repeating the behavior speeds its development, requiring less effort and willpower each time you perform it.
6. **Identify distractions:** Be aware of your potential distractions and what may hinder your progress. When you recognize and identify the things that can derail your efforts, you can plan around them and avoid interference.
7. **Reflect.**

WHAT IS A LEVEL THREE HACK?

A Level Three hack is changing the hard habit you have been wanting to change for a long time but can't seem to accomplish.

Examples include:

- establishing a regular weekly workout routine
- eliminating gluten or dairy completely from your diet
- meditating every day

THE NINE STEPS OF A LEVEL THREE HACK:

1. **Be aware.**
2. **Decide.**
3. **Plan.**

4. **Implement.**

5. **Repeat.**

6. **Identify distractions.**

7. **Be accountable:** Because this habit is identified as a difficult hack, it's advisable to have someone, besides yourself, to whom you feel accountable and who helps you to stay on track. Accountability is a huge aspect of remaining motivated toward your goal.

8. **Reflect.**

9. **Celebrate:** When it comes to habit changes, rewarding yourself when you are successful with the harder habit changes helps you stay motivated and excited.

This step-by-step procedure will not only provide you with the breakdown of habit development, it will also prepare you to stay on track and motivated as you progress through each "Habit Hack." With just a few easy steps, you now have a systematic plan that will allow you to implement positive change in your life! Just choose the hacking level, and hack away!

HOW TO USE THIS BOOK

After each chapter or section, make a list of all the habits that you wish to change. What are each of their triggers, routines and rewards? How can you alter a trigger, repeated behavior, or reward/punishment to get your desired outcome? What might this look like?

The following tables show examples of healthy habits to help paint a clearer picture. A template worksheet is available to download online to help you implement the hacks you are learning in each chapter:

www.hackyourhealthhabits.com/worksheets

READY #HEALTHHACKER?
EXAMPLES OF LEVEL 1, 2 AND 3 HACKS FOR THIS CHAPTER

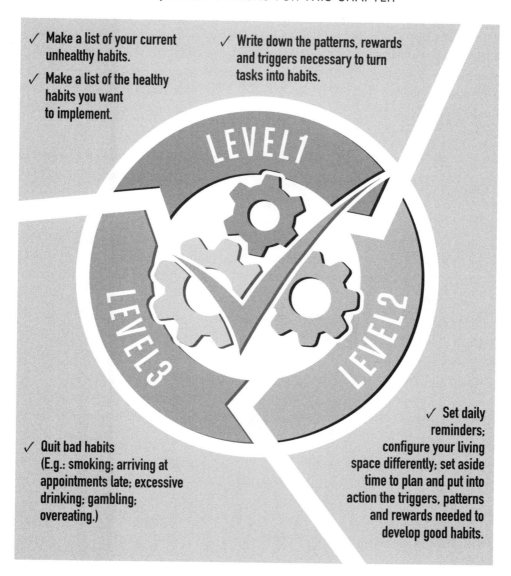

✓ Make a list of your current unhealthy habits.

✓ Make a list of the healthy habits you want to implement.

✓ Write down the patterns, rewards and triggers necessary to turn tasks into habits.

✓ Quit bad habits (E.g.: smoking; arriving at appointments late; excessive drinking; gambling; overeating.)

✓ Set daily reminders; configure your living space differently; set aside time to plan and put into action the triggers, patterns and rewards needed to develop good habits.

HACK YOUR HEALTH PROGRESS

CHAPTER 1

2 MOTIVATION
Are You Falling Short?

"Motivation is like food for the brain. You cannot get enough in one sitting. It needs continual and regular top-ups."

— Peter Davies

THINK IT OVER

- When in pursuit of a goal, are you identifying a strong enough "why" factor to keep you on track?

- Do you have a strong support system of people who will constructively encourage you toward your goal?

- Who are your role models, and what habits or behaviors can you adopt from them?

When asking people what their greatest challenge is in reaching their goals, the number one answer I get is *staying motivated*. People seem to have difficulties remaining focused on accomplishing what they have set out to do. After all, without consistent motivation, enthusiasm toward goals diminishes, along with the drive to accomplish them.

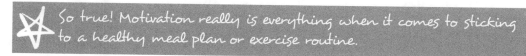

So true! Motivation really is everything when it comes to sticking to a healthy meal plan or exercise routine.

Motivation brings efficiency and productivity; it brings on the drive to create, to challenge ourselves and to change. It brings a desire to create the life we want and prepares us for whatever it takes to achieve our goals, regardless of obstacles. The truth is that many of us lack this drive in certain areas of our lives. However, that does not have to be the case. *You are not meant to be like everyone else.* You create your own goals, and, ultimately, your own accomplishments. The desire to change and create is implicit in goal-setting. It must be nurtured throughout the process in order to maintain motivation. Think of the difference between a person who jumps out of bed at the crack of dawn, fully motivated to start their day, versus the person who hits the snooze button continuously all morning. There are doers, and there are wishers!

Motivation requires a certain amount of emotion. Knowing something must get done is not enough to propel you into doing it. You must *feel* something on an emotional and physical level. This is what causes you to desire a certain outcome. As with any other skill, the more you practice and put it to use, the stronger you become at it, and the more easily it will come to you.

The term motivation describes *why* a person thinks, acts and behaves a certain way. Motivation causes us to act; it is the force that pushes us to do the things we do. When it comes to the source of motivation, we must have a big enough reason, motive, or *why* factor to keep us focused and determined to get it done. Our goals drive us only when they are important and valuable to us. When our *why* is big enough, we will figure out the *how*.

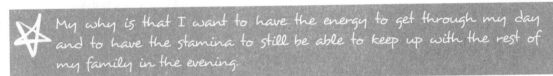

My why is that I want to have the energy to get through my day and to have the stamina to still be able to keep up with the rest of my family in the evening.

This *why* factor is affected by our locus of control—that is, whether we are driven by external factors (*extrinsic* motivation) as in rewards or punishments, or an inner drive (*intrinsic* motivation), such as an interest in or enjoyment of the task at hand. People are intrinsically motivated when they believe they possess the required skills to reach their goals. As a result, they become fully committed to mastering those skills and recognize their power to influence their performance. Extrinsic motivators include rewards that we are either offered or have set for ourselves. Both forms are necessary in order to persist and remain motivated in the long run.

When you feel as though you're not motivated, ask yourself:

- What is it that is stopping me?
- Is the task too difficult?
- Am I unclear about the outcome I want?
- Is my objective interfering with another goal?
- Do I believe that I truly have what it takes to get there?

It's important to identify and evaluate your personal goals, while being cognizant of the potential obstacles you will face and the intrinsic/extrinsic motivators that will help you stay on track to achieve your goals. The key is preparation; to succeed in achieving a particular outcome, you must identify realistic objectives required to move closer to the goal.

It also helps if the goal is something that is intrinsically motivating; that way, the effort expended will feel rewarding in itself. And finally, it is important to be aware that goals can change with time; as we go through various stages of life, our values, beliefs and personal goals will change.

However, people are often unaware of the value of setting personal goals. It's a natural human tendency to take the easy route, meaning we tend to choose paths that don't challenge us. We seek to avoid the pressure and the hurdles that, when overcome, actually serve to strengthen us.

> Goal-setting has played a huge role in my marriage. We started goal-setting together early on in our relationship, and I really credit it for getting us to where we are today.

One way of preventing this is to think like an entrepreneur. Entrepreneurs are almost always looking to grow and further expand their reach. Successful entrepreneurs are open to change because they know that change brings opportunity. The more they learn, the more they can earn; the more they acquire, the more value they can add to their company and deliver to their clients. The more successful they are, the more impact they have. If we could see ourselves through the eyes of a thriving entrepreneur and model our lives with similar planning and ambition, we, too, would strive to expand our own learning and performance in our daily life.

One key thing to keep in mind for goal-setting is that success and achievement are subjective. Success can come in many forms and mean different things to different people. For example, Elizabeth views success as becoming the youngest CEO in her company's history, while Margaret views success as raising three children to be productive members of society.

Learning a new skill, losing weight, or closing a business deal are all versions of success. First, we must define what success means to us and what accomplishments will bring us satisfaction. What are our priorities? When we sit back to reflect on our life in our golden years, what will make us proud?

The truth is, your future is contingent upon your immediate and long-term decisions and choices. You are in the driver's seat, and every thought, attitude and habit is a factor in determining your future. With positive affirmations and your own vision of success, you can plan and take action. The greatest challenges are embracing change, tolerating discomfort and resisting the need for immediate gratification in favor of later results. In facing these challenges, you become adaptable and persistent, accepting that, in reality, the only constant factor in life is change.

This is work. We don't always want to make sacrifices or be patient while waiting for results. Enter motivation. When we're motivated, our *why* exceeds our doubts and keeps us moving forward, despite the inevitable hard stuff that comes along the way. Fear of failure is often what may limit us from completing what we seek to accomplish. Or, we may fear success when we're unsure of what lies ahead. If you acknowledge that these limits are self-imposed and begin to master a motivated mindset, you'll find that excuses and distractions fade away.

You may have heard the saying: "Life is a marathon, not a sprint." This expression is supposed to show us how our journey through life takes time and constant effort. Do you feel overwhelmed when you read the word 'effort' in this context?

I see things differently. To me, life is not a marathon, or one steady-paced path. Instead, I see it as a series of sprints—bursts of motivation and productivity that slow down at times but always start again. We go through cycles, like anything else in life, and experience periods of highs and lows that shape our lives.

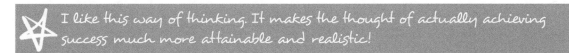

I like this way of thinking. It makes the thought of actually achieving success much more attainable and realistic!

Motivation and self-encouragement are similar; at times, we are motivated, driven and productive. At other times, we are not. It's important to understand that this is natural and acceptable. You will not always be on your "A" game. External factors, such as environment, relationships and even career, can impact your mindset. Internal factors, such as tiredness, doubt and the need for recognition, may also hinder your progress. It is how you get yourself back on track that matters! Success is not something that occurs overnight. It takes dedication, time, planning and effort to get results.

One exercise that may spark you to get motivated is to create a list of accomplishments of which you are proud. It can be anything that involves family, friends, your career, or business. The important thing to do is to document the things you've done or created that make you feel satisfied.

Look for patterns in all of those situations or experiences. Also, record the feelings you associated with each accomplishment. Then make a list of failures: projects you never completed, tasks that fell through, or a goal that you were never able to achieve. What feelings do you associate with those setbacks? The emotions that you experience while writing down your accomplishments and failures represent the intrinsic motivation that will help you stay on track. Remember how amazing it felt to reach that goal? Wouldn't it be wonderful to experience that joy and satisfaction again? You can!

So how does one remain motivated? Here are some tips:

- **Identify a specific goal** – It can be big or small, but you must be able to visualize it before taking action. Find what excites you. What is it that moves you? And don't forget—your *why* factor needs to be significant to see the value in realizing your goal. What are your objectives or the steps you must take to achieve it?

- **Prioritize** – Anything you want to accomplish in life will require you to commit yourself and focus your energy. Time and energy are limited resources. Properly managing your time will ensure that you are able to get things done. Set specific times to work on projects, and tackle the most challenging tasks first.

- **Take action** – The key to personal growth is pushing yourself to do things whether you feel ready or not. Anyone can set up a plan or a schedule, but it will be effective only with *action* and consistent effort.

Accomplishing important goals often takes time. However, as time passes, motivation can wane. It's like slowly letting the air out of a tire. Allowing this to happen may result in a cycle of *wanting* change, but not having the mental willpower to *actually* change.

Keeping your eye on the prize requires a strong mindset and consistent drive to action. Becoming the best version of yourself means going after the goals that support that vision. Remind yourself why you want this, what this goal means to you. What value will it add to your life? When it all seems too much, allow yourself to take some downtime. It's natural to have days where you'll be less productive. And that's OK. It's part of the process. You can be flexible in your methods, but never lose sight of working toward your goal.

To stay on track, there are a few things you can do to improve your overall mindset and keep a positive attitude. These are to:

1. **Create a positive environment that fosters your objectives** – Your environment can greatly impact your way of thinking. Be sure to surround yourself with people who encourage your growth and try to avoid negative influences as much as possible. Keep in mind that not everyone wants to see you succeed. It is important to distinguish between the encouragers and naysayers.

2. **Find someone you admire** – This should be someone who is an individual who has accomplished goals similar to yours, someone you can look up to as a mentor. Viewing situations from their perspective may help you make decisions congruent with your own goals. Ask yourself, *What would they do in this situation?*

3. **Plan out three actions for the day, week or month that you will fully dedicate yourself to accomplishing** – Choose three primary or minor actions that will help bring you closer to your goal, and enjoy the progress that your efforts generate.

4. **Create a mission statement** – Just as organizations have mission statements, create your own personal mission statement. What do you want to represent? What do you want to leave behind as your legacy? Having a clear idea of who you are and what you want will help drive your success.

If and when your motivation weakens, ask yourself, *Who is the ideal me?* Who do you envision yourself becoming? What are the habits and behaviors of that person within you? You *can* be who you want to be! The more you identify with the desired version of yourself, the bigger your *why* factor becomes, and the more likely you are to remain enthusiastic and motivated throughout the journey.

The following diagram shows examples of health habits with corresponding hack levels. To download the *Hack Your Health Habits Worksheet*, visit

www.hackyourhealthhabits.com/worksheets

READY #HEALTHHACKER?
EXAMPLES OF LEVEL 1, 2 AND 3 HACKS FOR THIS CHAPTER

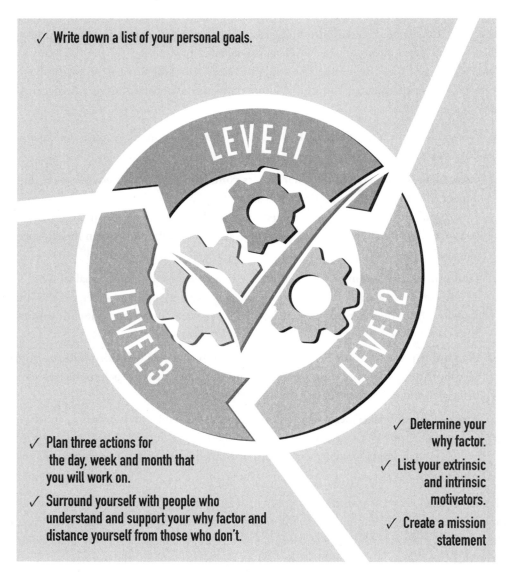

✓ Write down a list of your personal goals.

LEVEL 1

LEVEL 2

LEVEL 3

✓ Plan three actions for the day, week and month that you will work on.

✓ Surround yourself with people who understand and support your why factor and distance yourself from those who don't.

✓ Determine your why factor.

✓ List your extrinsic and intrinsic motivators.

✓ Create a mission statement

HACK YOUR HEALTH PROGRESS

CHAPTER 2

3
PRODUCTIVITY AND ENERGY MANAGEMENT

Are You Productive or Just Busy?

"'I don't have time' is the grown-up version of 'the dog ate my homework.'"

— Unknown

THINK IT OVER

- Do you follow your natural energy rhythm to maximize your productivity throughout the day?

- What are your biggest distractions? Do you have a strategy to get them under control?

- Are you making the healthy choices needed to keep your energy levels high?

To-do list after to-do list, an endless list of chores—the more tasks you check off your list, the more you add! No wonder it feels like you never accomplish anything. There's always something more to do. The cycle seems almost futile, doesn't it? You just can't get enough done. Sound familiar? That is why this chapter's focus is on productivity and the art of working smarter, not harder.

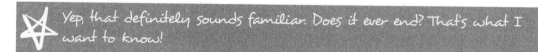

Yep, that definitely sounds familiar. Does it ever end? That's what I want to know!

You have probably heard the saying, *"We all have 24 hours in a day, but it's how we use those hours that count."* This is an undeniable truth. Everyone is busy. Between work, household duties, family obligations, children's activities, personal projects and our social lives, there is no doubt that time is a precious commodity. The beauty of it is this: We are in control of how we spend that time.

By setting priorities and focusing on the tasks that matter most to us, we become more productive and less "busy." Busyness creates stress, while efficiency creates fulfillment. Stress, in a way, is actually needed. *Eustress* (a term coined by Dr. Hans Selye) is the positive stress we feel that motivates us to get up and do what we need to do. *Distress* is the type of stress that is harmful to us. By learning to harness the power of *eustress*, we create conditions to set efficient time aside to do our work.

In his book *The Productivity Project: Accomplishing More by Managing Your Time, Attention, and Energy*, author Chris Bailey talks about a recent American Time Use Survey, which showed that the average person aged 25-44 with children spends 8.7 hours a day working, 7.7 hours per day sleeping, 1.1 hours on household chores, 1 hour eating and drinking, 1.3 hours per day caring for others, 1.7 hours on "other," and 2.5 hours per day on leisure.[1]

For most, leisure time involves watching television. According to Nielsen—a market research company—people can take back 13.5 years of their life by reducing the amount of television they watch. What's more, U.S. market research shows that 80 percent of 18- to 44-year-olds check their cell phones within the first 15 minutes of waking up, demonstrating an attachment to our devices.

With the evolution of technology and the Internet developing at a faster rate than our minds can handle, it is no wonder we fall victim to so many distractions. Time is of the essence, and, without proper time management, our lives can feel like an ongoing struggle to keep up with a fast-paced burden. While we try to keep it all together, sometimes it can feel like we are falling apart at the seams.

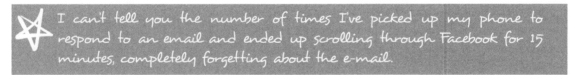

I can't tell you the number of times I've picked up my phone to respond to an email and ended up scrolling through Facebook for 15 minutes, completely forgetting about the e-mail.

Energy is an important aspect of time management and productivity. It is our capacity to do work, the fuel in our gas tank. However, our daily energy is limited. Our bodies have their own natural rhythms. When our physical, mental and emotional energies are taken care of, we are in tune with our natural rhythm and capable of keeping up with life's demands.

By taking care of our physical needs (movement, rest, nutrition, health), our emotional needs (self-love, acceptance, time for oneself, positive environment), and our mental needs (taking breaks, adopting relaxation techniques, constantly learning and engaging in what interests us), we are able to grow our mindset and perform at our best, and thus be more productive. The more we harness the power of our mind's energy, the less willpower we need to use to make good decisions.

So, what is productivity, and how do we maximize it? Productivity is how we organize our time and maximize our energy and attention to produce what we want to do. No matter what goal you have set, remain mindful of the importance that goal has to you. To justify making an effort, each task must have meaning.

As discussed in the previous chapter, in order to be motivated to do the things we do, we need a *why*—the reason for and the drive or desire to accomplish the task at hand. There are lots of ways to boost efficiency, limit distractions, and get stuff done! More time does not necessarily equal more productivity; studies show that productivity drops after 55 hours of work per week, so even if you put an extra 10 hours in, it may not always give you better results. It is not only the *quantity of time* we invest but, more importantly, the *quality* that determines our productivity.

Now, how do we do this?

- **Prioritize tasks in order of importance** – When we work on one goal at a time, we can laser-focus on the task and devote our best energy to it. This allows for more time-efficiency than dividing attention among numerous tasks. Sorry, multi-taskers! Studies show that multitasking is not conducive to optimal performance. When we scatter our attention over several simultaneous tasks, we are prone to distraction and inefficiency.

- **Tackle important tasks during "Prime Time"** – Research shows that the prefrontal cortex, the decision-making part of the brain, is the most active in the morning when we wake up. For most people, this is often when their willpower is strongest and they feel the most motivated. Thus, accomplishing our objectives and tackling our biggest and most complex tasks of the day while we are in this state will enhance our productivity. Everyone has their own time of day where their energy and motivation is highest, or their "prime time." Biologically, for most people, it's in the morning, but for some, it may be after lunch, or after their late-morning workout. Your mind switches between wandering mode (i.e., when you are running or taking a shower) and execution mode (i.e., when you are deeply focused). Tune into when you feel most productive and use that time to your advantage. Working during your 'prime time' will allow you to get more done with less effort, so you work smarter, not harder!

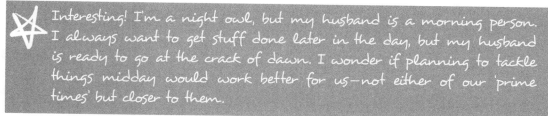

Interesting! I'm a night owl, but my husband is a morning person. I always want to get stuff done later in the day, but my husband is ready to go at the crack of dawn. I wonder if planning to tackle things midday would work better for us—not either of our 'prime times' but closer to them.

- **Know your distractions and avoid them at all costs!** – Making a list of triggers you *know* will distract you can be useful when trying to improve concentration. These can include: television, snacks, phones, Facebook, Pinterest, Twitter, email, and allowing your mind to wander. Write down your distractions and acknowledge how they detract from your productivity. Conditioning yourself to not 'give in' to the temptations of distractions trains your brain to recognize them as mere distractions so you can keep on working!

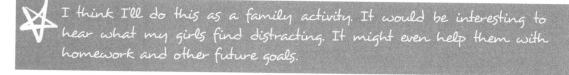

I think I'll do this as a family activity. It would be interesting to hear what my girls find distracting. It might even help them with homework and other future goals.

- **Log your time** – Along with writing down distractions, another effective method is to keep a time log journal that allows you to see how productively you spent your day and where you lost or wasted time. Was it necessary to watch that 30-minute sitcom? How long did you spend preparing dinner? How many hours of undisturbed work did you do? Don't rely on your memory as an accurate way of tracking time. When you physically write down your activities hour by hour, you will soon become aware of where you need to improve on time management and reducing distractions.

I should do this for a few days. It would be interesting to find out how much time my everyday duties take me.

- **Block out your time** – Once you are aware of your productive hours and your distraction triggers, you will be able to set up blocks of time dedicated solely to uninterrupted work. You may work in 30-, 60-, or 90-minute blocks before moving onto something else or giving in to the urge to check your phone. Setting a timer is a good way to stay on track. For myself, I have bought a fun "cube timer" that works in increments of 15, 30 or 60 minutes that I set to monitor my time. I call it my *productivity cube*. I play a game with myself that I won't do anything else but the task at hand for the time that I determine. No interruptions! It's amazing how much more efficient I am since using this tactic. Planning is key to productivity. Set a time to start each task, and you will be more likely to complete them rather than waiting until you feel like it. Decide on three crucial tasks to accomplish each day, and organize your time and energy around that. Make a list of pending projects and prioritize them according to your short-term or long-term goals.

- **Work on strengths and delegate weaknesses** – Don't spend endless hours doing work that doesn't interest you or that you do poorly when you can give it to someone else. A common mistake we make is taking on everything ourselves and wanting to do it our way. Yes, you, the perfectionist—you know what I'm talking about! In reality, it's not useful to expend energy on tasks that drain or don't interest you. You are more likely to procrastinate, make excuses and ultimately do a less-than-stellar job on them. I do believe you should challenge yourself to try new things, but it's a better use of your energy to pass on certain tasks whenever possible. Learn to refuse tasks that you know you will do poorly and pass them on to someone who you feel will do a better job and be more efficient with their time.

- **Take time to rejuvenate** – It is easy to get caught up in the hustle and bustle of our busy lives. Our brains need time for rest and rejuvenation to function optimally. Our bodies have a natural rhythm that allows us 90-minute intervals of productivity before it requires a break. Take breaks from work to meditate, work out, or write in your journal. Give yourself a mental break and return to tasks with a fresh mind. A good night's sleep helps improve attention and focus; when the mind and body are well-rested and alert, we are less likely to fall victim to distractions. Try keeping one day of the week free and use it as a 'catch-up' day to work on any of your unfinished projects.

- **Be congruent with your values and beliefs** – When the tasks we assign ourselves are not in line with our mindset, it causes an internal conflict within the subconscious mind. We call this *cognitive dissonance*. This occurs when we cannot identify with what we are doing. Without passion, drive, or a reason why we are doing what we do, our productivity falls. That's why it is so important to practice our strengths, follow our interests and perform tasks that are consistent with our values, as they all contribute to our purpose. The discussion of this topic continues later, in **Chapter 59: Life Purpose—Are You Living Yours?**

The following diagram shows examples of health habits with corresponding hack levels. To download the *Hack Your Health Habits Worksheet*, visit

www.hackyourhealthhabits.com/worksheets

READY #HEALTHHACKER?
EXAMPLES OF LEVEL 1, 2 AND 3 HACKS FOR THIS CHAPTER

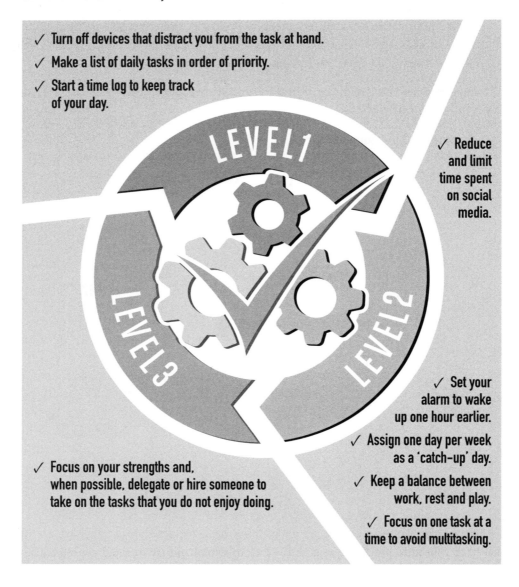

✓ Turn off devices that distract you from the task at hand.

✓ Make a list of daily tasks in order of priority.

✓ Start a time log to keep track of your day.

✓ Reduce and limit time spent on social media.

✓ Set your alarm to wake up one hour earlier.

✓ Assign one day per week as a 'catch-up' day.

✓ Keep a balance between work, rest and play.

✓ Focus on one task at a time to avoid multitasking.

✓ Focus on your strengths and, when possible, delegate or hire someone to take on the tasks that you do not enjoy doing.

HACK YOUR HEALTH PROGRESS

‖‖‖|||||||||||||||||||||||||||||||||||||||||||||||||

CHAPTER 3

4
PERSONAL PRIME TIME
Are You Setting the Stage for Your Day?

> "The only person you are destined to become, is the person you decide to be."
>
> — RALPH WALDO EMERSON

THINK IT OVER

- Do you have planned morning rituals that set you up for a productive and less stressful day?

- What habits or actions can you incorporate to make your mornings run smoother?

- Do you take time daily to nurture your physical, mental and emotional or spiritual development?

I want you to think of your morning routine. How does your day begin? If you're like most people, it may consist of a series of snooze buttons followed by a quick shower and a cup of coffee while you pack your kids' lunches. You rush the kids to school and try to avoid getting stuck in traffic. You make it to work by 9 a.m. and remember your daughter has an appointment right after school. Just as you go to call your spouse, your boss asks for the report you accidentally left on your counter while running out the door. Sound familiar?

Believe it or not, your morning rituals set the tone for your entire day. Whether you want to be productive, in a good mood, or just feel relaxed throughout the afternoon, how you begin your day is crucial to your mindset. Someone once asked me, *"How do you get so much done in a day?"* My answer was simple: *"I go to bed early and wake up a couple of hours before I need to start my day."*

A couple hours may seem like a long time, especially for those who love sleeping in, but waking up early allows me to start my day on the right foot. I prioritize myself in the wee hours of the morning.

✸ *Eek, getting up early has always been difficult for me.*

Many years ago, I noticed that most of my uber-successful mentors all had one major thing in common. They all took time in the morning to "work" on themselves. I decided to follow their lead and came up with my own morning rituals to suit my needs. I take this time to establish my goals for the day, to meditate, exercise, read, and to ease into the flow of the day without any rush or panic. I call this my "Personal Prime Time." It refers to tending to our physical, mental, emotional and spiritual needs before undertaking the tasks we've planned for the day.

From a productivity standpoint, it may seem counterintuitive. Why not just get straight to work? Why waste two hours of my time when I could be getting things done? The answer to that is: Personal Prime Time is *why* I get so much done. When I take care of myself, I focus better, and my decisions are less emotion-driven. I have a clearer outlook on situations and a better sense of self.

Easing into the day keeps your adrenal glands functioning as they should, instead of going into overdrive (more on this in Section 7, which covers hormones). This gentle approach also helps prevent your body from automatically entering the fight-or-flight mode throughout the day. As a result, you will feel calmer, more in control of your time and more organized!

Personal Prime Time may involve different things for different people and vary from day to day. The idea is to develop daily rituals that promote our well-being. In this day and age, we are constantly bombarded with information and expectations. We are expected to do more, be more and have more—all at a faster pace. With technology at our fingertips, distractions are everywhere. With so much to accomplish in a day, most of us even have a sense of guilt when taking time for ourselves. Yet, we need to realize that, in order for us to continue growing, we *need* to prioritize ourselves. We cannot pour from an empty cup. Once we prioritize our needs and have them taken care of, we can effectively tend to others' needs.

✸ *I've never really thought of it like that. I also have to teach my girls that it is important to take care of oneself; I have to lead by example!*

It's important to set a time for these rituals and integrate them into our daily routines. This might mean going to bed earlier or waking up earlier. It takes a conscious effort to put ourselves first. With time, established rituals can develop into habits. You will no longer have to think much about them; your body and mind will know what it needs to function optimally.

So, what can you put into your Personal Prime Time? There are three things I would like to suggest: physical development, mental development, and emotional or spiritual development. Let's take them one at a time.

PHYSICAL DEVELOPMENT

Movement can be a key component of your morning routine. The increased circulation and release of endorphins—feel-good hormones that rise following exercise—can help you feel positive and energized throughout the day. Early morning workouts use your hormones in your favor since, while you sleep your body releases Human Growth Hormone (HGH) and testosterone. In the morning, these hormones are at an elevated level, contributing to better performance and increased muscle usage during exercise. Early morning exercise can also help boost your metabolism, allowing you to burn more calories throughout the day. This phenomenon is called Excess Post-exercise Oxygen Consumption, or EPOC.

Furthermore, exercise increases your focus on your next activity due to the aroused state of your body. Whether you are headed to the office, school, or other important tasks, one of the advantages of working out in the morning is that you're more alert and focused throughout the day. Working out in the morning also removes the chance of distractions that may sabotage a later workout, such as less motivation, fatigue, going out for dinner, a sick child, or an overdue report for work or school.

If you've completed your workout in the morning, you can simply roll with whatever obstacles come up later in the day without feeling bad that you missed another day. You're far more likely to be consistent with your training if you get it done early in the day rather than waiting for later.

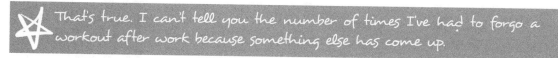

That's true. I can't tell you the number of times I've had to forgo a workout after work because something else has come up.

Try a morning kickboxing class, some Zumba, or even running a few laps around the block. Whatever activity you choose, it should be one that gets your body moving and gets that heart pumping! Your workouts do not even need to consist of heavy training in the gym. A simple bodyweight circuit routine in your own home will yield the same benefits.

STRETCH YOURSELF

Another great option to get moving, strengthen your core and stretch is yoga. Yoga or low-impact movement/poses will help increase your circulation and make your body feel rejuvenated. Yoga has the added benefit of relaxation, enabling a calmer mindset. It will help you expand your focus and attentiveness when embarking on other tasks. Yoga helps prevent injuries and strains by increasing flexibility and easing muscle and joint pain. It assists in reversing the effects of prolonged sitting, stimulates the lymphatic system and can reduce adrenal exertion.

MENTAL DEVELOPMENT

Your brain is most ready to learn, plan and execute first thing in the morning. This is because our pre-frontal cortex (the part of the brain responsible for planning, judgment and impulse control) is most active right when we wake up.[1] That's why it is important to nurture your mental development before taking on your obligations. Consider incorporating activities like goal setting, prioritizing, planning, budgeting and learning into your Personal Prime Time. Listen to podcasts, read a book, write down goals for the week, prioritize your tasks for the day, plan your finances, or brainstorm project ideas. The morning is also a great time to practice a skill, such as learning a new language or playing an instrument. These kinds of activities will get your neurons firing, harnessing the power of your brain.

Due to this increased activity in our prefrontal cortex, morning is a good time to take on our biggest or most important tasks. As suggested in the previous chapter, completing the larger tasks first, while you have the most energy and willpower, will not only help you to accomplish these priorities, but will likely leave you feeling more satisfied. Establishing this way of efficiently using your energy and not depleting your "prime time" with minor tasks will go a long way toward increasing your productivity.

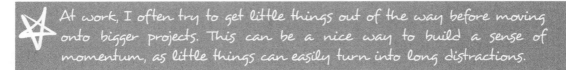

At work, I often try to get little things out of the way before moving onto bigger projects. This can be a nice way to build a sense of momentum, as little things can easily turn into long distractions.

EMOTIONAL AND SPIRITUAL DEVELOPMENT

Emotional and spiritual development is another important aspect of Personal Prime Time. Most people, upon awakening, have a clear undisturbed mind. Incorporating meditation, positive self-talk and journaling are great ways to become mindful of the present and nurture our emotional needs. Meditation has been practiced for centuries, but it has only recently become a more popular practice in the West. For many of our busy, wandering minds, sitting and doing nothing may seem like an impossible task. Meditation is more than just sitting cross-legged with your index finger and thumb connected. It's about silencing your mind and letting go of worry, negative thoughts and anxiety.

Meditation trains you to be mindful and fully aware of the present, of your surroundings, and your own inner peace. As you focus on the rhythm of your breath, your mind and body become more focused and relaxed. The benefits of meditation are profound: It calms the nervous system, improves cognitive function, memory, emotional control and concentration, and even helps to improve immunity and resistance to pain and illness.

See if you can meditate first thing in the morning after your alarm goes off. Instead of immediately jumping out of bed, take 10 to 15 minutes to relax and take deep breaths. Really focus on each breath. Visualize yourself in the moment. As you do, you will become one with the calmness of your body and mind. Easing into your day this way will get you started on a calmer, more self-aware note.

Positive self-talk and affirmations are another way to emotionally and spiritually connect with yourself. The science behind positive affirmations shows that the more you repeat something to yourself, the more your subconscious mind starts to believe it. Start the day with some encouraging words! Tell yourself that, despite setbacks, you will continue to persist with your goals; that no matter what the obstacles, you are in control of the outcomes. Remind yourself that you are a strong-minded, healthy and happy individual and that you truly believe in yourself.

Keeping a gratitude journal or memoir can also help keep you on track. Start the morning by writing down what you are thankful for, who you appreciate and what you are proud of. Express your state of mind and jot down your goals, feelings and ideas. Getting your thoughts on paper is therapeutic and can help clarify your aspirations.

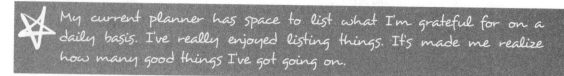

My current planner has space to list what I'm grateful for on a daily basis. I've really enjoyed listing things. It's made me realize how many good things I've got going on.

Prayer, contemplation and visualizations are other ways to meditate and grow spiritually. Contemplate your life purpose, imagine your growth and think of how you would like to improve your relationships. What do you need to let go of? What can you improve upon? Set intentions for yourself. These reflections will help nourish your outlook with composure and serenity. A big part of the idea behind practices like meditation and prayer, traditionally, is to cultivate qualities like compassion and care for others—to enlarge our view beyond ourselves, which, in a fortuitous paradox, is good for us.

You may choose to add an activity to the list mentioned above.

The specifics of your Personal Prime Time may vary on a daily basis, depending on how you feel. On some days, you may feel upbeat and energetic while on other days, you may feel more relaxed. The idea is to establish a daily self-management ritual, setting intentions for each day will help you become more connected with yourself and honor your personal needs. As you get in the habit of putting yourself first and taking care of your physical, mental and emotional needs, you will radiate wellness and energy to the people around you.

PERSONAL PRIME TIME EXAMPLES

If you're not sure what your Personal Prime Time could look like, here are some examples to inspire you:

Example One – 75 minutes

1. 60-minute fitness class (like CrossFit or Kickboxing) with warm-up and cool down
2. 15-minute guided meditation

Example Two – 60 minutes

1. 20 minutes of interval training on a bike
2. 20 minutes of yoga stretches and deep breathing
3. 20 minutes of reading

Example Three – 45 minutes

1. 15 minutes of learning a new language
2. 20 minutes of core and functional movement exercises
3. 10 minutes of meditation or prayers

Example Four – 30 minutes

1. 10 minutes of high-intensity intervals

2. 10 minutes of lower body mobility exercises

3. 10 minutes of monthly goal-setting

One hour of Personal Prime Time seems reasonable. Maybe I will finally become a morning person! I'll have to shift some stuff around, but I can definitely start setting my alarm clock a little earlier and packing lunches the night before. I can even iron my outfit in the evening to save more time. It'll be weird prioritizing myself, but I think it could be worth it.

The following diagram shows examples of health habits with corresponding hack levels. To download the *Hack Your Health Habits Worksheet*, visit

www.hackyourhealthhabits.com/worksheets

READY #HEALTHHACKER?
EXAMPLES OF LEVEL 1, 2 AND 3 HACKS FOR THIS CHAPTER

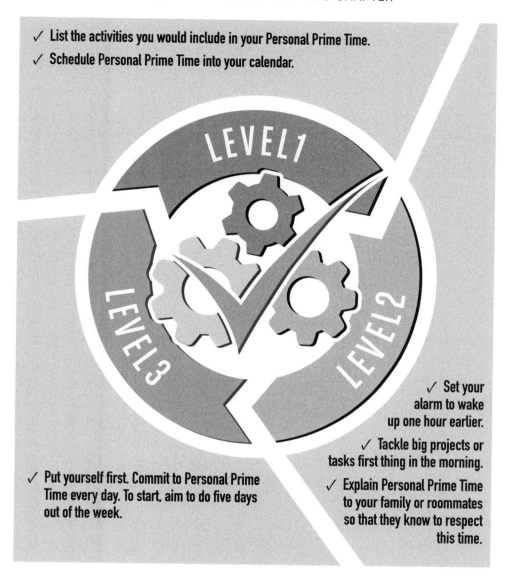

✓ List the activities you would include in your Personal Prime Time.

✓ Schedule Personal Prime Time into your calendar.

LEVEL 1

LEVEL 2

LEVEL 3

✓ Set your alarm to wake up one hour earlier.

✓ Tackle big projects or tasks first thing in the morning.

✓ Explain Personal Prime Time to your family or roommates so that they know to respect this time.

✓ Put yourself first. Commit to Personal Prime Time every day. To start, aim to do five days out of the week.

HACK YOUR HEALTH PROGRESS

CHAPTER 4

SECTION 2

Get Back to Basics—Understand the Foods to Consume to Keep Your Body Performing at Its Best

Do you really know what's fueling your body? Section 2 discusses everything from macronutrients—proteins, carbs and fats—to deciphering food labels, and from why to choose organic food matters, to eating the colors of the rainbow.

FATS

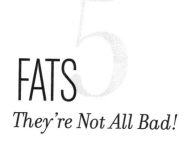

They're Not All Bad!

"Keep calm and eat
avocados."

— Unknown

THINK IT OVER

- Can you distinguish between the four different types of fat?

- Do you consume enough of the good fats in your diet?

- Do you know which fats are best for cooking and which are best consumed at room temperature?

Are you confused about fats? Not sure which are good, and which are bad? I don't blame you—there is a lot of conflicting information out there. One of the most troublesome myths is that eating fat will lead to weight gain. While recent studies show that this is not true, we still see books and articles advocating low-fat diets for fast weight loss.

The truth is, eating fats can actually play a major role in weight loss and overall optimal health. They help absorb other nutrients, balance hormone levels, maintain cell structure and much more. That being said, this is not the case for every type of fat. Eating bad fats (i.e. trans fats and hydrogenated oils) can lead to inflammatory diseases like heart disease, diabetes and arthritis—and can even lead to weight gain.

DEBUNKING THE "FAT-FREE" TREND

In the past, saturated fats were demonized because they were believed to increase Low Density Lipoprotein (LDL) cholesterol and atherosclerosis (plaque buildup in the arteries), leading to an increase in heart attacks. New research has debunked this way of thinking, showing that the risk for heart attacks and strokes can actually be increased by over-consumption of refined sugars, carbs and trans fats. According to recent research, eating foods with saturated fats—like grass-fed meats and coconut oil—actually have very little effect on your blood cholesterol levels and cardiovascular health.

 Yay!

So, why was it that we were told to replace our butter with margarine and our sour cream with skim milk? Trends have to start somewhere, and the low-fat, high-carb diet surfaced in the late 1970s and early 1980s when North America, particularly the United States, saw a spike in deaths caused by heart disease.

At that time, it was wrongfully found that saturated fats increase LDL cholesterol. Due to limited scientific knowledge back then, people didn't understand the complex role that saturated fat plays in our body, and all the good it does. However, from that point on, saturated fat was deemed an evil villain and blamed for weight gain, heart disease and high cholesterol. People were then told to reduce their fat intake and increase their "good" carbohydrate consumption. They were brainwashed into thinking fat was bad. But, instead of increasing whole grains, fruits and vegetables as suggested, it was unfortunately commercially packaged products, sugar and simple carbohydrates that surged. And so, the fat-free revolution began!

That would explain why "low-fat" is ingrained in my mom's head.

Even today, more than 20 years later, you can still buy a fat-free version of pretty much anything. The funny thing is, fat is flavor, so, to keep products tasting good, manufacturers replaced fat with sugar. Instead of eating full-fat yogurt for breakfast, people are eating low- or no-fat yogurt loaded with sugar. And, instead of bacon, people are choosing sugary cereals and low-fat muffins. Fats have been swapped out for something that is much worse…sugar! And, this is horrible when you think of the havoc that sugar wreaks on the body. It contributes to obesity, Type 2 Diabetes, weakened immune systems and provides a hospitable environment for disease to flourish.

The truth is, our bodies *need* saturated and unsaturated fats from animal or plant sources. Fats provide a multitude of health benefits, including:

- better muscular recovery
- better exercise endurance
- lower levels of acute and chronic stress
- improvements in insulin function

- increases in sex-hormone production
- reduced inflammation
- positive effects on depression when taken with a vitamin D supplement

HOW DO WE KNOW WHICH FATS ARE GOOD OR BAD?

There are four types of fatty acids:

- **Saturated Fatty Acids (SFA)** – such as animal fats, dairy and coconut oil
- **Monounsaturated Fatty Acids (MUFA)** – such as olive oil, avocado and nuts
- **Polyunsaturated Fatty Acids (PUFA)** – omega-3 and omega-6
- **Trans Fatty Acids (TFA)** – contained in foods like margarine, cookies, crackers and deep fried foods

Trans fat is truly the "bad guy." It is to blame for elevated blood triglycerides, obesity and Type 2 Diabetes. On the flip side, saturated fat provides structure to our cell membranes and tissues, strengthens our immune system, helps in the production of hormones, supports the nervous system and facilitates the absorption of vitamins and minerals.

When it comes to polyunsaturated fats balance is key. Typically, a low omega-6 to omega-3 ratio is recommended (1:1 to 4:1).[1] Unfortunately, this ratio can be hard to achieve. This is especially true in North America, where our diets tend to be much higher in omega-6. Imbalances have been shown to suppress immune system function, contribute to weight gain and cause inflammation. But, more on this later!

WHAT KIND OF FATS SHOULD I INGEST?

The following is a list of foods with good fats that should be introduced to your diet, if not already present:

- avocados
- nuts – such as walnuts, almonds, pecans and macadamia nuts
- seeds – such as pumpkin, sesame, chia, hemp and flax
- fatty fish – such as sardines, mackerel, herring and wild salmon
- extra virgin olive oil
- organic olives
- grass-fed animal products such as butter and ghee
- coconut oil
- hemp or flax seed oil – best used in dressing or when not heated

It's important to note that some good fats become 'bad' when heated, and should not be used in cooking, perhaps. When you're cooking with high heat, you want to use oils that do not oxidize or go rancid easily. The amount of saturation of the fatty acids in the oil determines its resistance to oxidation when exposed to heats. The higher the saturation, the more resistant it is to heat. The best sources of saturated fats are coconut oil, butter, ghee and animal fats from grass-fed livestock. These fats react well to high heat and will not easily oxidize. Polyunsaturated and monounsaturated fats are best consumed in salad dressings or at room temperature. These fats include olive oils, flaxseed oil, sustainably-sourced palm oil and nut oils.

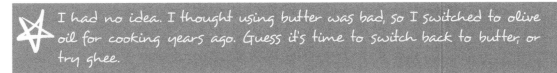

I had no idea. I thought using butter was bad, so I switched to olive oil for cooking years ago. Guess it's time to switch back to butter, or try ghee.

Industrial seed and vegetable oils are also on the "no-no" list. Not only should you not cook with them, you should probably avoid them altogether. They tend to be highly processed and way too rich in omega-6 fatty acids. Thought vegetable oil was safe? Vegetable and seed oils are often promoted as heart-healthy. However, new data links these oils with many serious diseases, including heart disease, elevated blood pressure, blood triglycerides and cancer.

Try your best to avoid these highly processed culprits:

- soybean oil
- cottonseed oil
- sunflower oil
- peanut oil

- corn oil
- canola oil
- safflower oil

WHAT ABOUT CHOLESTEROL?

The idea of reducing cholesterol was the main reason why butter and eggs were once treated as enemies. The truth is, you *need* cholesterol. That's right, this fatty substance is found not only in your bloodstream, but also in every cell in your body, where it helps to produce cell membranes, hormones, vitamin D, and the bile acids that help you to digest fat. Since your brain is 60 percent to 70 percent fat, cholesterol also helps in the formation of your memories and is vital for neurological function.

Today's research shows that there is very little correlation between the cholesterol that one consumes and the body's cholesterol production. Instead, the liver gets triggered to produce fat and cholesterol in response to excess sugar and carbohydrates. High-carb diets increase the production of triglycerides, lower the "good" cholesterol (High Density Lipoprotein, or HDL) and increase "bad" cholesterol (Low Density Lipoprotein, or LDL).

Now, let's talk about the elephant in the room, LDL. In recent years, LDL has been deemed the 'bad' cholesterol, but it's not that simple. There are small and large LDL particles, and this is where it gets more complex. The bad LDL is the small particles that can build up as plaque in arteries; however, the larger, fluffier LDL particles are essential in many areas such as hormone production, cognition and mood. Therefore, the 'good' and 'bad' are not that clear-cut. Healthy fats actually promote the production of these large LDL particles, whereas sugar and refined carbs trigger the production of the small, more dangerous ones.

The real concern is not so much the amount of cholesterol in your blood, but rather the oxidation of that cholesterol, which is a contributing factor to the formation of plaque in the arteries—which has been shown to lead to coronary heart disease.

What about statin drugs? Anyone who has been scolded by their doctor for high cholesterol levels will know that statin drugs are the drug of choice when it comes to lowering cholesterol. It is estimated that statin sales worldwide will approach $1 trillion by 2020. But, recent research is showing that statin drugs do not actually have a great impact on heart health. Another concern with statins is that they decrease levels of coenzyme Q10, selenium, omega-3 fatty acids, fat-soluble vitamins, carnitine and free T3.

As *The New York Times* reported:

- Participants taking the drug saw their LDL levels fall to an average of 55 milligrams per deciliter, from 84. Their HDL levels rose to an average of 104 milligrams per deciliter, from 46. Yet, 256 participants had heart attacks, compared with 255 patients in the group who were taking a placebo.

- Ninety-two patients taking the drug had a stroke, compared with 95 in the placebo group. And, 434 people taking the drug died from cardiovascular disease, such as a heart attack or a stroke, compared with 444 participants who were taking a placebo.[2]

These results are pretty shocking. What's even more shocking is that statins continue to be prescribed left, right and center, despite their proven ineffectiveness and numerous side effects. Side effects include muscle pain and cramps (I see this often with my patients), liver damage, kidney failure, Type 2 Diabetes, dementia, erectile dysfunction, cancer, and, in extreme cases, death. Knowing this, why would someone stay on them? Side effects for women are often worse, as cholesterol is the building block of hormones, and statin use can result in hormonal imbalances. If you are a woman taking a statin drug, I suggest you rethink your strategy.

 I wonder if my family knows this? Many of my relatives are taking statin drugs.

HOW MUCH FAT?

Now, back to fats. How much fat should we be eating? The amount of fat needed will vary for each person, however, here are some general guidelines for recommended daily amounts.

- **Consume 1-3 tsp. of PUFAs daily** – such as fish, krill, hemp and flax (unheated).

- **Consume 1-3 tbsp. of MUFAs daily** – such as extra virgin olive oil, macadamia oil and avocado oil (safe at low heat).

- **Consume 1-3 tbsp. of healthy saturated fats daily** – such as coconut oil, butter and ghee.

- **Reduce intake of highly processed omega-6 fats** – limit processed foods and vegetable oils in order to keep an optimal ratio of omega-6 or omega-3.

- **Say no to *all* trans-fats.**

As you will hear in many other chapters, nutrition is complex and personal. Every person is biochemically different, and what works for one person may not work for the next. I know it may be difficult for some to accept or understand that fat is good and that our bodies need it, especially if they have lived their whole life thinking the opposite. I ask you to research further if you're still not convinced. Change can be hard. Hang in there—and order that side of guacamole!

> I'm definitely making my mom read this chapter.

The following diagram shows examples of health habits with corresponding hack levels. To download the *Hack Your Health Habits Worksheet*, visit

www.hackyourhealthhabits.com/worksheets

READY #HEALTHHACKER?
EXAMPLES OF LEVEL 1, 2 AND 3 HACKS FOR THIS CHAPTER

✓ Write in a food journal for a week to determine the types of fat you're consuming and what kind.

✓ Toss any low-fat products you have in your fridge or pantry.

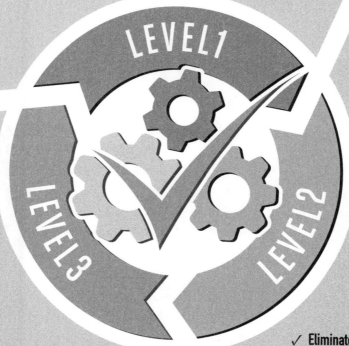

LEVEL 1

LEVEL 2

LEVEL 3

✓ If on statin drugs, consider working with a Natural Health Professional to focus on lifestyle changes to lower your cholesterol, instead.

✓ Eliminate trans fats from your diet.

✓ Cook with only heat-safe fats.

✓ Limit use of industrial seed and vegetable oils.

HACK YOUR HEALTH PROGRESS

||||||||||||||||||||||||||||||||||||||||||||||||||||||||||||||||||||||||||||||||||

CHAPTER 5

CARBOHYDRATES
What's The Deal?

"It's not just about low-carb,
it's about low-crap!"

— Unknown

Carbohydrates have caused a lot of controversy amongst health and nutrition professionals in recent years. Although the 2017 Canadian Food Guide suggests 6-7 servings of carbohydrates —in the form of grain products per day—and the American Food Guide suggests 6-11 servings per day for females between 19 and 50 years of age, new research contradicts this recommendation.

Wow, that's a lot of servings, and that doesn't even include fruit and vegetables, which I know are also a source of carbs.

For years, we've believed that carbohydrates are *the* ideal source of energy for the body, due to the fact that they can be converted more quickly into glucose. However, studies show that a diet too high in carbs can cause serious health implications. Carbohydrates can upset the delicate balance of your body's blood sugar level, resulting in fluctuations in energy and moods that leave you feeling irritated and tired.

Not sure what to believe? This chapter tells you why less is more when it comes to carbs.

WHAT ARE CARBOHYDRATES?

The three dietary carbohydrates are:

- **Sugars** – Sweet, short-chain carbohydrates; examples include glucose, fructose, galactose and sucrose.

- **Starches** – Long chains of glucose molecules, which eventually get broken down into glucose in the digestive system.

- **Fiber** – Humans cannot digest fiber, although the bacteria in the digestive system can use some of them to produce fatty acids for the body to then use as energy. This is why it's important to consume prebiotic foods that aid in digestion.[1] (More on this in **Section 8: Get Your Gut and Immune System Performing Optimally**).

All three carbohydrates are made from molecules of sugar. Sugars, or simple carbohydrates, contain just one or two molecules of sugar, whereas the complex carbohydrates consist of many molecules of sugar. Complex carbohydrates are generally better-quality carbohydrates. They contain other key nutrients like fiber (that helps keep you feeling fuller, longer), vitamins A, B and C, and iron. On the other hand, simple carbohydrates include refined and sweet foods such as fruits, juice, table sugar, corn syrup, honey, soft drinks, pastries, breads and pastas. Although they provide the body with energy, they rarely provide any other beneficial nutrients to our health and should be limited in consumption. They also tend to cause major spikes in blood sugar levels, which leads to a subsequent crash that can trigger hunger and cravings for more high-carb foods. This is the "blood-sugar roller coaster" with which many people are familiar.

BLOOD SUGAR AND CARBOHYDRATES

Carbohydrates can also be classified according to the glycemic index (GI). High GI indicates simple carbs, while low GI indicates mostly high fiber and complex carbs. The glycemic index is a scale that indicates how quickly certain foods get converted into sugar that then enters our bloodstream. Digestion breaks down and transforms carbohydrates into the simple sugar glucose, which is then transported everywhere by the blood to power everything our body does.

High GI foods cause spikes and drops in blood sugar levels, which can also cause insulin secretion to fluctuate. When insulin cannot metabolize that amount of sugar, our body is bombarded with excess glucose, which is turned to glycogen and stored in the liver or as fat around the body. This can also cause less stable energy levels throughout the day.

The GI sets sugar at 100 and scores other food against that number:

- **Low GI** score is considered to be under 55.
- **Moderate GI** score is considered 56-69.
- **High GI** score is considered 70+.

The goal should be to choose more food from the low GI index to avoid a spike in your insulin levels, as insulin is an important hormone in regulating fat storage. However, the combination of foods consumed together will also have an effect on glucose absorption and stabilization. Moreover, other factors such as consuming foods that our body is sensitive to—in other words, has an immune reaction to—can also affect blood-sugar levels as well.

The bottom line, though, is that tracking food GI is a good way to reduce foods that are greater stressors to the blood-sugar stabilization system.

HORMONES INVOLVED IN METABOLIZING SUGAR

When your body needs more energy, the pancreas secretes a second hormone called glucagon. This converts the stored glycogen back into glucose, which can be released into your bloodstream for cells to use. This means the body's glucose metabolism is a cycle of glucose, insulin and glucagon reactions. The slower the release of glucose and hormones, the more stable and sustainable the energy levels of the body. The more refined the carbohydrate (such as in flours, breads, pastas, jams, pastries etc.), the faster the glucose is released into your blood. Complex carbohydrates provide a slower and more sustained release of energy than simple carbohydrates.

High levels of insulin could lead to unwanted stress on your pancreas, which can lead to diabetes. Research shows that one out of three North Americans are now being diagnosed with Type 2 Diabetes, and more than 90 percent of those cases could be avoided with lifestyle changes.[2] Insulin secretion can also have an impact on cancer development as it triggers the release of Insulin Growth Factor (IGF), which stimulates cell growth. Therefore, it could potentially increase the number of cancerous cells.[3] Insulin and IGF also promote inflammation in the body, which can lead to other inflammatory diseases such as cancer, arthritis and heart disease.

FIBER

Fiber is important because it moves food through your digestive system, absorbing water and making elimination easier. Fiber also has a high-satiety quality to it, so eating high-fiber foods will fill you up faster. The average intake of daily fiber is 8-15 grams, when the recommended daily intake of fiber is actually 25-40[4] grams. Be aware that too much fiber may decrease your body's absorption of some vitamins and minerals. If you take a fiber supplement, do not take it at the same time as vitamins or prescription medication for this reason.

Oh wow, I never knew that! I take everything at the same time.

There are two types of essential fibers:

- **Soluble fibers** – These fibers are soft and sticky, and absorb water to form a gel-like substance inside the digestive system. Soluble fibers help soften stool so it can slide through the gastrointestinal tract more easily. They have also been shown to decrease cholesterol levels and help control sugar levels. Sources include gluten-free oatmeal, oat bran, steel-cut oats, baked beans, lentils and cereals.

- **Insoluble fibers** – These fibers contribute to stool bulk, as they do not dissolve in water. They are commonly called 'roughage.' Insoluble fiber isn't broken down by the gut and absorbed into the bloodstream. Sources include sprouted bran, fruits with seeds, broccoli, cauliflower, carrots, mushrooms and eggplant.

There are many benefits of increasing fiber intake. More fiber:

- slows transit in small bowel
- increases stool bulk
- holds onto water
- forms gels
- binds minerals and organic substances
- stimulates good bacterial growth
- metabolizes into Short-Chain Fatty Acids (SCFA)
- promotes anti-inflammatory activity

A DIFFERENT PERSPECTIVE

As we've already discussed, Western society hopped on the low-fat bandwagon years ago. However, despite eating less fat, the rate of obesity increased. Simply put, we replaced fats with carbs, which wasn't much of an improvement after all. Excess carbs raise our insulin levels and are converted into fat. Add to that the poor quality of many available carbohydrate sources, and it's a recipe for nutritional disaster. Countless studies over the years have refuted the notion that carbohydrates should be our primary source of energy. These studies show that the body actually thrives on burning fat for fuel, rather than the glucose provided by carbs. As a matter of fact, low-carb diets are much more effective than the standard low-fat diet that has been recommended for fat loss. They are able to lower bad cholesterol and triglycerides and prevent conditions such as diabetes and metabolic syndrome.

Many supporters of a high-fat/low-carb lifestyle claim that carbs are not even an "essential" nutrient. If you think about it, there are *essential* amino acids and *essential* fatty acids, but no *essential* carbohydrates. The body can function with very little amounts of carbohydrates in the diet. When we eat only small amounts of carbs, the brain can use ketones for energy, which are produced when the body utilizes fat. Additionally, protein can be turned into glucose for fuel when there is a surplus of protein, via a process called gluconeogenesis, making it another source of immediate energy when needed. This idea will be discussed in much greater detail in **Chapter 14: The Ketogenic Diet—A Way to Stay Lean & Prevent Disease.**

Other benefits of lower carb diets include:

- weight loss

- regulated blood pressure

- decreased blood glucose

- improved cardiovascular function

- enhanced cognitive function

- more sustainable energy

PROCESSED VS. WHOLE FOOD SOURCES

It's true that added sugars and refined carbs are linked to increased obesity. But, consuming small amounts of fiber-rich, whole-food sources of carbohydrates—such as the ones found in vegetables—do not yield the same outcome. Humans have been eating complex carbs for thousands of years, in some form or another. What they all had in common was that they ate real, unprocessed foods. It wasn't until recently that issues such as diabetes and obesity have become an issue.

- Blaming new health problems on a simple macronutrient simply doesn't make sense. However, populations that eat a lot of *refined* carbohydrates, sugars and processed foods tend to be sick and unhealthy. And in North America, this is unfortunately the case. Your toast and cereal for breakfast, that sandwich or wrap for lunch, and lasagna or pizza for dinner all contain high amounts of refined carbs, which then get quickly broken down to sugar in the body. And, what does sugar cause? Weight gain and inflammation! It is no wonder that this has become such a serious epidemic.

This makes me think of the Facebook post that went viral, the one that showed the amount of sugar in everyday snacks. It was shocking.

With this in mind, opting for a diet that is lower in simple carbs and greater in healthy fats and protein may be the best option to prevent future illnesses and treat current ones. To be considered a low-carb food, it is recommended to stick to a carbohydrate intake of no more than 50-70 grams per day, coming from complex carbs and foods that are high in fiber. To give you an idea of what that may look like, consider this list of carbohydrates in ordinary foods:

- Celery, raw (1 stalk) .... 1 g

- Broccoli, chopped raw (250 ml) .... 6 g

- Sprouted Bread, (1 slice) .... 16 g

- Apple with skin (medium) .... 19 g

- Banana .... 27 g

- Potato, baked, skin (medium) .... 34 g

- Plain bagel (10 cm in diameter) .... 38 g

- Rice noodles, cooked (250 ml) .... 46 g

- Brown rice, long grain, cooked (250 ml) .... 48 g

 Hmm, just a bit of rice equates to your daily intake. I will often eat double that amount in a day. I'm going to have to pay more attention to my servings!

The starchier the item, the higher the carb content. It is best to get your complex carbs from vegetable sources. Also, try to avoid wheat products as much as possible as they are highly refined or have been through a process of hybridization. There will be more on this in **Chapter 41: Food Sensitivities—Is Your Body Angry with What You Are Eating?**

Recommended carbohydrate intake varies from person to person, depending on their health background, activity level and even genetic makeup. Some thrive on little to no carbs while others need a little extra to get through the day. It is best to play around with your carbohydrate intake, increase your fat and protein intake and see how your body feels. How is your energy level? Are you gaining or losing weight? Are you retaining water weight? Is your brain as sharp? Test it out!

CARB CYCLING FOR FAT LOSS

Carb cycling has gained great popularity amongst health and fitness professionals who attempt to maintain healthy hormone levels, low body fat and lean muscle tissue. The idea behind carb cycling is to vary the amount of carbs consumed during the week to optimize energy metabolism and the body's use of fat stores, to keep fat cells from growing while keeping energy levels high. To do this, limit carbohydrate intake for 3-5 days a week and resume a higher carb intake for 1-2 days a week to replenish glycogen stores and accelerate fat loss.[5] This protocol can go well with intermittent fasting, which will be introduced in **Chapter 13: Intermittent Fasting—Could You Benefit from It?**

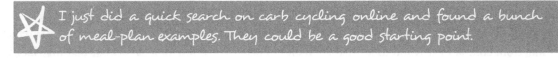 *I just did a quick search on carb cycling online and found a bunch of meal-plan examples. They could be a good starting point.*

The following diagram shows examples of health habits with corresponding hack levels. To download the *Hack Your Health Habits Worksheet*, visit

www.hackyourhealthhabits.com/worksheets

READY #HEALTHHACKER?
EXAMPLES OF LEVEL 1, 2 AND 3 HACKS FOR THIS CHAPTER

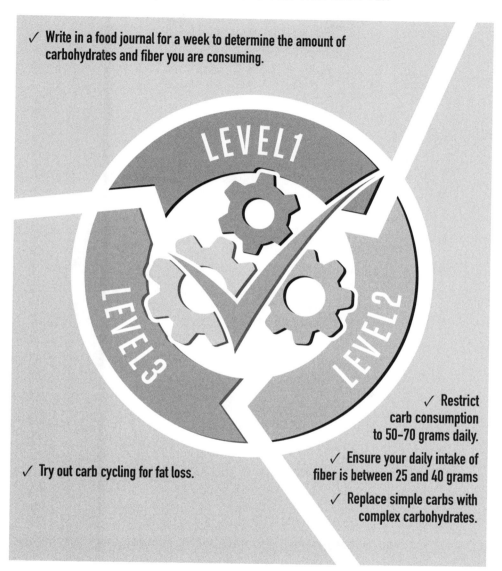

✓ Write in a food journal for a week to determine the amount of carbohydrates and fiber you are consuming.

LEVEL 1

LEVEL 2

LEVEL 3

✓ Restrict carb consumption to 50–70 grams daily.

✓ Ensure your daily intake of fiber is between 25 and 40 grams

✓ Replace simple carbs with complex carbohydrates.

✓ Try out carb cycling for fat loss.

HACK YOUR HEALTH PROGRESS

CHAPTER 6

PROTEIN
You Do Need Some!

"Food is fuel.
Use it wisely."

— DR. NATHALIE BEAUCHAMP

PROTEIN 101

Think protein is just for bodybuilders and athletes? Think again! Protein is the building block of life. It is found in muscle, bone, hair and virtually every other tissue and part of the body. It is essential for cell growth and tissue repair.

It is also responsible for building:

- red blood cells that provide oxygen and nutrients to your cells
- hormones that help build lean muscle and burn fat
- immune cells that fight off bacteria and viruses
- neurotransmitters
- muscle tissue to support exercise and general health[1]

Protein is made up of various compounds called amino acids. Amino acids link together to form the protein molecules that create enzymes, hormones, muscles, organs and other tissues in the body.

Protein relies on two types of amino acids:

- non-essential amino acids, which are made by the body
- essential amino acids, which cannot be made by the body and must be consumed through food

The protein we find in food is considered a thermogenic nutrient, meaning energy is needed to break it down after eating it.

THE IMPORTANCE OF PROTEIN IN THE DIET

Protein is an essential building block, so it's important that we consume enough of it. Not only will adequate amounts of protein help with cell growth and tissue repair, but also those who consume protein also report:

- improved satiety
- the ability to preserve and build lean muscle mass
- improved cholesterol and cardiovascular health
- accelerated fat loss

In all, you want to keep your refined carbohydrate levels low, healthy fats high and proteins at a moderate amount. In Section 3, we will discuss in greater detail the recommended amounts of each macronutrient, depending on one's choice of diet, activity level and health goals. For optimal health, it is said that most adults need about 0.8 to 1 gram of protein per kilogram of lean body mass, or 0.5 grams of protein per pound of lean body mass. Note that lean body mass is not the same as your total body weight.

If you are unsure of exactly how much protein you should be consuming, Dr. Joseph Mercola proposes a formula that can help us calculate exactly how much protein is required for our unique needs. In order to calculate this, first, you must determine your lean body mass. To do that, subtract your body fat percentage from 100. For example, if you have 30 percent body fat, then you have 70 percent lean body mass. Then, multiply that percentage (in this case, 0.7) by your current weight to get your lean body mass in pounds or kilos. As an example, if you weigh 170 pounds; 0.7 multiplied by 170 pounds equals 119 pounds of lean body mass. Using the "0.5 gram of protein" rule, you would need 59.5 or just under 60 grams of protein per day.[2]

100 – percent of body fat = percent of lean mass

percent of lean mass x actual weight = lean body mass

lean body mass x 0.5 gm protein = total grams of protein recommended

SOURCES OF PROTEIN

Now that we have a better idea of how much protein to eat, let's talk about what kind of protein you should consume. There are two main sources of protein: animals and plants. When it comes to which is the best, a case can be made for both. Animal proteins are a complete protein that contain all nine of the essential amino acids, and therefore, have a high absorption rate. They are the richest source of branched-chain amino acids and creatine (a nitrogenous organic acid), both of which are critical in building muscle, burning fat, improving energy and upgrading general health. This type of protein is found in meat, poultry, fish, dairy products, eggs and whey protein supplements.

However, there can be some drawbacks with animal protein consumption. One of the biggest drawbacks is the increased exposure to antibiotics, hormones and heavy metals. Because cattle are typically fed modified grain and corn products to help them gain weight faster, they have larger fat stores than grass-fed cattle. This isn't a good thing. The more fat cells an animal has, the more synthetic hormones and heavy metals they will store. So, if and when we consume fatty meat, we expose ourselves to hormones and heavy metals. Making matters worse, the vast majority of this meat comes from animals raised in Concentrated Animal Feeding Operations (CAFOs), where the overall quality of meat produced is inferior to organically raised, pastured, or grass-fed meats.

ANIMAL PROTEIN SOURCES

THE IMPORTANCE OF GRASS-FED MEAT

For those who eat meat regularly, I strongly suggest you choose grass-fed over grain-fed animals. Cattle are meant to graze on grass; they are not adapted to digest grains. Even though a grain-based diet promotes faster weight gain for the animal, it often generates the need for antibiotics. This is because the feeding of grains results in alterations in the natural flora of their gastrointestinal tract, often leading to inflammation and infection. When they tested samples of ground meat, *Consumer Reports* found that 18 percent of the samples taken from conventional beef were contaminated with dangerous antibiotic-resistant bacteria. In comparison, only 9 percent of the samples from sustainably produced beef were deemed contaminated.[3] Quite the difference!

In addition, meat from grass-fed cattle has more omega-3 fatty acids, vitamin E and conjugated linoleic acid—all good for human health. Incidentally, organic beef isn't necessarily grass-fed, as they are fed organic *grains*, which we now know cattle cannot digest well, and results in creating inflammation in their bodies—therefore in ours, too. To avoid this, select organic, grass-fed meats from local and sustainable farms.

For many people, the higher cost of grass-fed beef is a concern. According to *Consumer Reports,* grass-fed beef costs shoppers an extra $2.50 per pound, and grass-fed organic beef is priced about $3 higher per pound than conventional beef from the supermarket. This averages out to an additional $260-$300 per year if you buy two pounds of ground beef each week. The reason for the higher cost is the time it takes a producer to get a grass-fed animal to slaughter—up to a year longer than a conventionally raised one. *Consumer Reports* also found that grass-fed cattle tend to be smaller at slaughter than conventionally raised animals, so there is less meat for producers to sell per head.[4]

 I've been trying to buy more organic and grass-fed meat. It is more expensive but I've started making a few vegetarian meals a week to balance out the cost. It's nice to know the reason behind the cost.

Using grass-fed livestock as a food source is also substantially better for the environment. Grass-fed animals are the exception to the frequent vegetarian assertion that meat is bad for the planet. When you feed grain to animals, you are taking food that could potentially feed humans and using it much less efficiently than if you fed it straight to humans. This is mostly since the animal uses up a bunch of it to support its own life; so you need to use many times the amount of a GMO and pesticide-ridden annual-based grain to get the same caloric end result for humans. But cows and other ruminants are extremely efficient at converting low-protein, low-energy, hard-to-digest but perennial plants (i.e. grasses) into high-protein, high-energy and human food (i.e. meat and milk). Therefore, grass-fed farming short-circuits the argument that consuming meat is 'bad' for the environment. Also, *pastures* by definition are a naturalized, low-intensity form of farming.

Based on all this information, we should also focus on purchasing dairy products that are organic and from grass-fed cows, since what a cow consumes essentially becomes what we consume through the dairy they produce.

WHAT ABOUT FISH, POULTRY AND EGGS?

When it comes to eating meat, we're often told to consume white meats (fish and poultry) and limit consumption of red meats (beef, lamb and pork). Though many consider white meat a healthier option, be warned. Just because you choose a chicken breast over a juicy steak doesn't necessarily mean you've made the better choice. Truth be told, the fish and poultry industry have their own flaws, which we're about to uncover.

Fish has been identified as a very good source of healthy fat and has even been recommended for consumption at least once or twice a week. Although it is true that fish is a good source of omega-3, the quality of the fish and where it came from may be an even more important factor. While fish farming (known as aquaculture) has been in place for centuries, its popularity has exploded in recent years because of the continued high demand for fish and seafood.

To some, farming fish sounds like a great idea, since the thought of the exposure to mercury and pollutants in the wild is not as desirable as a clean, confined fish in a tank. However, in reality, the industry is plagued with many of the same problems that are found in CAFOs, including pollution, disease and even decreased nutritional quality of the meat.

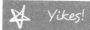 **Yikes!**

Farmed fish are kept in tanks where they are fed genetically modified corn and soy. The close quarters where farmed fish are raised combined with their unnatural diets means disease can spread quickly. Studies have consistently found levels of pollutants, such as polychlorinated biphenyls (PCBs), dioxins, toxaphene, dieldrin, and mercury, to be higher in farm-raised fish than wild fish.

Furthermore, farm-raised fish, like conventional meat, is pumped full of antibiotics, hormones and even chemicals to change their color. Due to the lack of nutrients and the lack of filtration of fish feces, farmed salmon are surrounded by uneaten food and waste. They typically turn out to be a pale gray color, so they are given chemical dyes to resemble the fresh pink color we are used to seeing. What's more, it has been shown that the omega-3 content of farmed fish can be reduced by up to 50 percent.[5]

All right, so farmed fish is a no-no. But, what about the pollutants that wild fish are exposed to? It is true that wild fish found in certain areas of the ocean have had their health severely compromised—such as the Atlantic Ocean, which has been plagued with oil spills, and the Western Pacific Ocean that is currently filled with radiation leakage from Japan as a result of the 2011 earthquake that damaged the Fukushima nuclear reactor. But, there is still hope in finding good-quality wild fish in the North. Wild Alaskan sockeye salmon is far less likely to contain these pollutants, therefore making it the healthier option. You can usually tell the difference between sockeye salmon and farmed salmon just by looking at it. The latter is larger, paler in color, and has more visible fat within the layers. Sockeye salmon has a rich pink color and is visibly leaner. Opt for wild sockeye salmon when consuming fish, and your body will thank you for it!

Now to tackle the chicken and the eggs. No, I don't know which one came first. But, you may have seen the People for Ethical Treatment of Animals' (PETA) videos of chickens stored in tiny cages, being overfed and sitting in their own feces, and thought, *I will not be consuming caged poultry and eggs again!* We have been told that going for cage-free eggs is the healthier, more ethical option, but is this really the case?

Turns out, cage-free isn't always better. Cage-free chickens are still confined in tight, uncomfortable spaces where diseases can spread like wildfire. Antibiotics are given to these chickens to prevent serious infections, and when we consume their meat, we consume these antibiotics, too. Again, similar to CAFO cattle and fish, chickens are fed a modified grain- and soy-based diet, *and* are given many doses of synthetic hormones to accelerate their growth, making the quality of their meat and eggs less than desirable, as well. The best option would be to opt for free-range eggs and poultry from your local farmers' market, where the hens are allowed to forage freely outdoors and are safe from synthetic hormones.

PLANT-BASED PROTEINS

Plants have protein, too! Examples of plant-based proteins include nuts, seeds, legumes, grains, vegetables and fermented organic soy. However, those refraining from meat due to ethical or health reasons should keep in mind that not all plant-based proteins contain all essential amino acids. It is for this reason that many vegetarians or vegans find themselves deficient in some essential nutrients. Plant sources such as quinoa, buckwheat, hemp and amaranth are complete proteins—meaning they have all nine essential amino acids—and therefore it is important to include a variety of these sources when thinking of refraining from animal products.

Sprouted grain and seed proteins are increasing in popularity due to dairy and wheat allergies. Known as hypo-allergenic proteins, these plant-based products can be digested without problem or irritation. While they do offer a variety of essential amino acids, they contain lower concentrations of branched-chain amino acids and creatine, making them inferior to whey, in regards to performance and recovery. Those taking plant-based protein should consider taking branched-chain amino acids and creatine separately to reap their full benefits.

If you choose to stick solely to plant-based protein sources, I would strongly suggest adding a mix of different protein sources to each meal to ensure you are consuming all essential amino acids. Also, it is important to be taking high-quality supplements, such as B6, B12, and iron, as most vegetarians or vegans find themselves deficient in these specific nutrients.

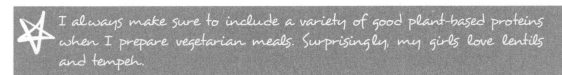

> I always make sure to include a variety of good plant-based proteins when I prepare vegetarian meals. Surprisingly, my girls love lentils and tempeh.

WHEY PROTEIN: THE "WHEY" TO GO?

Grass-fed whey is considered best when it comes to protein supplements. It is a by-product of cheese-making, where milk is separated into whey (20 percent) and casein (80 percent, which is used for the basis of the cheese). There are different forms of whey protein that serve different functions. Whey *isolate* has the highest biological value and is considered the number one choice. Why is that?

Whey isolate contains a high concentration of leucine, the branched-chain amino acid that triggers muscle protein synthesis. It's also a rich form of glutathione, your body's most potent antioxidant, detoxifier and liver supporter. In addition, it supports cardiovascular function and lowers blood pressure. It is ideal to consume isolate before, during, or right after exercise as it is quickly absorbed into the bloodstream. It is also ideal to consume in the morning when your body is in negative nitrogen balance after a long night's sleep—unless you do intermittent fasting, but more on that later.

Whey *concentrate* is the most widespread form of protein out there. It usually has higher concentrations of vitamins, minerals and immune-boosting nutrients, especially if it comes from grass-fed milk. However, it has less protein and is more difficult to digest than the isolate for those with dairy sensitivities. On that note, whey protein may cause some minor issues for those with a dairy sensitivity. Bloating, cramping and gas may occur, making it not suitable for everyone.

In any case, try selecting *grass-fed* whey if you want to give it a shot!

HOW DO WE GO WRONG WITH PROTEIN?

- **Not enough protein in your first meal** – Inadequate protein supply when you break your fast can lead to a number of negatives, including lower levels of dopamine (the feel-good hormone) and leptin (the satiety hormone), blood sugar spikes and drops and increased cravings for carbohydrates. Make sure to start your day with plenty of protein to avoid this.

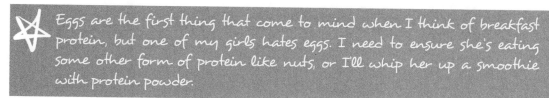

Eggs are the first thing that come to mind when I think of breakfast protein, but one of my girls hates eggs. I need to ensure she's eating some other form of protein like nuts, or I'll whip her up a smoothie with protein powder.

- **Too little protein and too much carbs** – Blood sugar and insulin will rise rapidly with a high-carb diet without enough protein to slow the release of sugars, keep insulin levels low and balance your appetite throughout the day. More on this in **Chapter 37: Blood Sugar— How Is It Impacting Your Weight and Your Health?**

- **The wrong kind of protein** – Sandwich meats, low-quality meats and cured meats are high in antibiotics, hormones, nitrates and preservatives that are more detrimental to your health than beneficial. Try to stick to organic, free-run poultry, grass-fed beef, wild fish and nitrite-free lunch meats. These options will improve the quality of protein absorption in your diet.

- **Too much protein** – Yes, too much protein may be a bad idea, as well. You see, when you consume more protein than your body needs, your body must remove more nitrogen products from your blood, which may put extra stress on your kidneys. As a result, you may be chronically dehydrated and have higher levels of acidity, throwing off your pH balance. In addition, because the body cannot store protein, any amount consumed in excess may be converted into glucose (a process known as gluconeogenesis) and raise blood glucose levels. Too much protein can also inhibit the body from burning fat as its main source of fuel instead of burning sugar, which will be discussed in greater detail in **Chapter 14: The Ketogenic Diet—A Way to Stay Lean & Prevent Disease.**

The following diagram shows examples of health habits with corresponding hack levels. To download the *Hack Your Health Habits Worksheet*, visit

www.hackyourhealthhabits.com/worksheets

READY #HEALTHHACKER?
EXAMPLES OF LEVEL 1, 2 AND 3 HACKS FOR THIS CHAPTER

✓ Write in a food journal for a week to determine how much protein you are consuming.

✓ Figure out how much protein you should be eating using the formula suggested.

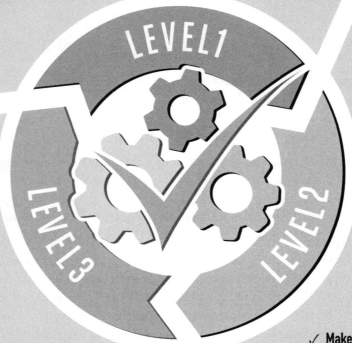

✓ Find local sources for organic, grass-fed meats and make those your priority source of protein.

✓ Make sure to eat protein at your first meal of the day.

✓ Include a source of protein with every meal or snack.

✓ Find a quality protein powder.

HACK YOUR HEALTH PROGRESS

||||||||||||||||||||||||||||||||||||||||||||||||||||

CHAPTER 7

FOOD LABELS AND ADDITIVES
Do You Know What You Are Eating?

THINK IT OVER

- Do your meals and snacks consist mostly of food with labels?

- Can you identify some of the names that are used in place of sugar?

- Are you able to spot misleading claims on food packaging?

We all know that the best thing for us to eat is fresh, organic food made from scratch. Yet, many people opt for processed and packaged foods instead. I get it. It's a challenge to make time to cook meals every day. Plus, organic produce can be expensive, especially during winter months if you live in a cold climate area. When it comes down to it, processed and packaged foods can make mealtime easy. They also don't break the bank. But, what exactly are you eating when you choose packaged food over fresh food?

WHAT IS PROCESSED FOOD?

To put it simply, if food travels to a manufacturer before making it to your home, then it is processed. Processed food is any food that is not in its original, natural form. This means that nutrients or substances have either been added or taken away. Food processing is done for a few reasons: to change the look of a food, to increase its shelf life, to enhance the flavor, color, or texture and to make it more "nutrient-dense."

The following substances are used when processing foods:

- **Antimicrobial agents** – These inhibit the growth of bacteria, fungi and viruses. Although this may sound good, these agents are creating "superbugs," which are highly adaptable microbes resistant to antimicrobial agents.

Well, that's terrifying!

- **Artificial colors** – Many foods are dyed to make them look more appetizing. Some of the dyes used have been linked to A.D.D. and A.D.H.D. in children.

I heard something about red dye being particularly bad.

- **Artificial flavors** – These are chemicals that mimic natural flavors. They are just that—chemicals that serve no nutritional purpose.

- **Bleaching agents** – These are substances used to whiten foods such as sugars, salts, flours and cheeses. More chemicals!

- **Nutrient additives** – You'll often see "fortified with calcium" or "added vitamin C" on boxes. These vitamins and minerals are usually derived from genetically-modified foods that your body has a hard time absorbing. It's best to get your vitamins and minerals from whole foods or a high-quality supplement.

I thought I was doing the right thing in buying foods like this, especially kids' snacks!

- **Preservatives** – These are man-made or natural substances/chemicals added to foods to increase their shelf-life and prevent them from spoiling.

- **Thickening or stabilizing agents** – When food lacks the "right" consistency, chemicals are used to thicken or stabilize. That's right, more chemicals, yet again.

WHY YOU SHOULD AVOID PROCESSED FOOD

We keep hearing processed foods are bad for us. But, what exactly do they do to our bodies? With high amounts of chemical additives, salt, refined sugars, grains and trans fats, a diet high in processed foods has been linked to several health conditions and illnesses. Those who regularly consume processed food are more likely to suffer from obesity, Type 2 Diabetes, heart disease, cancer, poor immunity, gastrointestinal issues and even cognitive defects.[1] The reason for this lies in the ingredients.

We talked about bad fats in the previous chapter and will talk about the detrimental effects of refined sugar later on in this book. To put it as simply as possible, processed foods contain chemicals and toxins that can compromise the immune system's ability to fight illness. In addition to this, most processed foods contain sugar and carbohydrates that lead to the storage of fat, resulting in weight gain and insulin resistance.

HOW TO READ FOOD LABELS

Another way to tell if food is processed is if there is a nutritional label on it. That being said, not all processed foods are terrible for you. There are many healthy snacks on the market. It's important to learn how to read nutrition labels so you can decipher between the healthy and not-so-healthy choices. Visits to the grocery store may become a bit longer when reading labels, but knowing exactly what is in the food you buy is an important step on your path to wellness.

Here is a breakdown of what you would usually find on the back of a food label, and some things to consider before adding something to your shopping cart:

Serving size – This one gets most people; the numbers shown on the Nutrition Facts apply only to the serving size listed on the label. For example, a bottle of orange juice may say 20 grams of sugar, but it may be per 250 ml in a 2 L bottle. Be sure to check to see per how many millilitres (etc.) that number applies to.

Yes, this gets me all the time!

Calories – Not all calories are created equal, and a calorie is a unit of energy, not a fat, a protein, or a carb! The number of calories per serving is simply how much energy you are getting from that food.

Percentage Daily Value (DV) – This number is based on the key daily nutrients you should consume based on a diet of 2,000 calories. Depending on your BMR (basal metabolic rate) and daily energy output, you may need more or less of the recommended nutrients.

Total fat – This is the amount of saturated, monounsaturated, polyunsaturated and trans fats in the food.

Saturated fats – For years, we have been told to keep saturated fats low, but as discussed in the chapters on fats, not all saturated fats are bad.

Polyunsaturated fats – Be wary of these types of fats! They become unstable when exposed to heat and oxygen, creating unwanted free-radicals.

Trans fats – *Avoid at all costs*. They raise small LDL cholesterol particles, which lead to arteries getting clogged.

Cholesterol – Cholesterol has a bad rap, but most people don't realize that the body manufactures most of our cholesterol; food adds only a small amount. The body needs a certain amount of cholesterol to produce hormones, to keep the brain functioning properly and to maintain a healthy heart. Concern yourself more with the types of fat that you are eating.

Sodium – The U.S. food agency recommends consuming less than 2,400 mg of salt per day. This number is 2,300 mg in Canada. This number may vary if you are physically active and lose sodium through your sweat. The type of salts you consume are also important, as conventional table salt is known to raise blood pressure and cause coronary issues. Be aware that processed foods contain very high amounts of unhealthy salts, usually hidden in vegetable juices, soups, sauces, seasonings, and can take the names of monosodium glutamate (MSG), baking powder, baking soda, disodium phosphate and sodium bisulphate. Stick to sea salt and, more specifically, Celtic sea salts or pink Himalayan salts when cooking. Try to avoid table salt whenever possible.

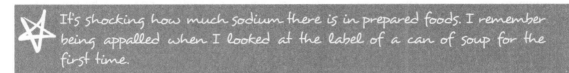

It's shocking how much sodium there is in prepared foods. I remember being appalled when I looked at the label of a can of soup for the first time.

Total carbohydrates – This is the total amount of all sugar, starch and fiber in a food. What is important here is the type of carbohydrate. Aim to consume complex carbs (e.g. brown rice, quinoa, oats) and stay away from refined ones (e.g. white bread, white pasta). Refined carbs will show up on the label as sugars.

Fiber – Any food with at least four grams of fiber per serving is good. The higher, the better!

Sugar – Try to keep this number under five grams or less per serving. According to the World Health Organization (2015), the recommended daily intake of sugar should be no more than 25 grams (or six teaspoons) per day. This should equal about 5 percent of your daily caloric intake.[2] Our diets are already high enough in sugar as is, therefore it's important to keep added sugars on the low side. When checking the ingredients, look for words such as fructose, glucose, sucrose, sucralose, lactose, galactose, maltose, molasses, cane sugar, syrup, high fructose corn syrup, corn syrup, liquid sugar, dextrose, dextrin, maltodextrin, isomalt, lactitol, mannitol, maltitol, sorbitol, aspartame and xylitol. These are all fancy words for sugar! Some are a little less harmful than others—like the fructose and glucose naturally found in fruits and vegetables. Regardless, keep sugar consumption to a minimum, and avoid High Fructose Corn Syrups (HFCS) and aspartame at all costs.

Protein – This is usually mentioned in grams. The recommended amount per day varies from person to person depending on level of activity and type of diet (e.g. paleo, vegan, keto, etc.). Always remember that the quality of protein matters; meaning grass-fed for animal sources and complete proteins for plant-based sources.

Vitamins and minerals – Calculations for vitamins and minerals are geared toward the prevention of deficiency and not for the promotion of optimal health. Whether the food contains added vitamins and minerals or not, a high-quality multivitamin is strongly suggested to obtain healthy vitamin and mineral levels for your body.

Ingredients list – The ingredients of certain foods are listed in order of quantity, from largest to smallest. Foods that contain sugars, enriched or bleached wheat flours, vegetable oils and anything that says "modified" in the first five ingredients should be put back on the shelf. These are the processed foods that cause the health problems discussed above!

BEWARE OF MISLEADING CLAIMS

Now that we've discussed the back of the box, let's discuss the front. The food industry knows that we're trying to make healthier decisions. They want us to think that their product is a healthy choice and often use clever marketing tactics to do so. They write things like "all natural," "low fat," or "no sugar added" on the front of the box to make us think that we are making the right choice. A quick read of the ingredient list, though, and we realize that's not the case. Here are a few more things to watch out for when shopping:

All natural – All natural doesn't mean organic. It doesn't even mean all natural. At this point in time, there are no restrictions on using the phrase "all natural." Unlike products that are labeled certified organic, a manufacturer that labels their product "all natural" can still have ingredients that are genetically modified, contain antibiotics and growth hormones or have toxic pesticides.

> This is absurd. So many people are getting tricked by these kinds of marketing tactics! How is this allowed?

Made with/from real fruit – Manufacturers are required by law to list ingredients based on the amounts used. As mentioned earlier, the first few ingredients on the list makes up the bulk the product, whereas those at the end of the list may be included in only tiny amounts. This means that a company can make a product containing only 0.5 percent of actual fruit and slap on a label saying it's "made with real fruit!"

Fat-free, sugar-free, or low-sodium – I put these three together for the simple fact that they are almost always linked together in products. If you have something that is labeled low-fat or fat-free, the manufacturer will usually add more sugar and sodium to enhance the flavor. Conversely, if a manufacturer has labeled something as sugar-free, then the fat and sodium content will likely go up. You'll also notice that other chemical ingredients will also be added, and most of the time these other ingredients—such as monosodium glutamate (MSG) or carrageenan, a hidden source of MSG, which come with a host of negative side effects.

The 'less than 100 calories' gimmick – As consumers started to become more aware of their caloric intake, the food industry figured out ways to work around this problem. By adjusting the size of a single serving, they could make their products seem healthier. For example, a bottle of cola can claim "100 calories per 250 ml" when their bottle actually holds 500 ml. This can mislead the person into believing they are only consuming 100 calories without realizing that the claim was only made for half the serving size.

A LAST WORD OF ADVICE

Always read the label. You know the old saying, "Never judge a book by its cover?" Well, never judge a product by its packaging! Check out the ingredients list and remember that if you cannot pronounce it, chances are you should not eat it. Becoming more aware of what you put in your body and taking action toward better choices will bring you one step closer to attaining the healthy body you deserve.

 I shop in the health aisles of my regular grocery store or at my local health food store. I figure processed foods in these places are pretty safe, and I don't really bother to look at their food labels. But maybe I should, especially considering all of the marketing tricks out there.

The following diagram shows examples of health habits with corresponding hack levels. To download the *Hack Your Health Habits Worksheet*, visit

www.hackyourhealthhabits.com/worksheets

READY #HEALTHHACKER?
EXAMPLES OF LEVEL 1, 2 AND 3 HACKS FOR THIS CHAPTER

✓ Clean out your pantry and throw out all food containing high fructose corn syrup.
✓ Read labels when shopping.
✓ Pay attention to serving sizes.

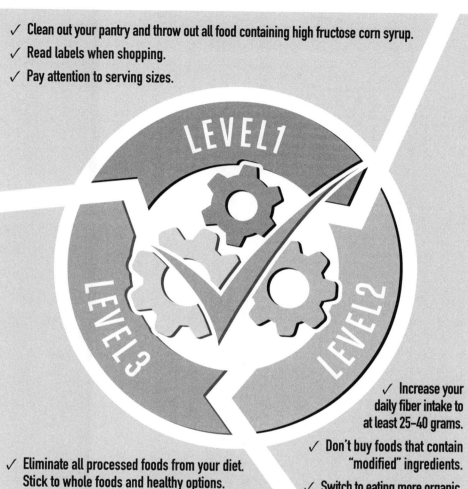

LEVEL 1

LEVEL 2
✓ Increase your daily fiber intake to at least 25–40 grams.
✓ Don't buy foods that contain "modified" ingredients.
✓ Switch to eating more organic.
✓ Eliminate refined sugar from your diet.

LEVEL 3
✓ Eliminate all processed foods from your diet. Stick to whole foods and healthy options.

HACK YOUR HEALTH PROGRESS

||||||||||||||||||||||||||||||||||||||||||||||||||||||||||||||||||||||||||||||||||||||||

CHAPTER 8

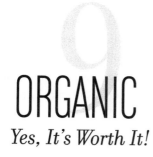

ORGANIC
Yes, It's Worth It!

"Eating organic is not
a trend. It's a return to
tradition."

— UNKNOWN

THINK IT OVER

- When doing groceries, can you identify the fruits or vegetables that are conventionally grown versus the ones that are genetically modified?

- Are you aware of the health effects of the herbicide glyphosate on your health?

- Do you know the "dirty dozen and clean fifteen" fruits and vegetables?

I t is said that today we do not consume real food, only food-like items. The majority of things we eat are heavily altered, modified from their natural form to grow quicker, larger, and be resistant to disease. To some, this may sound like an awesome advancement in agricultural engineering. But what if I told you that these advancements come at the expense of our health: wreaking havoc on our digestive health, harming our body's microbiome, impeding our ability to detox, and even disrupting our hormones?

WHY ARE GMOs THE NORM?

Genetically modified organisms (GMOs) and pesticide- and herbicide-latent foods are growing exponentially, all over North America. The debate between consuming organic and conventional foods has been going on long enough for the evidence to have become clear. Study after study is showing the effects of genetically-engineered foods on our bodies, making organic foods well worth the modest extra cost.

One would like to believe that our governments are taking the right measures to protect us against anything that is not good for our health. Unfortunately, this is not always the case. Many government agencies, as part of their mandate, promote GMOs. How can this be? GMOs are deemed "safe" by the same industry that produces them—corporate agriculture. They are responsible for testing the safety of their own products and sharing the test results with government organizations. This is a huge flaw in the current system, and it makes it very difficult to know if the food on our shelves is actually safe for consumption.

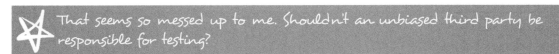

That seems so messed up to me. Shouldn't an unbiased third party be responsible for testing?

Due to strict patents, independent scientists are unable to validate the safety of GMOs.

Oh, that's why!

And the food industry—that makes billions off GMO foods—is not likely to jeopardize its business by admitting to safety issues.

In addition to issues with self-governance, there often lies a conflict of interest between Big Agriculture and government regulatory agencies. With Big Ag's incessant lobbying, too often there is a revolving door between industry executives and lawmakers. This, in turn, creates a flawed system, as companies now have a great influence on laws governing our agriculture.

The fact of the matter is that the "faster, bigger, cheaper" approach to food is slowly draining our resources and compromising our health. According to experts, the earth's soil is depleting at more than 13 percent the rate that it can be replaced, and 75 percent of the world's crop varieties have already been lost over the last century. Additionally, over the past ten years, we've had about 100 million tons of herbicides dumped onto our crops, polluting our soil and streams.[1] To make matters worse, genetically-engineered crops are now speeding up the destructive process by completely altering the composition of soil bacteria in the fields where such crops are grown.

WHAT IS ORGANIC FOOD?

Keeping the above in mind, there is a growing trend worldwide toward organic foods. While some consumers are making an effort to purchase high-quality organic foods, many are still wary about spending the extra money or taking the extra time to find such foods. Organic certification is a detailed process for organic food producers and includes standards that stretch above and beyond standard government regulations that apply to non-organic producers. Requirements vary from country to country but generally involve a set of production standards for growing, storing, processing, packaging and shipping.

Organic standards generally include:

- avoidance of most synthetic chemicals—fertilizers, pesticides, antibiotics and food additives

- a ban on the use of genetically-modified organisms

- production on farmland that has been free from chemicals for at least three years

- random and periodic on-site inspections

Your local farmers' market can be a great source of fresh products even if they are not certified organic. Many small producers cannot afford certification, but still use organic growing methods. (Certification is most useful for farmers who are selling to commercial establishments like groceries and restaurants.) Also, one of the great advantages of going to a market is that you can talk to the farmer directly, ask questions, and hear how they grow their food. Any good grower will welcome visits to their farm if you want to dig even deeper. The food will be fresh and locally grown and will, therefore, not have been subject to a lengthy transport schedule.

> I live at the farmers' market in the summer! I pretty much buy all my produce from there. And, I actually save money!

You'll feel good about supporting your community, as well as taking part in reducing transportation pollution. Otherwise, a variety of organic products are carried in urban supermarkets and grocery stores that contain far less harmful toxins than their conventionally grown counterparts.

For example, in Canada, any agricultural product that's labeled organic—including food for human consumption, livestock feed and seeds—is regulated by the Canadian Food Inspection Agency which introduced the Canada Certified Organic label in 2009. If a producer wants to use the Canadian Organic logo on their product, or if a producer wants to sell a product labeled organic, that producer is subject to the following rules under the Organic Products Regulations:

- Only products with at least 95 percent organic content may be labeled as organic or bear the organic logo. These products must be certified, and the name of the certification body must appear on the label.

- Multi-ingredient products with 70 percent to 95 percent organic content may have the declaration: "contains xx percent organic ingredients." These products may not use the organic logo or the claim to be organic. These products must be certified, and the name of the certification body must appear on the label.

- Multi-ingredient products with less than 70 percent organic content may use organic claims only in the product's ingredient list. These products do not require certification and may not use the organic logo. However, the organic ingredients contained within these products must be certified.[2]

WHAT ABOUT IMPORTED ORGANIC PRODUCTS?

As mentioned previously, organic standards vary by country and are tailored to local climate and growing conditions. Generally, producers who want to sell their products in a foreign country must certify their goods to the standard of that country. In addition, certain countries have mutual agreements recognizing each other's standards. Canada has such an agreement with the U.S. This means products certified as organic by the U.S. Department of Agriculture—whose standards are quite similar to those of Canada—are automatically considered organic in Canada and vice versa.

THE ORGANIC DIETARY DEBATE

NUTRIENT VALUES

The nutrient content of foods has *dramatically* declined since the introduction of mechanized farming in 1925. For example, as explained by Dr. August Dunning, chief science officer and co-owner of Eco Organics, *"In order to receive the same amount of iron you used to get from one apple in 1950, by 1998, you had to eat 26 apples."*

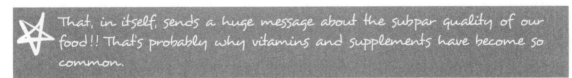

That, in itself, sends a huge message about the subpar quality of our food!! That's probably why vitamins and supplements have become so common.

On several occasions, the media has reported that there are no significant differences in nutrient values between organic and conventionally-grown produce. However, this is virtually impossible if you consider what organic farming actually entails. In a study conducted by Virginia Worthington, organic crops had higher nutrient levels and lower levels of toxicity in 56 percent of the 1230 published comparisons between organically grown and conventional crops. [3]

The nutrients mentioned, when comparing conventionally grown and organic foods, are mostly essential nutrients such as water, fiber, proteins, fats, carbohydrates, vitamins and minerals. Among the differences cited between conventional and organic foods are notable differences in the amount of *secondary* nutrients, called phytonutrients, which are more concentrated in organic foods. (There will be more on phytonutrients in the next chapter.)

Organic foods were also found to contain a high level of potent antioxidants called phenolic compounds, which are ten times more efficient at mopping up cancer-causing free radicals than conventional foods. According to some findings, organic fruits and vegetables can contain anywhere from 18 percent to 69 percent more antioxidants than conventionally-grown varieties. The healing effects of these organic foods are associated with the superior secondary nutrient content and quality.

So, organic really is better!

IMPACT ON PROTEIN QUALITY

One of the largest studies on organic food, the Haughley Experiment, found that cows that were fed organic products ate less, but consistently produced more milk. This is believed to be a result of the quality of the protein in the grass. Protein quality is dependent on the range of amino acids composing it. This, in turn, depends on the soil quality and the conditions in which they are grown. Plants are dependent on trace minerals in the soil, and their availability, in turn, is dependent on soil microorganisms.

These essential microorganisms may be depleted as much as 85 percent in conventionally farmed soils, usually as a result of chemical fertilizers, herbicides and fungicides.[4] The proteins in the plants growing in the depleted soil are thus inferior.

In addition, livestock that are fed conventional grains are at an even higher risk for developing inflammatory illnesses due to an inability to digest grains. Grain requires a completely different set of enzymes for digestion and a completely different digestive process to unlock the nutrients inside it. The grass-digesting microbes in the cow's stomach are not able to crack the tough outer shell of grain and extract the nutrients from it. How does this affect their health? Well, the cow's diet—grass-dominant or grain-dominant—determines the type of fat in beef. Meat from animals raised on a high-grain diet is much higher in omega-6 fatty acids and much lower in omega-3 fatty acids, which can be an inflammatory ratio.[5] And once again, guess who inevitably inherits this imbalanced ratio when beef is ingested? To avoid this, look for locally grown, grass-fed beef and dairy to ensure you are getting high-quality animal proteins and fats.

HORMONES AND ANTIBIOTICS

Over the past two decades, chickens have grown 25 percent bigger in less time and on less food. Meanwhile, the average cow produces 60 percent more milk, all due to synthetic hormones. Producers reap big, but at the cost of our health.

Also, antibiotics, which are put in animal feed and are present in non-organic animal products, increase antibacterial resistance in humans, creating "superbugs" and major health concerns in the long term. It is said that 60 percent of the antibiotics produced in the United States are administered to livestock to prevent illness from occurring due to living conditions in which they are raised.[6] The antibiotics they consume are then ingested by consumers, and the adverse effects of said antibiotics then take their toll on the person, as well. Livestock raised in confined animal-feeding operations (CAFOs) are routinely fed genetically-engineered feed—typically corn and soy—which destroys the animal's gut bacteria and promotes disease.

EFFECTS OF PESTICIDES

Pesticides are a controversial topic. Because of pesticides, the average farmland yields 200 percent more than it did before they were introduced 70 years ago—quite an incentive for some people to ignore the potential health hazards. The Environmental Protection Agency (EPA), however, considers 60 percent of herbicides, 90 percent of fungicides and 30 percent of insecticides to be carcinogenic.[7] Pesticide exposure has been shown to have many negative effects on our health, such as non-Hodgkin's lymphoma, endocrine disruption, general developmental problems and cognitive deficits in infants and children, low birth weight and smaller brain, reproductive problems, asthma and poor respiratory health, increased risk of obesity and diabetes and infertility.[8]

That's a lot of health conditions linked with pesticides.

HERE ARE SOME MORE FACTS ON PESTICIDES:

- More than 1 billion pounds of pesticides are used annually in the U.S.

- 71 percent are used in commercial agriculture.

- 15 percent are used in the home and garden (including golf courses) and 14 percent in forestry.

- The EPA has approved more than 350 different pesticide ingredients to be used on the food we eat.

- Only 0.1 percent of pesticides reach the intended pest. The remainder contaminates the environment.

GENETICALLY MODIFIED FOODS

Genetically modified foods began hitting grocery shelves only in 1995. Now, a whopping 90 percent of an average person's grocery budget in the western world is spent on processed foods, and 70 percent of that food has been genetically modified in some way or another.[9]

 It's hard to avoid buying processed foods especially during harsh winter months when organic produce is minimal. Hopefully, organic options will continue to become more popular, so the price becomes less expensive!

Monsanto, the company that brought us Agent Orange (the chemical defoliant used to terrible effect in the Vietnam War) has a lot to do with this recent problem. Monsanto's scientists pioneered the development of genetically-engineered crops. Having also invented the common pesticide Roundup (glyphosate), the company started making their GM crops dependent on its use. Roundup has been in the news as it continues to lose many court cases around the world because of irrefutable research that conclusively points to Roundup as a known carcinogen.

In addition, genetically modified crops have far higher concentrations of pesticide use, as they are engineered to withstand massive amounts of exposure.

GLYPHOSATE—AVOID AT ALL COSTS!

When farmers spray glyphosate on their fields, not only are they destroying the fertility of the soil, they're also promoting chemical resistance in the field *and* antibiotic resistance in the human food chain. Indeed, weeds have developed resistance to glyphosate, making the weed problem an ever-worsening one. Monsanto claims glyphosate is safe for humans because it acts on a mechanism present only in plants but not in animals or humans. However, it turns out the same mechanism is present in the bacteria in our gut. Glyphosate's deadly impact on our natural gut bacteria has substantial negative consequences.

Glyphosate is a chelator, which means it binds to vital nutrients such as iron, manganese, zinc and boron in the soil, preventing plants from absorbing them. This is problematic, as these minerals are essential to the function of many important metabolic pathways in our bodies. One of these pathways, the shikimate pathway, is used by gut bacteria to produce essential amino acids.

Amino acids are precursors for the production of serotonin (our mood regulator), melatonin (our sleep hormone) and dopamine (our euphoria generator). Knowing that our gut is responsible for about 80 percent of the production of serotonin, inhibiting this ability can become a grave problem. As the building blocks for these essential neurotransmitters are destroyed, we face issues such as anxiety, insomnia and pain. To make matters worse, glyphosate does more damage to beneficial bacteria than pathogenic organisms—leaving behind extremely harmful colonies in their wake.

Next, exposure to glyphosate stunts the body's ability to produce vital digestive enzymes, which can contribute to serious digestive dysfunction and compromise as digestive enzymes are required for the proper breakdown and absorption of nutrients. Aside from malnutrition, the absence of digestive enzymes provides a food source for pathogenic bacteria and yeast.

WHAT DISEASES ARE ASSOCIATED WITH GLYPHOSATE-INDUCED BACTERIA BREAKDOWN?

When good bacteria are affected by glyphosate, they release ammonia into the bloodstream, setting up the body's system for the following diseases:

- liver disease
- type 2 diabetes
- multiple sclerosis
- Parkinson's disease
- irritable bowel syndrome
- cancer
- infertility
- depression
- Alzheimer's disease
- obesity
- cardiovascular disease
- autism
- dysbiosis
- encephalitis
- fatty liver
- allergies
- chronic inflammation

WHERE IS GLYPHOSATE?

It is important that readers understand that glyphosate is used on GMO crops and conventional crops. However, Roundup carcinogens are much higher in genetically-engineered crops when compared to conventional crops. The exposed produce is systemically infused with chemicals such as glyphosate, and they cannot be washed off. Such harsh chemicals and genetically-engineered foods have been deemed unfit for human consumption in numerous European countries. That's right. It's unsafe for people in those European countries, but it's OK for people in the United States and Canada. Our only healthy choice, in this case, is to consume organic produce as often as we can to avoid the harmful effects of GMOs and glyphosate on our systems.

NOT DANGEROUS ENOUGH? WELCOME BT TOXIN TO THE MIX!

Did you know that certain types of pesticides are not even counted when researchers assess pesticide contamination on food? The soil bacteria *Bacillus thuringiensis (Bt)*, produces Bt toxin—a pesticide that breaks open the stomach of certain insects and kills them. This pesticide is actually permitted in organic farming, where it's applied topically. Monsanto has consistently claimed that Bt toxins would harm only insects; meaning that Bt toxins produced inside the plant would be completely destroyed in the human digestive system and would not have *any* impact at all on consumers.

These claims have since turned out to be false. Shocker! In 2011, doctors at Sherbrooke University Hospital in Québec found Bt-toxin in the blood of:

- 93 percent of pregnant women tested
- 80 percent of umbilical cord blood in their babies
- 67 percent of non-pregnant women[10]

The mechanism by which Bt toxin works on an insect is the exact same way it interacts with humans. The toxin literally punches holes in the lining of the digestive tract—which is arguably the most important line of defense for the immune system—making it more permeable. What does this put us at risk for? Leaky-gut syndrome! This occurs when toxins that are meant to remain in our digestive tract for elimination escape through these little holes into our bloodstream, wreaking havoc on our lymphatic and immune systems. Yikes!

As you can see, the extent to which non-organic and genetically-modified foods affect us are far greater than imagined. You can help prevent the adverse effects by buying organic and locally grown as much as possible.

Tip: To spot a genetically-modified fruit or vegetable, look at the little sticker that shows the Price Look-Up code (PLU):

- PLU code for a conventionally grown fruit consists of four numbers (i.e. 1022)
- PLU code for an organically grown fruit is five numbers, beginning with the number 9 (i.e. 91022)
- PLU code for a genetically-modified fruit is five numbers, beginning with the number 8 (i.e. 81022)

Some of the most common "Roundup Ready" crops are:

- soy and corn
- canola
- sugar beets
- cotton
- alfalfa

New GMOs that are increasing in popularity:

- apple
- potato
- zucchini
- papaya
- yellow squash

It is best to purchase these items organic and buy locally as much as possible!

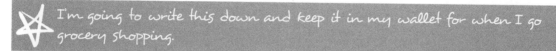

I'm going to write this down and keep it in my wallet for when I go grocery shopping.

BETTER FOR THE ENVIRONMENT

From the soil up, organic farming is better for the environment as a whole. It was the way we survived for thousands of years. Modern "advances" in farming such as chemical fertilizers, pesticides and genetic modifications result in the destruction of soil, plants, animals, and, eventually, the humans that depend on them.

Does this mean you have to buy everything organically? It would probably be best if you could but if it is not possible, the Environmental Working Group (EWG) has come up with a list. Updated every year, it shows which produce has become most contaminated by herbicides, pesticides, and fungicides, and should be bought organic as often as possible, and which ones could be bought that are grown conventionally. As of 2017, here are the dirty dozen and the clean fifteen lists:

THE DIRTY DOZEN

1. Strawberries
2. Nectarines
3. Peaches
4. Cherries
5. Celery
6. Bell Peppers
7. Spinach
8. Apples
9. Pears
10. Grapes
11. Tomatoes
12. Potatoes

Bonus: Hot Peppers

THE CLEAN FIFTEEN

1. Sweet corn
2. Pineapples
3. Onions
4. Papaya
5. Mango
6. Honeydew melon
7. Cantaloupe
8. Cauliflower
9. Avocados
10. Cabbage
11. Sweet peas (frozen)
12. Asparagus
13. Eggplant
14. Kiwi
15. Grapefruit[11]

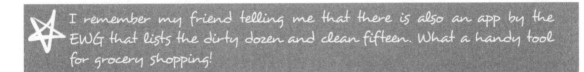

I remember my friend telling me that there is also an app by the EWG that lists the dirty dozen and clean fifteen. What a handy tool for grocery shopping!

THE "GRAY ZONE" OF ORGANIC

There are products, however, that even if bought organic, may not be beneficial or may even have a negative impact on your health. Such items include:

1. **Seafood** – You'd be surprised to hear that there are no official standards for organic seafood in the U.S. Be aware that seafood labeled as organic may be farmed, not wild-caught.[12]

2. **Cosmetics** – Although everything you put on your body is absorbed through your skin, due to lax laws, any cosmetic product can call itself natural but can still be synthetic, as well. To evaluate the products that you're using, log on to www.ewg.org (see **Chapter 18: Your Skin— What Are You Soaking Up?**).

3. **Organic milk** – Buying organic milk is better than non-organic milk, as it will be pesticide-free, hormone-free, and antibiotic-free, but pasteurization can still be a concern. The process of pasteurization destroys the good enzymes, reduces vitamins, dramatically reduces protein content, and is associated with allergies, increased tooth decay, colic in infants, growth problems in children, osteoporosis, arthritis, heart disease and cancer. Clean raw milk can be an alternative, depending on where you live, as it is illegal in some states or countries. Visit www.rawmilk.com to learn more about it.

4. **Organic grains** – Like regular grains, organic grains are quickly metabolized to sugar. So, even if you are purchasing organic whole-grain bread, for example, it may still disrupt insulin levels if eaten in a large quantity.

5. **Organic sugar** – Sugar, even if organic, is not the best choice to make for your health—regardless of the organic label. So, again, don't be fooled by great marketing strategies trying to sell you organic, when the food is essentially bad for you. A box of organic cookies is still a box of cookies, and you don't need the sugar, period.

> ✦ Well said. I know so many people who confuse organic or gluten-free foods with healthy options.

DO YOUR BEST!

You might be thinking that going organic is too much work—that you don't have the resources, the time, or the money. Indeed, healthy eating is a commitment, but eating organic food is better for you. Not to mention the way it tastes and the way it will make you feel should have you converted in no time. Hopefully, with the demand for organic foods skyrocketing, getting these foods will become easier and less expensive over time. It's nice to see some companies even investing in organic farmlands and livestock raising to be able to provide better-quality organic foods. Just do your best; start by changing the way you eat gradually—and feel good about it! There are now a growing number of organic food services that will deliver to your door! "Ding dong! Your fresh organic food is here..."

The following diagram shows examples of health habits with corresponding hack levels. To download the *Hack Your Health Habits Worksheet*, visit

www.hackyourhealthhabits.com/worksheets

READY #HEALTHHACKER?
EXAMPLES OF LEVEL 1, 2 AND 3 HACKS FOR THIS CHAPTER

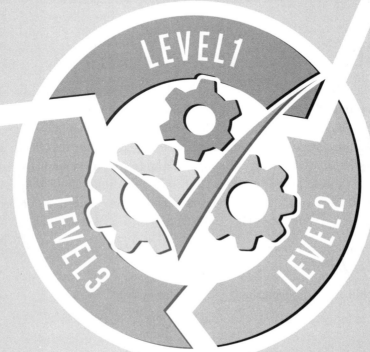

✓ Use your dirty dozen app the next time you are doing groceries to make more health-conscious choices about your produce.

✓ Aim to have 80 percent of all your food intake come from organic sources.

✓ Shop around for organic (or grass-fed) meats, eggs and poultry from your local farmers' market or butcher.

HACK YOUR HEALTH PROGRESS

|||||||||||||||||||||||||||||||||||||||||||||||||||||||||||||||||||||||||||||||||||||||||||||

CHAPTER 9

10
PHYTONUTRIENTS AND ANTIOXIDANTS
Are You Eating by Color?

"The colors of a fresh garden salad are so extraordinary, no painter's pallet can duplicate nature's artistry."

— DR. SUNWOLF

THINK IT OVER

- Is the food you're eating mostly processed and packaged?

- Are you eating the colors of the rainbow in fruits and vegetables every day?

- Do you consume enough antioxidants daily to fight cellular aging?

If you're looking for a way to eat better, lose weight, prevent illness and slow down the aging process, one easy thing to do is eat more whole foods. Whole foods are foods in their natural state, meaning they are unprocessed, unrefined and unpackaged prior to consumption.

While this may sound like a no-brainer, stop and think for a second. How many whole foods do you actually eat in a day? Fruits, vegetables, legumes, nuts, seeds and grains are considered whole because they haven't been altered from their natural state. Hmm, maybe you aren't eating as many whole foods as you thought. Don't worry, you aren't the only one.

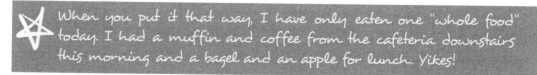

When you put it that way, I have only eaten one "whole food" today. I had a muffin and coffee from the cafeteria downstairs this morning and a bagel and an apple for lunch. Yikes!

These days, people are busy! Pre-made, pre-packaged foods have become a way of life. From granola bars to pre-wrapped sandwiches and frozen dinners, convenience seems to trump whole foods. Unfortunately, this can have a big impact on our health. Most processed foods are heavily altered from their natural form, and riddled with additives and preservatives to keep them fresh. These chemicals can build up in the body and cause an array of side effects. As the saying goes: "*The longer the shelf life, the shorter yours!*"

WHY CHOOSE WHOLE FOODS?

Whole foods contain a wide variety of nutrients. These nutrients include vitamins, minerals, phytonutrients, essential fatty acids, fiber and antioxidants. Antioxidants are especially important, and we will go into why a little later. Eating whole foods doesn't have to be difficult. There are so many delicious, natural options available that are easy to prepare.

Some of my favorite health swaps are:

- replacing store-bought potato chips with baked sweet potatoes, sprinkled with Himalayan sea salts
- replacing processed mayonnaise with guacamole or hummus
- replacing sweetened fruit juice with a real piece of fruit
- replacing instant flavored oatmeal with whole-grain steel-cut oats (which really don't take that much longer to make)
- replacing your morning sugary cereal with a chia seed pudding with a piece of fruit and some nuts

When you buy your groceries, focus on shopping in the organic and fresh-food aisles, which are usually on the outside perimeter of the stores. Try to stay away from center aisles, where you will find mostly processed foods. If your supermarket doesn't have a wide variety of organic options, try your local health food store. And during the warmer months, consider a visit to your local farmers' market.

THE MAGIC OF ANTIOXIDANTS

When it comes to natural healing, antioxidants are the closest thing to magic there is! Countless studies show that the antioxidants found in many whole foods are key in the prevention of disease. There are literally thousands of antioxidant compounds out there, but the most common ones are vitamins A, C, and E, beta-carotene, carotenoids, selenium, flavanol, resveratrol and lycopene—all of which can be absorbed when eating rich, colorful foods such as fruits, vegetables and herbs. In a nutshell, antioxidants help prevent cell damage caused by dangerous free radicals known as oxidants.

WHAT ARE FREE RADICALS?

Free radicals are atoms or molecules that contain unpaired electrons. Due to this, they are highly reactive. In many cases, oxidants will attack the nearest stable molecule so that they can steal its electron.

When the "attacked" molecule loses its electron, it becomes a free radical, itself, and the cycle repeats. Our bodies actually create free radicals to help ward off dangerous viruses and microbes, so they aren't all bad. However, an overabundance of free radicals can lead to health issues. An increase in free radicals can be caused by daily exposure to things like air pollution, cigarette smoke, processed foods and alcohol. Similar to how oxidation rusts metal, it also "rusts" our cells.

Cell damage caused by free radicals is assumed to be a major contributor to aging and disorders, such as:

- cancer
- cognitive decline
- autoimmune disorders
- cardiovascular disease
- weakened immune system

HOW DO ANTIOXIDANTS HELP?

Antioxidants are the first line of defense against trouble-making oxidants. They stop oxidants from stealing electrons from healthy cells and repair cells that have been damaged. This minimizes the risk of cancer, heart disease and other serious diseases. To prevent the biological rust that oxidation causes to our cells, stick to a diet rich in antioxidants.

WHICH ANTIOXIDANTS ARE BEST?

When it comes to antioxidants, there is no set Recommended Daily Intake (RDA) or Daily Value (DV). The number of antioxidants a certain food contains can be evaluated by its ORAC Score (Oxygen Radical Absorption Capacity). This score tests a plant's power to absorb and eliminate free radicals. The following measurements were developed by the National Institute On Aging and are based on 100 grams of each food or herb.

Top-rated foods include:

- goji berries – 25,000 ORAC Score
- wild blueberries – 14,000 ORAC Score
- dark chocolate – 21,000 ORAC Score
- pecans – 17,000 ORAC Score
- artichoke – 9,400 ORAC Score
- elderberries – 14,000 ORAC Score
- kidney beans – 8,400 ORAC Score
- cranberries – 9,500 ORAC Score
- blackberries – 5,300 ORAC Score
- cilantro – 5,100 ORAC Score[1]

Wow! Dark chocolate is almost right up there with goji berries.

EAT YOUR COLORS!

Phytonutrients refer to the several thousand healthful, non-nutritive compounds found in plants. These compounds are referred to as 'non-nutritive' because they do not supply calories like proteins, carbohydrates, or fats do. Despite this, they benefit the body in several ways. Studies show that people who eat more phytonutrient-containing plant foods have a reduced risk of chronic diseases such as diabetes, heart disease and cancer.

Phytonutrients provide many functions in the plant, itself, such as providing protection from pests and environmental stressors, along with imparting color and distinctive tastes and smells. In the human body, phytonutrients stimulate enzymes that help the body get rid of toxins, boost the immune system, improve cardiovascular health, promote healthy estrogen metabolism and stimulate the death of cancer cells.

Fruits and vegetables are rich sources of phytonutrients, along with whole grains, legumes, herbs, spices, nuts, seeds and teas. Phytonutrients in food come in all different colors—red, orange, yellow, green, blue-purple-black and white-tan-brown. To promote good health, it is important to eat fruits and vegetables of varied color each day. Aiming for one to two of each color per day is a healthy goal. While darker-colored plants are generally higher in phytonutrients, fruits and veggies from the white family do have potent contributions to make.

WHAT DO THE SIX DIFFERENT COLORS MEAN?

Red foods contain phytonutrients that may help reduce the risk of certain cancers and protect the brain, heart, liver and immune system. Examples of these foods include beet, bell pepper, blood orange, cranberry, cherry, pink grapefruit, goji berry, grape, onion, plum and pomegranate.

Orange foods help protect the immune system, eyes and skin. They also help reduce the risk of cancer and heart disease. Examples of these foods include apricot, bell pepper, cantaloupe, carrot, mango, nectarine, orange and papaya.

Yellow foods are beneficial because they contain compounds that are anti-cancer, anti-inflammatory, and protect the brain, heart, vasculature, eyes and skin. Examples of these foods include apple, Asian pear, banana, bell pepper, star fruit and squash.

Green foods contain compounds that are anti-cancer, anti-inflammatory, and protect the brain, heart, vasculature, liver and skin. Green foods that help with liver function also help balance hormones. Examples of these foods include avocado, asparagus, green apple, bell pepper, bean sprout, bok choy, broccoli, zucchini, okra, cabbage, celery, spinach, kale and cucumber.

Blue/Purple/Black foods contain compounds that are anti-cancer, anti-inflammatory, and protect the brain, heart and vasculature. It is interesting to note that out of all the colors, this is the category of which most people eat the least. Too little blue/purple can result in issues with the brain, as these foods protect it from damage and promote healthy cognition and memory. Examples of these foods include berries, eggplant, fig, plum, prune and raisins.

White/Tan/Brown foods – When thinking of white/tan/brown foods, processed foods may come to mind—foods like bagels, cereals, breads, pastas, cakes, cookies and crackers. Focus on those that are beneficial like nuts, fruits, vegetables, legumes, spices, seeds and whole grains that are beneficial to your health. The compounds in these earthy-colored foods are anti-cancer and anti-inflammatory. Additionally, like green foods, there are certain compounds that can assist with liver and hormone health. Examples of these foods include ginger, apple, cacao, onion, garlic, coffee, coconut, date, mushroom, nut, bean and tea.

Unfortunately, in the U.S. and Canada today, there exists what is called a "phytonutrient gap," meaning more and more people are not getting enough of their colors throughout the day. More specifically:

- 69 percent fall short in green
- 78 percent fall short in red
- 86 percent fall short in white
- 88 percent fall short in purple/blue
- 79 percent fall short in yellow/orange

EASY WAYS TO EAT YOUR COLORS

Start by observing the colors you eat. As we have discussed, humans are creatures of habit, and, as creatures of habit, we tend to eat the same foods over and over again. This does our body a disservice. In order to get more phytonutrients and antioxidants into your diet, you are going to have to mix things up!

It has been estimated that 80 percent of people are missing one or more of the phytonutrient colors in their diet.[2]

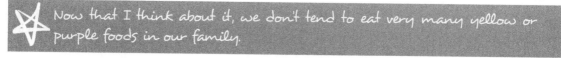

Now that I think about it, we don't tend to eat very many yellow or purple foods in our family.

This is likely because most people stick to eating processed foods that are brown, yellow, or white. For example, think of a typical breakfast menu—waffles, pancakes, ready-to-eat cereal, sausage and eggs. This doesn't provide very many phytonutrients now, does it? Opting for a smoothie with blueberries, apples, raspberries, spinach and carrots would be much more beneficial. That's five of the six color categories right there!

Here are some other simple ways to jump-start getting more whole foods and phytonutrients into your diet. When implementing this way of eating, keep in mind that fruits contain sugar. Even though it's a natural form of sugar, fruits can still spike insulin levels so be sure to load your cart with heaps of colorful vegetables and just a few fruits.

- Make it your goal to try one new plant food (fruit, vegetable, nut, seed, or legume) per week. Explore ethnic stores for greater variety.

- Stock up on organic frozen vegetables for easy cooking, or organic berries as they tend to retain their phytonutrients well.

- Keep fruits and vegetables where you can see them so you will remember to eat them.

- Keep a bowl or container of fresh-cut vegetables on the top shelf of the refrigerator, within easy reach.

- If you must eat something sweet after dinner, choose a fruit for dessert—fruit kabobs, berry compotes, fruit salads, etc.

- Have dishes with lots of vegetable variety (e.g., soups, stir fry).

- Choose darker vegetables over lighter to maximize nutrient content.

- Make a switch from mashed white potatoes to sliced carrots or mashed cauliflower.

- Toss in red pepper, tomato sauce, garlic, onions, mushrooms, or broccoli in omelets.

- Add rinds of oranges or lemons to your water.

- Try a little bit of every color at a salad bar.

- Be generous with your use of herbs and spices.

- Devote some time at the start of your week to preparing your meals and recipes. This will make eating whole foods throughout the week so much easier!

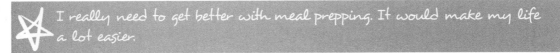
I really need to get better with meal prepping. It would make my life a lot easier.

One more tip. To make things easier for myself, I re-arranged my fridge to emphasize the food colors. Forget separating fruits and vegetables, I now separate things by color. It has made preparing my meals and shakes so much easier. I open the fridge and grab at least one or two items from each group. It's a good reminder to add variety to my dishes, and it looks pretty! It's also a great way to teach kids about the importance of healthy, colorful foods. Make them choose which colors they want to eat. Try making it into a little game, or have a color chart that they can check off each day to make sure that they are eating all the colors of the rainbow.

That's a great idea! I should also start bringing the kids with me to the grocery store to help me buy all the different colors of fruits and vegetables.

After reading this chapter you might be thinking, *Who knew eating food could be so complex?* Trust me, it's not that hard. A few changes to your grocery list and dedicating time for meal prep on Sunday, and you'll do great! When it comes to free radicals, antioxidants and phytonutrients, just go back to the basics: less prepared and packaged foods and more whole foods. My Grandpa was a farmer, and I often think to myself, *What would Grandpa eat?* He was always so proud of his garden, and he should have been! Opt for whole foods, eat all sorts of colors, and you should be covered. The food industry might have made things more convenient for us, but it comes at the sacrifice of our health. Keep food simple and enjoy!

The following diagram shows examples of health habits with corresponding hack levels. To download the *Hack Your Health Habits Worksheet*, visit

www.hackyourhealthhabits.com/worksheets

READY #HEALTHHACKER?
EXAMPLES OF LEVEL 1, 2 AND 3 HACKS FOR THIS CHAPTER

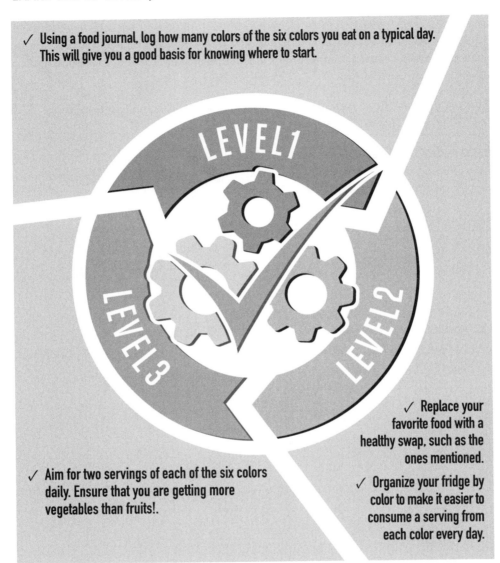

✓ Using a food journal, log how many colors of the six colors you eat on a typical day. This will give you a good basis for knowing where to start.

LEVEL1

LEVEL2

LEVEL3

✓ Replace your favorite food with a healthy swap, such as the ones mentioned.

✓ Organize your fridge by color to make it easier to consume a serving from each color every day.

✓ Aim for two servings of each of the six colors daily. Ensure that you are getting more vegetables than fruits!.

HACK YOUR HEALTH PROGRESS

||||||||||||||||||||||||||||||||||||||||||||||||||||||||||||||||||||||||||||||

CHAPTER 10

SECTION 3

*Get Fueled with the Right Foods
and Figure Out the Diet That
Works for You*

Want to say goodbye to fad diets once and for all?
Section 3 presents a full overview of some of the
most popular diets on the market, and which one
may be best suited for you. You will also learn that
food is information, food is energy, and determine
why the right fit is essential when it comes to
personalizing your diet.

NUTRITION
Who Should You Believe?

> "The worst thing about being lied to is knowing you weren't worth the truth."
>
> — Unknown

THINK IT OVER

- Are food politics having too much of an impact on food guidelines?

- How often are the food guidelines actually revised?

- Can you identify what recommendations in the current food guideline might have a negative impact on your health?

Disclaimer: We realize some of our readers may live elsewhere, but for the purposes of this book, I will be discussing the recommended food guidelines of the United States and Canada. Also, don't forget that the standard American Food Guide and Canadian Food Guide Pyramid are subject to change over the years, and the statements made in this chapter are based on the guidelines as of 2017. For the purposes of this chapter, I will use the general term "Food Guide," which applies to both countries' published dietary recommendations.

According to Health Canada, four out of five Canadians are at risk for developing cancer, heart disease, type 2 diabetes, and a plethora of other health issues as a result of unhealthy eating.[1] And, the cause of obesity and other chronic conditions can be linked directly to poor eating habits, which, in turn, can put a considerable burden on the health-care system. But, how does that fit with the famous food guide recommendations we grew up with, that told us what foods we should eat and how many servings of each type of food we should consume in a day?

Until 2017, guidelines stated that we should be consuming mostly carbohydrate and grain sources, followed by fruits and vegetables, followed by meats and dairy, and then fats, which are to be eaten sparingly. It was only recently that Health Canada decided to update its food guide to include fruits and vegetables before grains and starches.

Although the changes were made in an effort to keep up with new research on healthy eating, recent studies have shown that the key to weight management, illness prevention, and overall health lies in a food regime that is still very different from what the food guide recommends, which will be discussed in further detail in the rest of this section. So, why then is the government still endorsing guidelines that are not keeping up with the latest research and that are not in the best interests of our health?

The food guide recommendations released in both the United States and Canada have catapulted us into the worst epidemic of obesity, diabetes and cardiovascular illness in history. Before we get into how this happened, let's first take a look at why these guidelines came to be.

During the 1970s, when it became evident that obesity and heart disease were on the rise, concerned politicians held hearings to discuss how to advise citizens about diet, health and preventing heart disease. In 1977, D. Mark Hegsted, a nutrition professor at Harvard, led a study addressing the connections between food consumption and heart disease. The group issued the very first set of Dietary Guidelines distributed by the U.S. Federal Government.

Among its findings, Hegsted's report recommended Americans to consume 55 percent to 60 percent of their total daily calories from carbohydrates and to only consume 30 percent to 35 percent of their calories from fat, to help decrease the risks of heart disease.[2] This first guideline suggested avoiding saturated fats entirely and eat only low-fat foods

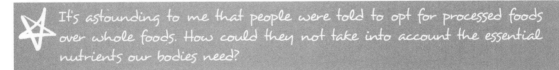

It's astounding to me that people were told to opt for processed foods over whole foods. How could they not take into account the essential nutrients our bodies need?

Since their inception, the guidelines in the United States have been revised roughly every five years. In the 1980s, a follow-up called the American Food Guide Pyramid was released. Unfortunately, it was even worse than its predecessor. At the base of the pyramid were refined carbohydrates such as breads, pasta, rice and cereals, of which we were told to eat six to eleven servings a day.

Whoa! I don't think I'd be able to eat that many carbs even if I tried.

Think back to our chapter on carbohydrates; six to eleven servings is a lot. We now know that carbohydrates break down into sugar, and easily stored in the body as fat. We also know that consumption of refined carbs creates inflammation, which triggers most chronic diseases, including diabetes and obesity (or "diabesity," a term coined by Dr. Mark Hyman), heart disease, cancer, dementia and depression.[3] As previously discussed, eating sugar and other refined carbohydrates turns on our metabolic switch, spiking insulin (our fat storage hormone) and causing unwanted and dangerous belly fat.

Following the American and Canadian government's guidelines, the food industry started what is now known as the "low-fat craze." They created everything from low-fat salad dressing to fat-free yogurt and even "light" desserts. Fat became the enemy, and processed foods became healthy alternatives to the whole foods we knew and loved. As good citizens, we listened wholeheartedly, not understanding why our bellies and health problems continued to grow. While recommendations in the current food guide regarding carbs and fats are the most prominent problems, there are other issues:

- **Dairy is overemphasized** – Although calcium is important, it's more about how much we absorb rather than how much we consume. The calcium absorption rate from milk is about 32 percent, whereas some leafy green vegetables have a calcium absorption rate of more than 50 percent.[4] What's more, many people have developed allergies and sensitivities to dairy products, which contributes to poor health. More on this in **Chapter 41: Food Sensitivities—Is Your Body Angry with What You Are Eating?**

- **Quality Matters** – There is no differentiation made between good sources and not-so-good sources of protein, good sources and not-so-good sources of carbs, and good sources and not-so-good sources of fats. An avocado (which contains good fat) is incredibly nutritious, whereas margarine (bad fat) has no real nutritional value.

- **"Sugar sugar"** – There is an issue with having fruits and vegetables grouped in the same category. For example, in the 2016 Canadian Food Guide, the suggested servings for fruits and vegetables for a female aged 19-50 is about 7-8 servings. If someone eats seven fruits a day and only one vegetable a day, think of the sugar! While natural sugars are fine in low doses, too much could send your blood-sugar levels on a roller coaster ride, if you're not careful.

Though the food guide meant well, it has come at a cost to our health. Could this be due to a conflict of interest? When it comes down to it, the food industry is a huge revenue generator, and many companies could be negatively impacted if the guidelines were modified to the detriment of the product that they sell.

Fortunately, when it comes to food, you have a choice. You can do your own research and make choices based on what feels right to you. Making healthy choices now will help push the food industry into the right direction.

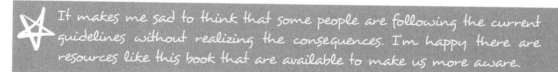

It makes me sad to think that some people are following the current guidelines without realizing the consequences. I'm happy there are resources like this book that are available to make us more aware.

TIME FOR A CHANGE—A NEW FOOD PYRAMID

As discussed in Chapter 5, fat is not completely the enemy but rather sugar is—and sugar can come in many forms such as in grains and even fruit. With this in mind, we need a new generation of our food pyramid; one that addresses the issues currently present in our food guidelines and that genuinely supports our health. With the benefits of fats, proteins, and phytonutrients in mind, I have put forth what I believe to be an improved food guide that can help decrease the chances of chronic inflammatory illnesses. My *Hack Your Health Habits Food Pyramid* would look something like this:

- At the very base of the pyramid, we would find non-starchy vegetables such as leafy greens like spinach, kale and Swiss chard. Eat these in abundance!

- Our next level would include healthy fats and fermented foods. We already know the benefits of a high-fat diet, and the importance of fermented foods will be discussed in greater detail in **Chapter 27: Probiotics—Keep Your Bugs Happy!**

- Following the fats and fermented foods, we have the proteins and grass-fed dairy. A moderate amount of protein is needed but should not overpower the amount of fat we consume. Grass-fed dairy is a good source of animal fat for those who are not sensitive to it; but, for those who have a dairy intolerance or sensitivity, dairy would *not* be a good option.

- Up next, we have the fruits and starchy vegetables. Notice we separated the starchy vegetables* (such as sweet potatoes, carrots and squash) from the non-starchy ones (such as kale, spinach and celery), as the former can cause an insulin response due to the higher carbohydrate content. Fruits are grouped into this category, as well, are high in fructose, and too much fruit can actually increase blood sugar levels and prevent weight loss.

- Sprouted grains and legumes* would be next as we approach the top of the pyramid, since they can often be labeled as 'good carbs' but are to be eaten sparingly, again, because of their higher sugar and lectin content. Sprouting removes phytic acid and enzyme inhibitors from beans, which can limit mineral absorption. Sprouting technically turns a grain or bean into a vegetable.

- And finally, at the very top of the pyramid, we would find the "sugars with *at least* some benefits," which include the occasional indulgence like dark chocolate or red wine. Although these do turn to sugar in the body, chocolate at least has the benefit of the cacao bean and red wine of resveratrol.

*Note: These foods can be completely omitted for some people who choose to try a lectin-free diet (discussed in the next chapter). Nightshades and certain seeds would also be avoided on this diet.

You can download the *Hack Your Health Habits Food Pyramid* at

www.hackyourhealthhabits.com/hyhhfoodpyramid

The following diagram shows examples of health habits with corresponding hack levels. To download the *Hack Your Health Habits Worksheet*, visit

www.hackyourhealthhabits.com/worksheets

READY #HEALTHHACKER?
EXAMPLES OF LEVEL 1, 2 AND 3 HACKS FOR THIS CHAPTER

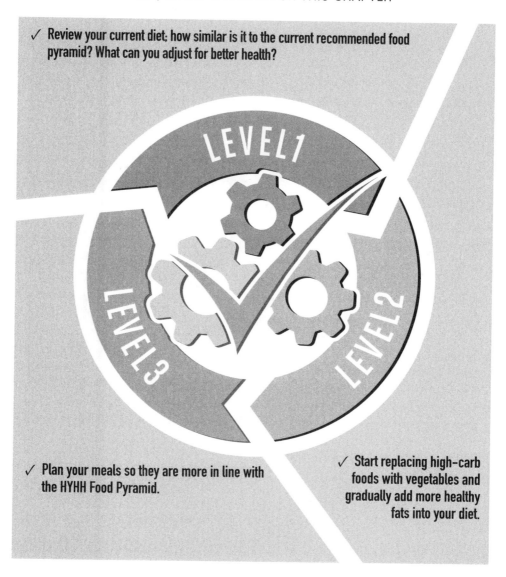

✓ Review your current diet; how similar is it to the current recommended food pyramid? What can you adjust for better health?

✓ Plan your meals so they are more in line with the HYHH Food Pyramid.

✓ Start replacing high-carb foods with vegetables and gradually add more healthy fats into your diet.

HACK YOUR HEALTH PROGRESS

||||||||||||||||||||||||||||||||||||||||||||||||||||||||||||||||||||||||||||||

CHAPTER 11

DIETS 101
Which One is Right for You?

12

> "I am not dieting, I am changing my lifestyle."
>
> — Unknown

THINK IT OVER

- Have you ever tried a fad diet? How did it make you feel? Did you achieve the results you expected?

- Do you think that there is a one-size-fits-all way of eating?

- Can you identify which diet plan may work best for you?

Your co-worker looks great these days. She's changed her eating habits, has started working out and has lost 20 lbs. You wonder what she's doing and gather the courage to approach her and ask her about it. *What's your secret?* you ask, eagerly awaiting her answer. Her response: *I've been following the _____ diet! It has been working great!*

You go home, read about the diet online, print recipes, meal plans and grocery lists; you are ready to do this! The first few days are tough, but you get the hang of it within a couple of weeks. After a month, you step on the scale, excited to see your results. To your disbelief, you've lost only a few pounds, despite following the diet to a T! Though the results are disappointing, you decide to stick with it. At month two, you hop on the scale again to see similar results: You're losing some weight, but not nearly as much as your co-worker. *This sucks*, you think to yourself. *What am I doing wrong?*

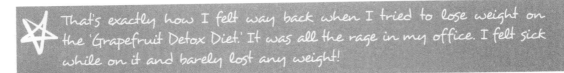

That's exactly how I felt way back when I tried to lose weight on the 'Grapefruit Detox Diet.' It was all the rage in my office. I felt sick while on it and barely lost any weight!

This is, unfortunately, a very common occurrence. Someone tells you about a "revolutionary" new product, diet, or fitness regime, and you try it for yourself, only to realize that it's not working for you. You wonder what all the hype is about and question whether you're doing something wrong.

Here's the thing. Just because something doesn't work for you doesn't mean it doesn't work at all. When it comes to diets, no two people are the same. No diet is a one-size-fits-all solution. There are a lot of diets, quick fixes, and "solutions" out there, and, in this age of information, the pure volume of ideas can be staggering. How do we know which diet will work for us? How do we know which diets are healthiest?

The right diet for you will make you feel great and keep your energy steady throughout the day. It will allow you to stay at a healthy weight, not feel bloated, and help you avoid blood-sugar spikes and dips. Most people will have to tweak their diet every now and then, depending on their level of physical activity, age, health goals and stress levels. You may even have to try a few different diets before finding the one that is best suited for you, but it's worth the effort.

Eating the right foods to fuel your body will have a huge impact on your overall health and well-being. Your health goals may also be different from someone else's, meaning, if you have arthritis, allergies, or cardiovascular issues, you may need to be on a more anti-inflammatory diet. If you have hormone issues, you may do better on a slightly different diet to rebalance your hormones. Or, for philosophical reasons, you may decide that you don't want to eat meat. We all have different goals and different needs! To make things a little easier for you, I have created a summary of some of the most popular diets today. Although these diets don't fully follow the HYHH Food Pyramid per se, they are still valid food plans that can yield good results depending on individual needs.

POPULAR DIET OPTIONS

1) PALEO

This hugely popular diet is based on foods our ancestors ate in the Paleolithic or "caveman" period. It proposes that human health is best served by the foods humans originally evolved to eat. To make it simple, the Paleo diet consists of foods that you can find in their natural forms, such as meats, plants, nuts and seeds. It excludes grains, legumes, dairy and anything processed. This diet is often followed by athletes and performance coaches as they believe it provides them with the ideal fuel to perform at their highest level.

What to Eat	What to Avoid	Pros and/or Cons
Meat and seafood	Grains	Emphasizes whole foods and is fairly easy to follow
Vegetables and some fruit	Dairy	Helps reduce overeating through increased fats and protein consumption
Fats	Beans and legumes	Can be expensive
Nuts and seeds	Processed foods and sugar	Phytonutrients from beans, legumes and whole grains are not included

2) VEGAN DIET

The vegan diet is pretty simple to describe. It doesn't include any animal products—only plant-based foods. This means no dairy, eggs, seafood, or foods derived from animals. Even honey is not allowed. The vegan diet rests on the premise that humans should not exploit animals by using them for food, and that this is a healthier and more environmentally responsible diet. Vegans believe it is because we are consuming animal products, that illness and disease have become so prevalent in our society today. This diet consists mainly of vegetables, nuts, seeds, grains, legumes and soy products (preferably fermented soy; more on this later).

What to Eat	What to Avoid	Pros and/or Cons
Fruits and vegetables	All animal products	High plant content = a diet rich in fiber, antioxidants and phytonutrients
Whole grains, beans and legumes		Studies show vegans have lower cholesterol, blood pressure and blood lipids
Nuts and seeds		Very restrictive
Soy products		Eliminating animal products from diet increases risk of nutritional deficiencies (in particular vitamin B12)

3) KETOGENIC DIET

A ketogenic diet involves following a high and healthy fat, moderate protein and low-carb food plan. The goal of the diet is to achieve a metabolic state called nutritional ketosis, which is when the body burns fat instead of glucose as fuel. The ketogenic diet is recommended for those with autoimmune disorders, cognitive impairments and for those with metabolic conditions. It consists primarily of meats, seafood, non-starchy vegetables, lots of healthy fats, and excludes grains, legumes and processed foods. We will cover the ketogenic diet in great length in **Chapter 14: The Ketogenic Diet—A Way to Stay Lean & Prevent Disease.**

What to Eat	What to Avoid	Pros and/or Cons
Moderate amount of animal protein and seafood	Grains and starchy vegetables	Emphasizes whole foods
Lots of fats including full-fat dairy	Pasteurized low-fat dairy	Studies show that a ketogenic diet can help reduce body weight and BMI
Non-starchy vegetables	Beans and legumes	Helps improve cholesterol, triglycerides and blood glucose
Nuts and seeds	Processed foods and sugar	Huge mind shift for those used to following a low-fat diet

4) ADRENAL RESET DIET

According to Dr. Alan Christianson, author of *The Adrenal Reset Diet,* when our bodies shift into survival mode (also known as adrenal stress), we gain weight. Survival mode disrupts sleep and raises our reactions to stress. Processed foods, pollutants, and the pressures of daily life trigger this physiologic pattern. Typical weight loss efforts like eating less and exercising more only make the problem worse. The book states that by cycling carbohydrates, repairing our circadian rhythms and raising our mental clarity, we can make ourselves resistant to survival mode, lose weight and thrive.

What to Eat	What to Avoid	Pros and/or Cons
Low carb and protein in morning	Fructose and processed meats	Emphasizes whole foods
High carb in afternoon	Carbs in the morning	Focuses on healing the adrenal glands in line with the three stages of adrenal fatigue
Focuses on daily detox and targeted tonics to repair circadian rhythm		Focuses on decreasing life stressors (environmental, work, relationships and finances)
		Also suggests natural ways to help adrenals

5) THE HORMONE RESET DIET

When weight loss is your goal, you often don't think that your hormones may be the culprit for your inability to lose weight. But when you develop resistance to any of the major metabolic hormones, your body will adjust by down-regulating your metabolism, unfortunately impeding your ability to reach optimal weight.

The solution is to reprogram your hormonal levels by repairing hormone receptors and growing new ones. In *The Hormone Reset Diet*, Dr. Sara Gottfried uses cutting-edge research to craft a weight-loss and energy program that will reverse hormone resistance in just 21 days. As a result, you will boost your metabolism and calorie-burning by growing new and fresh thyroid receptors, increase your weight loss by re-balancing estrogen and progesterone receptors, and reverse aging by resetting glucocorticoid receptors, for better cortisol processing.

What to Eat	What to Avoid	Pros and/or Cons
High fiber and slow carbs	Meat and sugar	Designed to reset your hormones to promote weight loss
1 pound of vegetables per day	Most fruits	Restrictive diet
Healthy fats	Caffeine and alcohol	Boosts fat-burning and helps reduce inflammation
"Clean" protein	Grain and dairy	Promotes good gut health
Suggested supplements	Toxins	Decreases body's overall toxic load

6) GLUTEN-FREE

Consumption of grains has been linked to various emerging disorders such as cognitive decline, high cholesterol, elevated blood glucose and high blood pressure. The goal of a gluten-free diet is to eliminate wheat and all other gluten-containing grains such as rye and barley. There are many different versions of this style of eating as the ones described in the books *Wheat Belly* by William Davis, MD, and *Grain Brain* by David Perlmutter, MD. Gluten-free diets often emphasize whole foods, lean proteins, healthy fats and veggies. This diet is similar to the Paleo diet.

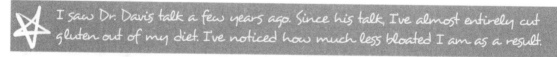

I saw Dr. Davis talk a few years ago. Since his talk, I've almost entirely cut gluten out of my diet. I've noticed how much less bloated I am as a result.

What to Eat	What to Avoid	Pros and/or Cons
Non-starchy vegetables	Anything containing gluten including wheat, rye, barley	Emphasizes whole foods
Low glycemic fruit	High carbohydrate foods	May help reduce digestive issues
Nuts and seeds		Studies show that a gluten-free diet may reduce inflammation and boost mood and energy
Lean meats, seafood and eggs		Gluten-free doesn't automatically mean healthy; don't fall for clever food packaging

7) THE PEGAN DIET (PALEO + VEGAN)

The Pegan diet is a modified version of the Paleo and Vegan diets, which may sound like an oxymoron at first. The Paleo diet is known as the "caveman" diet because it's high in meat, fish, eggs, vegetables and fruits. Meanwhile, the vegan diet bans consumption of all animal products, focusing on a diet high in vegetables, fruits, grains, nuts and seeds. The Pegan diet is a medley of the two, minimizing the consumption of animal products and sticking to a gluten-free diet, which is high in fat.

What to Eat	What to Avoid	Pros and/or Cons
Focus on more protein and fats. Nuts (but not peanuts), seeds (like flax, chia, hemp, sesame, pumpkin)	Stay away from most vegetable oils such as canola, sunflower, corn, and, especially, soybean oil	Focuses on the glycemic load of your diet—it's beneficial to stabilize sugar levels
Eat the right fats: coconut, avocados and olive oil	Avoid dairy	Emphasizes whole foods
Some saturated fat from grass-fed or sustainably raised animals	Avoid gluten and eat gluten-free whole grains sparingly	Emphasizes organic meats
Eat mostly plants – lots of low glycemic vegetables and fruits (This should be 75 percent of the diet and the food on your plate)		Eat meat or animal products as a condiment, not a main course
		Vegetables should take center stage, and meat should be a side dish

8) THE PLANT PARADOX PROGRAM

If you want to focus on a diet that aims to decrease inflammation and the possibility of developing an autoimmune disease, then the plant paradox program may be something of interest to you. Curated by Steven Gundry MD, the program strives to put an end to conditions like leaky gut syndrome, weight gain, brain fog and many other chronic ailments for good. The program claims that even "health" foods like fruit some vegetables, grains and legumes can actually do your body harm, as they contain a protein called lectin. Much like gluten, when lectins invade our bodies, they can cause some serious inflammatory responses that wreak havoc on our health. For this reason, his program consists of a fairly restrictive but targeted method of eating that aims to repair and restore the gut, improve cellular communication, and have you feeling at your very best.

What to Eat	What to Avoid	Pros and/or Cons
Leafy greens and non-starchy vegetables	Animal meats and fats—to be eaten sparingly (and only grass-fed)	High plant content = a diet rich in fiber, antioxidants and phytonutrients
Dairy from goats or sheep and wild-caught seafood	All grains	Lesser chance of leaky gut, cellular miscommunication and molecular mimicry
Nuts and seeds (with the exception of pumpkin, chia and sunflower seeds)	Nightshade vegetables	Restrictive and requires extensive planning and preparation

Omega-3 fats from fish oil, flaxseed, avocado, walnut, olive, MCT, or macadamia	Out of season fruits	Can be difficult for people who live in colder climates as it encourages eating produce that are only in season
Sorghum and millet	Soy and legumes	Limitation in animal products may increases risk of nutritional deficiencies (in particular iron and B12)
In-season fruits	All sweeteners (with the exception of stevia or sugar alcohols)	Helps decrease inflammation, improve immune function and resistance to illness

THE BOTTOM LINE

There are many different conventional diets out there. As previously mentioned, one size doesn't fit all. We are all different. What works for one person may not work for you. Also, keep in mind that our needs or goals may change as we shift through the various stages of life. We might have loved to have one steak per week in our younger years, but now prefer to follow a more plant-based diet. Become a food detective. Experiment with some of the different approaches to eating and keep track of your results in a food journal. Monitor things like digestion, mood, energy, sleep and weight. Over time, you may start to notice some patterns and be able to modify your eating to achieve the desired results.

The following diagram shows examples of health habits with corresponding hack levels. To download the *Hack Your Health Habits Worksheet*, visit

www.hackyourhealthhabits.com/worksheets

READY #HEALTHHACKER?
EXAMPLES OF LEVEL 1, 2 AND 3 HACKS FOR THIS CHAPTER

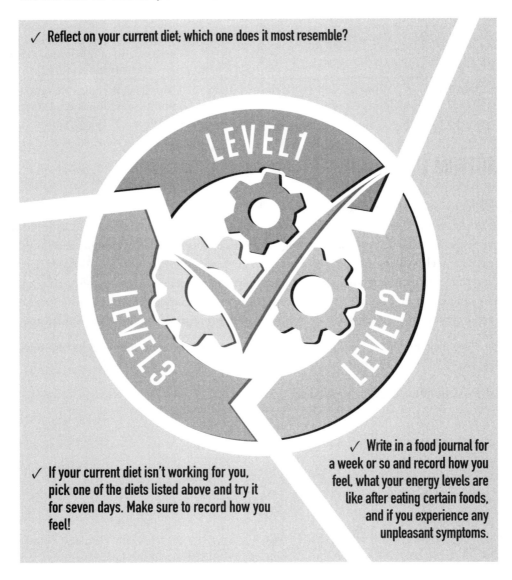

✓ Reflect on your current diet; which one does it most resemble?

✓ If your current diet isn't working for you, pick one of the diets listed above and try it for seven days. Make sure to record how you feel!

✓ Write in a food journal for a week or so and record how you feel, what your energy levels are like after eating certain foods, and if you experience any unpleasant symptoms.

HACK YOUR HEALTH PROGRESS

IIIIIIIIIIIIIIII

CHAPTER 12

INTERMITTENT FASTING
Could You Benefit from It?

"Fasting is like spring cleaning for your body."

— JENTEZEN FRANKLIN

THINK IT OVER

- Have you ever tried any type of fasting before?

- What is your current "eating window?"

- Do you know the health benefits of intermittent fasting?

For thousands of years, ancient cultures around the world have used fasting as a means of healing the body during times of sickness. To this day, some cultures continue to believe that restricting food intake is a path to obtaining mental clarity and spiritual awakening. In Western society, intermittent fasting, a modern spin on the concept of fasting, has created a buzz among health professionals. Some claim it to be the breakthrough to fat loss, while others believe it's just another fad diet. But, what does the evidence say? And, who can really benefit from it?

Intermittent fasting relies on the notion that the timing of food intake is crucial to how your body will use that food. It claims that restricting your *eating* window to 6-8 hours, thereby extending your *fasting* window to 16-18 hours, will yield tremendous benefits for fat loss, hormone balance, energy and insulin stabilization. Also, since food activates the parasympathetic nervous system—the "rest and digest" part of the nervous system—if you eat more during the day, you will be more tired as your body busies itself processing the food. It is better to eat more toward the end of the day so that the food you eat does not take energy from you during digestion.

> ★ I pretty much eat from the time I wake up in the morning to the time I go to bed. My eating window is almost 16 hours right now.

From an evolutionary standpoint, researchers say that our ancestors went through periods where food was abundant at certain times and less available at others. This *feast and famine* pattern conditioned the human body to burn stored fat as its primary source of energy when food was scarce. As well, many ancient religions observed some forms of fasting as a way of cleansing and creating mental alertness.

There are several ways to go about intermittent fasting, depending on your lifestyle and personal preferences. The most commonly used method is the 16:8, which consists of 16 hours of fasting and an 8-hour window for eating. Although 16 hours of fasting may seem like a bit much, keep in mind that sleep will generally occur for seven to nine of the fasting hours. An example of this would be breaking your fast at 11 a.m. and eating your last meal at 7 p.m.

Another intermittent fasting approach is the Warrior Diet, consisting of a 20-hour fast and 4-hour eating cycle. Ori Hofmekler, the author of *The Warrior Diet*, suggests: *"There is a dual relationship between your feeding and innate clock. And, as much as your innate clock affects your feeding, your feeding can affect your innate clock. Routinely eating at the wrong time will disrupt your innate clock and devastate vital body functions, and you'll certainly feel the side effects as your whole metabolic system gets unsynchronized."*[1] This method is not for everyone and would need to be developed gradually, as 20 hours of fasting may be quite difficult for some. An example of this would be breaking your fast at 2 p.m. and having your last meal at 6 p.m., allowing for 20 hours of fasting in between.

Block fasting has also gained some popularity; it consists of a full 4-10-day fast done periodically instead of fasting intermittently on a daily basis. As block fasts can last for several days, one would rely solely on water or bone broth while the body completely cleanses and detoxifies itself. Block fasts, if done at least once a year, have been shown to reduce risk for developing cancer, break through weight-loss plateaus, balance hormones, help reach a state of ketosis quicker, improve insulin sensitivity and increase cellular energy. A 24-hour fast can even boost the human growth hormone (which stimulates cell growth and regeneration) by 1300 percent-2000 percent![2] To perform a block fast safely, you must start gradually. You don't run a marathon on the day you take up running; you ease into it slowly. The same thing applies to block fasting.

Finally, let's talk about the *alternate day* method, where most of the research on intermittent fasting originated. This system consists of intermittently fasting for two days out of the week and eating normally for the remaining five days. On the fasting days, you would have an eating window of eight hours and a fasting window of sixteen hours. This allows those who find it difficult to refrain from eating still reap some of the benefits of fasting. Liquids such as water, tea and coffee may be consumed during the fasting hours. Coffee also acts as an appetite suppressant, which may help you to get to that first late meal of the day.

Each of these methods is effective in its own way, and useful when done in accordance with one's schedule, lifestyle and health goals. It is important to note that intermittent fasting is not a calorie-restriction diet, nor does it count macronutrients or portion sizes. It works by limiting the window in which we consume food during the day. You are not eating *less* food, but rather eating *less often*. Changing your eating patterns may be challenging at first. Hang in there. It takes the body only a short time to adapt, and the benefits are well worth it.

THE PHASES OF FASTING

When you first begin to limit your eating window, your body will have to shift from food-burning mode to fat-burning mode, so, as the constant flow of food for energy stops, your body must rely on its own fat stores for energy. When this happens, a state of nutritional ketosis occurs, meaning that the body will burn fat for its primary source of energy rather than sugar (more on this later in the next chapter). This process may take a while, and hunger is likely, but once your body has adapted to this new shift, you will be using your own body fat for energy, without extreme feelings of hunger. Give your body a chance to adapt, and once it does, you will know it. Intermittent fasting will then become effortless.

THE BENEFITS OF INTERMITTENT FASTING

- Intermittent Fasting (IF) increases the body's ability to become fat-adaptive, resulting in greater fat loss. As your body fluctuates between periods of fasting and eating, it will start burning fat as fuel, instead of carbohydrates. [3]

- IF stabilizes insulin and leptin resistance. In one study, fasting dropped levels of leptin by 76.3 percent in obese males, resulting in massive weight loss. [4]

- It increases brain-derived neurotrophic factor (BDNF), which supports neural growth by 20 percent to 30 percent.

- It increases ghrelin, resulting in people feeling less hungry.

- IF reduces triglycerides, inflammation and free radicals.

- It helps decrease chances for metabolic syndrome (which involves high blood pressure, prediabetic blood sugar, cardiovascular disease, high LDL cholesterol, oxidative stress).

- IF boosts the human growth hormone (HGH), usually produced during sleep and exercise—potentially by up to 2,000 percent!

- IF increases insulin sensitivity; a study has shown that only 20 hours of water fasting is enough to increase insulin sensitivity.

- It leads to better muscle retention as intermittent fasting has shown to be more effective at preventing muscle loss than strictly caloric restriction.

- It decreases the risk for certain cancers. Fasting less than 13 hours per night was associated with an increase in the risk of breast cancer recurrence versus 13 or more hours per night.

In addition, each two-hour increase in the nightly fasting duration was associated with significantly lower hemoglobin A1c levels—a diabetes marker—and a longer duration of nighttime sleep, according to one study.[5]

- Exercise while fasting can boost testosterone (the muscle-building hormone) levels by up to 180 percent! Research shows that eating prior to exercise causes a significant drop in testosterone levels. According to the research, the worst times to eat are between 5:30 a.m. and 8:30 a.m., when testosterone levels are at their highest.[6]

- IF improved performance on behavioral tests of sensory and motor function, learning, memory—and was even associated with increased synaptic plasticity.

Still not convinced? Here are five huge reasons why intermittent fasting can aid in increasing lifespan:

- In a study of epigenetics, intermittent fasting has shown to turn on longevity genes and turn off inflammatory genes.

- Intermittent fasting inhibits glucose and insulin spikes, which are now known to be the underlying causes of inflammation and disease.

- Autophagy—the processes by which your body cleans out various debris, including toxins, and recycles damaged cell components—occurs within only 18 hours of fasting. This means that cancer cells have a hard time adapting and can eventually self-destruct.[7]

> *It's amazing how interlinked food and illness really are.*

- As fasting accelerates the process of entering ketosis, the body burns clean energy (explained in further detail in **Chapter 14: The Ketogenic Diet—A Way to Stay Lean & Prevent Disease**), lowering inflammation in the body, which can help heal the brain and positively influence DNA expression.[8]

- Intermittent fasting has also been shown to increase production of new neurons from neural stem cells.

HOW TO GET STARTED

If you are eager to test out the benefits of intermittent fasting yourself, here's how to get started. First, choose your eating and fasting window. For beginners, you can start the first week with eating for 12 and fasting for 12 and slowly decrease your eating window by 2 hours each week until you reach your desired schedule. Optimally, try to attain a fasting window of 16-18 hours and an eating window of 6-8 hours, as this will yield the best results. Or, you may choose to do a 24-hour fast once or twice a week and resume eating normally the rest of the week. You may want to warn your loved ones on the days you fast.

Let's say you chose to use the 16:8 method. In this scenario, you would have your first meal around 11 a.m. or 12 p.m. (typically when you would have lunch) and have your last meal around 7 p.m. or 8 p.m. You can choose to have 2-3 meals during your eating window, but beware of snacking too much!

Remember, the clock starts ticking when you consume your last bit of food, so if you finish your dinner at 8 p.m., but then have a handful of almonds at 9 p.m., then 9 p.m. is your start time. Ensure your meals are comprised of a good balance of healthy fats and proteins, with a variety of vegetables to get as much phytonutrients as possible. It is also important to eat your last meal "to full." You don't want your body to feel hungry and think that it is in famine mode, and then start storing fat as reserve in the event that adequate energy supply may not be available later.

When our eating window is complete, fluids such as tea and water are still OK to consume—and even necessary to keep you hydrated. If you are having trouble skipping breakfast, coffee mixed with a healthy source of fat such as grass-fed butter or coconut oil are perfect appetite suppressants. This may even help your body produce more ketones—which are produced when the body burns fat—while lowering blood glucose.

 Phew, I was worried coffee would be off limits.

DIET VARIATION: WHY IT IS SO IMPORTANT

When it comes to intermittent fasting, variation within the timing of meals is crucial for reaching optimal results. The body is a pattern-recognizing machine and adapts to changes in stimuli. To maximize the benefit of intermittent fasting, the body needs to be challenged periodically by manipulating meal timing and macronutrient intake. With this in mind, there is the 5-1-1 protocol, comprised of 5 days of intermittent fasting, 1 day of fast and 1 day of feast. For example, from Monday to Friday, you would stick to a 16:8 schedule. On Saturday, you would do a full 24-hour fast with water and bone broth. On Sunday, you could start increasing protein and carbohydrate intake significantly, compared to your intermittent-fasting days. This diet variation cycle is designed to push you into using your fat stores as fuel efficiently if you are having difficulty losing weight, have low energy and have hormone imbalances.

Another key aspect of diet variation is that our diets should not be maintained consistent all year round. Moreover, your diet should vary throughout the seasons, depending on your body's needs. Historically, ancient cultures were forced into dietary shifts by environmental factors, seasonal changes, or simply a lack of available food. Indigenous cultures survived harsh, North American winters by being in a state of ketosis, where relying on scarce animal meats, and fats was their only choice. However, in the summer, meat consumption was reduced substantially and consumption of greens and carbs were increased. We can mimic these dietary shifts, ourselves, weekly, monthly and seasonally. Ideally, a rotation between very low carb and higher healthy carb diets seasonally (i.e. every 3-4 months), should yield the best results.

FACTORS TO CONSIDER BEFORE FASTING:

- **Which strategy works best for you?** – Which is the most convenient for your daily schedule? You can create your own intermittent-fasting schedule, starting with a 12-hour eating window, and working your way down to a smaller eating window, as your body adapts to the change.

- **You *must* have healthy eating habits** – Intermittent fasting will not produce benefits if you are consuming processed food that is high in refined sugars and carbohydrates. You *must* be consuming a diet of whole foods, rich in vegetables and fruits, nuts, seeds, organic meats and healthy fats. Intermittent fasting on a junk food diet is *not* the way to do it!

- **Gender** – Due to hormonal activity, men can continue on an intermittent-fasting schedule longer than women. If you are female, consider trying it for a maximum of three months, then go back to regular eating for a while before restarting.

- **Sleep is crucial** – If you don't sleep well, intermittent fasting may not be the best option for you as you likely have disruptions in your circadian cycle, which is important to intermittent fasting.

- **Hypoglycemia or irregular sugar levels** – If you have hypoglycemia or irregular sugar levels, gradually introduce fasting to your diet, as it can cause drops in blood sugar and induce feelings of lethargy. Monitoring by a knowledgeable health-care practitioner is recommended while fasting.

- **Kids** – Fasting is not recommended for children unless it's for teenagers with serious weight issues. It's better to get children in the habit of choosing healthier and non-processed foods, as their growing bodies need more regular fueling.

- **Body image** – Intermittent fasting is not recommended for those with a history of, or who are prone to disordered eating.

Intermittent fasting is not a one-size-fits-all approach and may not be for everyone. Though many people trying to lose larger amounts of weight or trying to stabilize insulin levels may find it beneficial. People with inflammatory conditions such as arthritis, atherosclerosis, irritable bowel syndrome, and asthma may also experience great relief by adopting an intermittent-fasting approach. It may require practice, but for those who choose to follow it, it can yield great results.

If you decide to try intermittent fasting—or anytime you make major changes in your diet—be sure to be in tune with your body. How are you feeling? Are you tired or feeling energized? Is your blood sugar more stabilized? Are you sleeping better? Do you feel less sore? Food is fuel! It's important to figure out what works for you and your body. Intermittent fasting can be another great tool in your health toolkit.

The following diagram shows examples of health habits with corresponding hack levels. To download the *Hack Your Health Habits Worksheet*, visit

www.hackyourhealthhabits.com/worksheets

READY #HEALTHHACKER?
EXAMPLES OF LEVEL 1, 2 AND 3 HACKS FOR THIS CHAPTER

✓ Introduce intermittent fasting by starting with a fasting of 10 hours and increase slowly to 12 hours, for a minimum of 2 days during your week.

LEVEL 1

LEVEL 2

LEVEL 3

✓ Try a 24-hour fast with bone broth once a week.

✓ Aim to fast for 16 hours for a few days during your week.

HACK YOUR HEALTH PROGRESS

||||||||||||||

CHAPTER 13

THE KETOGENIC DIET
A Way to Stay Lean & Prevent Disease

"Don't blame the butter for
what the bread did."

— Unknown

KETOSIS—THE NOT-SO-NEW PATH TO GREATER HEALTH?

Trying to lose weight? Then you may have heard the words ketones, ketosis, or ketogenic being thrown around. People are calling the ketogenic diet a miracle method, the best way to shed pounds and get healthy. Think it's just a fad? Although the ketogenic diet is not very well understood in the health world, it has been used for years to deal with diabetes, epilepsy, heart disease, cognitive impairment, depression and even cancer. Could it be the answer to your health problems?

A ketogenic diet consists of eating a low amount of carbohydrates, a high amount of fat and a low-to-moderate amount of protein. It involves drastically reducing carbohydrate intake and replacing it with fat.

Really? I know not all fats are bad, but I still wouldn't think to consume a lot of them.

When glucose is available as fuel, the body will use it as a source of energy. In a ketogenic diet, the body will go into what is called nutritional ketosis and will burn fats as fuel, producing a by-product called ketones, a more-efficient fuel source for the brain and body. That said, fat is only the most efficient fuel source when there is little glucose available for use in the body.

So, what's the deal with using only glucose as fuel? Well, in a simplistic way, glucose is actually a dirtier fuel and creates inflammation in the body, while ketones are a much cleaner fuel and do not create remotely as much inflammation.

From an evolutionary standpoint, our Paleolithic ancestors spent most of their time in a state of ketosis. Their diets naturally consisted of high fats, some proteins and very low carbohydrates. Furthermore, they would often go through periods of feast and famine. During times when food was scarce, they would rely on their fat stores to provide ample energy. These fat stores allowed our ancestors to survive, even thrive, without food for long periods of time. This diet has provided us with a basic understanding of keto-adaptation and has greatly influenced research in the field. Based on our ancestors' eating patterns, researchers have recognized the need to transition away from sugar burning as a constant need for fuel.

BUT, DON'T WE NEED SUGAR FOR ENERGY?

As we eat our food, our body breaks down proteins into amino acids, carbohydrates into glucose, and fats into glycerol and essential fatty acids. These are then further broken down into energy units that the cell mitochondria use to produce energy.

To better understand the difference between sources of fuel to produce energy and their effect on the body, let's use the analogy of a fireplace. A fireplace that burns wood (i.e. glucose), produces smoke. This smoke goes up the chimney as best as it can, but often leaves behind a dirty residue that is difficult to clean. In this scenario, the wood fuel represents glucose, and the smoke represents inflammation in the body. Like wood, glucose is a dirtier fuel source. It produces waste that accumulates at a cellular level and causes unwanted aftereffects. In comparison, when a fireplace uses natural gas (i.e. ketones), less smoke is produced and little-to-no mess is made. This fuel is safe; it warms your house without undesired side effects.

Using ketones as fuel results in an increase in cellular energy and protection of the mitochondrial membrane. It also contributes to a reduction of inflammation and its markers. In addition, ketones can be used by neurons that cannot use glucose, making the brain (which is 70 percent fat) sharper and more efficient. While there are *essential* requirements for both fat and protein, we can live a perfectly healthy life without consuming large amounts of carbohydrates. The key is to train the body to use ketones, instead of sugar, as its energy source. This can be done through a ketogenic diet.

KETOSIS AND ILLNESS PREVENTION

Historically, the ketogenic diet has been used to treat conditions such as epilepsy, cancer, and cognitive and autoimmune disorders. These diseases are aggravated by toxins and other physical and chemical stressors that contribute to defective cellular energy metabolism. In other words, toxins damage the cell's mitochondria, which decreases the production of cell energy. To adapt, cells make up the energy difference by using glucose.

This goes back to our fireplace analogy: The waste created by burning glucose produces inflammation throughout the body, resulting in illness. Simply put, unhealthy cells will use glucose in the presence of oxygen for energy, instead of fat and ketones. In the case of cancer, recent research is pointing to the fact that the higher the glucose levels, the faster the tumor growth. As glucose levels fall, tumor size and growth rates fall.

So, what is the role of ketosis in all of this? As mentioned, by reducing your carbohydrate intake and replacing it with fat, our bodies slowly adapt to burning ketones (cleaner energy) instead of glucose (dirtier energy). However, recent research shows that being in ketosis on its own is often not enough to trigger the rise of ketones and the decrease of glucose. This is where the role of intermittent fasting comes into play; under food restriction, glucose levels drop and ketones rise, literally starving cancer cells of their main source of fuel.

> ✭ So, ketosis and intermittent fasting go hand in hand!

This causes cancerous lesions to shrink, excess fat to be burned, and damaged cells to repair. Without intermittent fasting, a drop in glucose may not occur and, therefore, ketones might be flushed out in the urine instead of being used as a source of energy. To explain this a little further, a study conducted on humans and mice concluded that there was no significant decrease in weight nor tumor size by simply being in a state of ketosis. Restriction, in the form of intermittent or block fasting, was absolutely crucial for the benefits of ketosis to kick in.[1] Therefore, the key is to combine a ketogenic diet with either an intermittent or block fast to see the best results in weight loss and reduction in inflammation. However, it is again important to mention that intermittent fasting is not recommended for people who have reactive hypoglycemia, as sugar levels need to first be stabilized before attempting to fast.

There are many benefits to ketosis:

- natural hunger and appetite control
- effortless weight loss and maintenance
- mental clarity
- more restful sleep
- normalized metabolic function
- stabilized blood sugar levels
- restored insulin sensitivity

- lower inflammation levels
- feelings of happiness and general well-being
- lowered blood pressure
- reduced triglycerides
- use of stored fat as fuel source
- endless energy
- eliminated heartburn
- improved fertility
- prevention of brain injury
- increased sex drive
- improved immune system
- slowed aging
- reduction in free-radical production
- improvement in blood chemistry
- optimized cognitive function
- reduced or eliminated acne
- faster recovery from exercise
- reduced anxiety or mood swings
- reduced need for medications

HOW WOULD YOU FEEL ON UNLIMITED ENERGY?

We eat for energy, or so we have been told. Another benefit of being keto-adapted is your ability to rely on your body's adipose tissue (or fat stores) for energy rather than needing a constant intake of food for energy. When we are reliant on glucose as fuel, constant hunger and snacking is needed to keep your body's blood glucose levels from spiking and dropping. When your blood glucose becomes low, you then have to tap into your glycogen stores as fuel. When doing so, you have maybe 2,000 calories of energy available to you.

However, when we are in ketosis, our body naturally uses our fat stores for energy and does not require the constant input of food for energy. When we rely on our own body fat as fuel, there can be up to 40,000-50,000 calories in our tank ready to be used. This is one of the reasons more and more endurance athletes are turning to a ketogenic diet. Ketogenic diets allow them to better sustain energy while active, without the negative effects of glucose burning (i.e. inflammation and oxidative stresses).

When blood glucose drops, sugar burners experience hunger, drops in mood, and an instinct to find food fast. However, as you adapt to burning ketones, your negative symptoms will dissipate and fasting will become easier. As a result, you will gain more sustainable energy and mental clarity.

WHY HAVEN'T I BEEN TOLD ABOUT THE BENEFITS OF A KETOGENIC DIET?

If there are so many benefits to eating a ketogenic diet, why aren't more doctors recommending it to their patients? Unfortunately, there is still a lot of controversy surrounding this subject. Certain misconceptions have led some health professionals to believe that ketosis can be dangerous and even serve as a precursor to conditions such as diabetes.

Why is this? Well, ketosis is often mistaken for diabetic ketoacidosis (DKA). In DKA, ketones are produced as a by-product of burning fat for fuel, and the buildup of ketones in the blood can make it very acidic. But, there is a huge difference between nutritional ketosis and diabetic ketoacidosis. DKA occurs in type 1 diabetics (who cannot produce adequate insulin), when elevated blood glucose and a lack of insulin prevents glucose from getting stored in cells, causing it to accumulate in the bloodstream. As blood glucose and ketone levels rise, the individual is at a risk of getting very ill. A key point that can be missed is the fact that the rise in blood ketone levels that leads to ketoacidosis in diabetics occurs *with* a simultaneous elevation of blood-glucose levels. However, when ketosis is used for therapeutic reasons in those who are not diabetic, blood-glucose levels actually stay stable, as their insulin does what it's supposed to do. It would be nearly impossible for DKA to occur to non-diabetics. As long as your body can produce insulin, ketosis can actually help prevent type 2 diabetes.

Another misconception surrounding the ketogenic diet stems from its resemblance to the Atkins diet, created by Dr. Robert Atkins in the 1970s, who proposed a diet high in both fat and protein, with almost no carbs at all. Although this diet incorporated some of the key concepts of the ketogenic diet, there existed a subtle, yet important, distinction. Nutritional ketosis, in which the body uses fat to generate ketones for energy, may be brought on only by a low-carb, high-fat, and *low-to-moderate* protein-based diet.

The Atkins diet focused primarily on restricting carbs, yet made almost no distinction between consumption of fat and protein, and it never proposed any practical or systematic ways to increase ketone production. For this reason, the overconsumption of protein may lead to some health issues and even prevent the body from going into a full fat-burning (keto-adapted) state, as excess protein gets converted by the body into glucose.

SO, HOW DO I BECOME KETO-ADAPTED?

Becoming a fat-burner as opposed to a sugar-burner is not a process that happens overnight. In fact, it may take up to several weeks for your body to adapt to this new and improved method of energy usage. Typically, when you begin, you want to decrease carbohydrate consumption to no more than 50 grams total per day. This can be quite the change as the average person usually eats 300 grams of carbs per day. Next, replace 65 percent to 80 percent of your daily calories with healthy fats.

Believe me, it does seem like a lot at first, but it's necessary! Proteins should be consumed moderately, meaning no more than half your lean body mass, at most. For example, if you have 70 pounds of lean body weight, your protein consumption should not be more than 35 grams per day. And, lastly, weekly diet variation, such as the 5-1-1 rule discussed in the chapter on intermittent fasting, is a key fat-adapting accelerator.

It is important to note that the first few weeks of consuming a ketogenic diet may be a bit of a shock to the system, and feelings of fullness, bloating, fatigue, and even digestive discomfort may occur. To relieve yourself of these negative symptoms, ensure that you are getting enough electrolytes, staying hydrated, and supplementing with magnesium and sea salts. Intermittent fasting also aids with this. After the initial first weeks of consuming a ketogenic diet and intermittent fasting, the feelings of lethargy should pass as the body becomes more aware of the need to burn fat for energy; this is when our energy comes back, our appetite decreases, and our pounds may even start coming off.

HOW DO I KNOW I AM KETO-ADAPTED?

There are three methods to test for ketones whose presence indicates the body is burning fat. You can test the breath for acetone levels, the urine for acetoacetate levels, or the blood for beta-hydroxybutyrate levels. Out of the three, testing the blood is the most accurate, and better yet, no lab is needed. You can do it yourself, in much the same way a diabetic would check their glucose levels using a strip. Ideally, you want to check your ketones first thing in the morning and then before your first meal. Ketones between 0.5 to 3.0 mmol/L indicate the body is in a state of ketosis. The breath and urine test can be purchased at any local pharmacy, however, the meter to measure blood ketone levels can be ordered online, along with the strips.

WHAT IF I AM NOT ADAPTING?

You think you're doing all the right things, but your body still isn't shifting into its fat-adapting mode. Don't worry, this happens sometimes. In his book *Keto Clarity*, Jimmy Moore explains why:

- **Too much protein** – Why is too much protein a bad thing? As mentioned earlier, we don't have ways of storing protein. When we consume more protein than needed, our body transforms that protein into glucose. This raises blood glucose, impeding on our ability to reach ketosis.

- **Testing urine ketones instead of blood ketones** – Blood ketone testing is the gold standard to measure ketones. When the body becomes keto-adapted, the urine test may give you inaccurate results. This is because urine ketones may disappear after a person is keto-adapted. Testing the blood before meals and exercise is the most effective way to see if you're in a state of ketosis.

- **Not eating enough mono and saturated fats** – You need to eat a variety of fats. Eating the same fats day after day can negatively affect ketosis.

- **Eating too often or too much** – If you are eating a sufficient amount of fat and are testing blood regularly, yet are still having trouble adapting, then it is an indication that more restriction is needed. In this case, consider applying the 5-1-1 protocol: 5 days of intermittent fasting per week (14-20 hours daily), 1 day of fasting (24 hours), followed by 1 day of feast (with three meals that are higher in protein and carbs as a refeed). Without proper restriction, blood glucose fails to stabilize and this, in turn, makes it more difficult for the body to enter ketosis.

- **Eating too many carbs** - As mentioned earlier, 50 grams of carbs is a good starting point. However, some people may have to drop to at least 20-30 grams per day when first trying to get into ketosis.

WHAT FOODS CAN YOU AVOID AND CONSUME?

To keep with the low-carb/high-fat/moderate-protein rule, certain foods must be avoided, and others should be increased. Generally, starchy, refined, and sugary foods must be avoided as much as possible, and a steady intake of healthy fats is recommended.

Avoid:

- sugary foods or artificial sweeteners
- grains and starches
- beans and legumes
- low-fat or diet products
- some condiments and sauces high in sugar or unhealthy fat
- alcohol
- processed foods
- fat replacements: vegetable oils, shortening, margarine etc.
- overly processed meats
- fruit overconsumption

Consume:

- red and white meats, preferably grass-fed or wild
- eggs, preferably organic and from your local farmer
- unprocessed, full-fat cheese, preferably from grass-fed animals
- nuts and seeds and their butters
- healthy fat-rich food like avocado, coconut, olive, etc.

- herbs and spices
- non-starchy vegetables (i.e. lots of greens)

SAMPLE KETOGENIC DIET, COMBINED WITH INTERMITTENT FASTING

So, what does a diet with little-or-no carbs look like? Here is an example of some of the meals you can eat to give you an idea of what to expect.

Breaking your fast:

- bacon, eggs and tomatoes
- breakfast "muffins" made with eggs, veggies and avocado
- a protein smoothie with whey, coconut milk, nut butter and chia seeds
- omelette with avocado, salsa, peppers, onions and spices
- nut butter and veggies
- assortment of nuts, cheese made from grass-fed animals and veggies
- breakfast "muffins" made with seeds, coconut flour (or any grain-free flour), protein powder and eggs

Ending your eating window:

- beef stir-fry cooked in coconut oil with vegetables
- chicken salad with olive oil and feta cheese
- meatballs, cheddar cheese and vegetables
- bun-less burger with bacon, egg and cheese
- wild salmon with asparagus cooked in butter (preferably from a grass-fed animal)
- shrimp salad with olive oil and avocado
- cheese and broccoli-stuffed chicken breast and roasted veggies

 Yum! All of this sounds delicious and not too restrictive.

WHAT ABOUT KETONE SUPPLEMENTS?

Depending on how carb-adapted an individual is, it can take several weeks for the body to switch into being fat-adapted and using fats and ketones efficiently for fuel. A little help from an exogenous ketone supplement may be worthwhile when trying to achieve nutritional ketosis. Though it is not recommended that one stay in nutritional ketosis for an extended period of time, taking an exogenous ketone supplement in times where diets are slightly higher in carbs may help individuals continuously experience the benefits of ketosis. Ketone supplements provide a multitude of benefits, ranging from performance enhancement, more efficient weight loss, illness prevention, cognitive improvement, anti-inflammatory properties and much more.

There are three different types of ketones that your body runs on: acetoacetate, beta-hydroxybutyrate and acetone. Beta-hydroxybutyrate is the active form that can flow freely in the blood and be used by your tissues, so it is the one that is most used in exogenous ketone supplements.

RECAP AND ADDITIONAL GUIDELINES

- Cravings for carbs can be satisfied with fat. Have some avocado and nuts, or consider supplementing with L-glutamine.

- Protein is an essential nutrient, but its consumption should be moderated. Fat intake should exceed that of protein.

- Saturated fats are the most satisfying.

- It may take up to 2-6 weeks before you enter a state of ketosis.

- Intermittent fasting will help increase production of ketones.

- Not getting adequate salt in your ketogenic diet can increase appetite; use Himalayan sea salts.

- To help with ketone production, if you are having difficulty, add avocados, coconut oil, butter, ghee or medium-chain triglyceride (MCT) oil.

- Make sure you're getting your electrolytes! Sodium and potassium are key! Little-known fact: A banana has 487 g of potassium, whereas an avocado has 975 g of potassium.

- Constipation on a low-carb diet can be remedied by increasing one's consumption of non-digestible fibers (prebiotic foods), magnesium, salt and water.

- Don't test your ketone levels after exercise—wait at least 2 hours; exercise will actually increase your blood sugar and decrease your ketones temporarily.

- It is possible that urination will increase. This happens because the kidneys will drop more water as glycogen is being depleted and excess water is being released—carbs cause fluid retention.

- Remember our chapter on phytonutrients? To ensure you do not become deficient in vitamins and minerals, make sure the vegetables you eat are all different colors. Remember, eating the colors of the rainbow helps ensure you are getting all the important nutrients your body needs.

- It is harder to get into ketosis with a vegan diet, but it is still doable.

- If you have had your gallbladder removed, you can still eat a diet high in fat. However, you may need bile salts to get your body used to digesting fats efficiently.

- As the liver is mainly involved in the processing of fats and production of ketones, it is imperative that it functions optimally. That said, it is important to note that prescription medications can tax the liver and slow down the process of ketosis. If you are currently on medication, some detoxifying might be required.

- Since alcohol needs to be processed by your liver, drinking alcohol will not only add sugar, but also stress your liver further.

- Ketones can decrease during menstruation! This is perhaps not the best time to test for ketones in your blood.

- Post-menopausal women tend to have to keep their carbs particularly lower to get into ketosis, but, once achieved, it is a great way to balance hormones.

- Some individuals are also genetically predisposed to have difficulty metabolizing high fats, therefore it would be beneficial to get tested. Genetic testing will be discussed in much further detail later on.

There you have it! Remember, as with any diet, it will work only if you are consistent and stick with it for the long term. It may be difficult to transition to a full ketogenic diet and/or intermittent fasting routine to start with, as some digestive discomfort and hunger may occur. But, soon enough, the benefits will kick in. The beauty of a ketogenic diet is that it excludes the idea of calories in versus calories out; instead, food quality is taken into account rather than quantity.

True. I've calorie counted on and off throughout my life, and fats tend to take up a lot of calories. I like the fact that this isn't about calories, but about eating good, whole foods.

The following diagram shows examples of health habits with corresponding hack levels. To download the *Hack Your Health Habits Worksheet*, visit

www.hackyourhealthhabits.com/worksheets

READY #HEALTHHACKER?
EXAMPLES OF LEVEL 1, 2 AND 3 HACKS FOR THIS CHAPTER

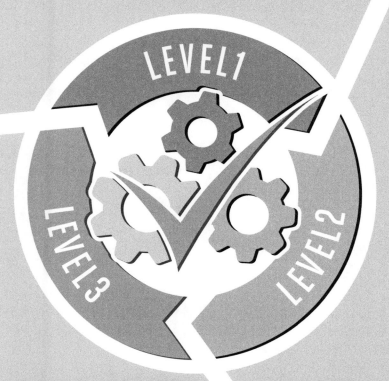

✓ Eat more good fats.
✓ Avoid processed foods, alcohol and sugar.

✓ Adopt a ketogenic diet and pair the diet with intermittent fasting.
✓ Test ketone levels regularly to determine if you are in ketosis.

✓ Focus on eating a low-carb, medium protein and high-fat diet.

HACK YOUR HEALTH PROGRESS

||||||||||||||

CHAPTER 14

15

pH BALANCE
Don't Be So Acidic!

"No disease, including cancer, can exist in an alkaline environment."

— Dr. Otto Warburg,
Nobel Prize winner for
cancer discovery

THINK IT OVER

- Why are pH levels important to overall health and well-being?

- Are the foods you eat acidic or alkaline?

- What are ways you can ensure adequate alkalinity in your body

ARE YOUR pH LEVELS IN CHECK?

When explaining the importance of healthy pH levels, I like to use the following analogy with patients. Imagine this: Cynthia just hosted a big dinner party. The kitchen is a mess, there is food everywhere, but instead of cleaning up, she leaves everything where it is and goes on vacation. When she comes home two weeks later, an awful stench greets her at the door, and she notices vermin and insects have taken over her household. Baffled, she calls an exterminator. The exterminator gets rid of the pests but warns her that if she doesn't clean up, the insects and vermin will return. Had Cynthia just cleaned her house in the first place, this even bigger mess could have been avoided altogether. What exactly does this analogy have to do with pH levels?

The sad truth is that a lot of people treat their body like a dumping ground. They make poor nutritional choices, smoke, drink and don't get an adequate amount of exercise. These types of habits are like the garbage littering Cynthia's house. If we do not get rid of the garbage (poor habits) in our house (body), we will attract pests (disease). We can try to get rid of the pests in different ways, but, ultimately, if we don't take out the trash, our problem will never really go away.

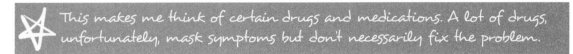

This makes me think of certain drugs and medications. A lot of drugs, unfortunately, mask symptoms but don't necessarily fix the problem.

Without addressing the root cause of imbalances, treating symptoms is exactly like getting rid of the pests without getting rid of the garbage. In this case, an overly acidic body can be one of the root causes of the onset of disease. In other words, over-acidic pH levels are like rotting garbage in our bodies. We need to learn how to create a harmonious, balanced pH level so that we can keep our body clean and free from disease!

> "There is only one disease—the over-acidity of the fluids and tissues of the body, which leads to an overgrowth of microorganisms whose toxic wastes produce the symptoms we call disease."
>
> — ROBERT O. YOUNG

WHAT ARE pH LEVELS?

Most people are familiar with acid rain and the damage it does to our environment. Acid has a similar effect on the internal human environment. Therefore, we need to become internal environmentalists and safeguard our internal health. pH stands for *potential of hydrogen* and is the measure of how acidic or alkaline a substance is. pH levels range from 0 to 14, with 7 being neutral. When our pH level decreases, it signifies that our body is more acidic, and when it rises, our body is more alkaline.

The normal pH levels of the body are:

- gastric (stomach) acid = 1.0 to 2.0
- normal urine = 6.0 to 6.5 in the morning and 6.5 to 7.0 in the evening
- saliva = 6.5 to 7.5
- blood = 7.4

Litmus paper is a simple tool that you can use to measure and monitor your pH levels. However, no research has confirmed the validity of saliva testing for pH—therefore, opt for the urine testing when checking for acidity. Litmus paper is available at natural health-food stores.

While I believe that the litmus test can provide a good baseline, it's important to note that test results can be variable. Several variables have to be taken into consideration when doing these kinds of tests. All ingested food and all stressors—physical, emotional or mental—can play a role on acidity or alkalinity levels.

ACIDITY

In general, people are more likely to have an acidity imbalance rather than an alkaline imbalance. The Western diet can be very acidic, with a lot of meat, sugar and processed foods. Tobacco, alcohol, coffee and low physical activity are also contributors to an acidic environment. While we could counter this, to some degree, by eating more alkaline-producing foods like vegetables, they aren't usually as abundant as they should be on our grocery list.

An acid-forming reaction refers to any changes in the body that produce a decreased ability to energize the system and leave an acid residue in the urine. Acid-forming minerals found in food are phosphorus, sulfur, chlorine, iodine, bromine, fluorine, copper and silicon.

When you have a highly acidic diet, it puts pressure on your body's regulating systems to work at achieving a neutral pH. This depletes your blood of the alkaline-forming minerals and can lead to chronic and degenerative illnesses. In addition, diseases—including cancer—thrive in acidic environments, which makes it easier for you to get sick and stay sick. In contrast, when your body is more alkaline, bacteria and viruses are less able to survive, and disease has less of an opportunity to occur.

Finally, recognize that the impact of stress on your body is as powerful as the foods you eat. Any major stress will leave its acid residue. Because of the body's fight-or-flight reaction when stressed, excessive hormones are secreted, and even foods that are alkaline will turn acidic.

Signs of an acid imbalance in your body include:

- weight gain, obesity and diabetes
- lack of energy and constant fatigue
- hormonal problems
- osteoporosis and joint pain
- slow digestion and elimination
- headaches
- tendency to get infections

Note that not all acids are bad. Hydrochloric acid (HCl) is an acid, for example, but is vital for digestion. It allows the stomach to break down food, and it maintains proper alkaline/acid balance. It becomes alkaline after its job is done. HCl is also our first line of defense against microbes that might enter our body with our food. Adequate HCl levels greatly decrease tissue acid-waste buildup.

ALKALINITY

Alkaline imbalance is quite uncommon compared to acid imbalance. Alkaline-forming reaction refers to any changes in the body that produce an increased ability to energize the system and leaves an alkaline residue in the urine. Alkaline-forming minerals found in food are calcium, magnesium, sodium, potassium, iron, manganese, boron, nickel and zinc.

pH OF COMMON FOODS

Below is a list of high acid-forming and high alkaline-forming foods. Some may surprise you. This information can be a little mind-bending, because some foods that we think of as "acidic" are, in fact, alkalizing once metabolized.

It's actually better to look at whether the food is acid-forming or alkaline-forming, not where the food itself falls on the pH scale. So, even though we think of citrus as acidic, fruits like lemons are alkalizing because, when they're consumed, they break down and donate alkaline mineral salt compounds like citrates and ascorbates. This is why it's a great idea to start your day with a glass of lemon water to help alkalinize your body in the morning.

HIGH ACID-FORMING FOODS

- Blueberries, cranberries, prunes and sweetened fruit juices
- Wheat, white bread, pastries, biscuits and pasta—anything with refined wheat
- Beef, pork and shellfish
- Conventional dairy products
- Peanuts and walnuts
- Beer, liquor and soft drinks
- Artificial sweeteners and chocolate

HIGH ALKALINE-FORMING FOODS

- Asparagus, onions, vegetable juices, parsley, raw spinach, broccoli, garlic and barley grass
- Lemon, watermelon, limes, grapefruit, mangoes and papayas
- Olive oil
- Herb teas and lemon water
- Stevia

The goal is not to become fully alkaline, as the body produces acidity as a result of the digestion of certain foods, and this is even required. Our skin needs to be slightly acidic in order to deal with environmental factors like bacteria and other toxins. Likewise, the vagina maintains an acidic environment to protect itself, and, when the pH is raised too high, infections like bacterial vaginosis and yeast infections can result. And, as mentioned earlier, the stomach and other parts of the digestive system require different levels of acidity out of biological necessity. The digestive acids are part of how we process and use the foods we eat as fuel. They are part of our internal combustion for nutrition.

HERE ARE SOME TIPS TO REDUCE ACIDITY IN THE BODY:

- **Cut out refined sugar** – Try to avoid any refined sugar like high fructose corn syrup and artificial sweeteners like aspartame.

- **Eat raw, organic, fresh vegetables as much as possible** – Most vegetables are alkaline-forming.

- **Avoid toxic fats like trans fats** – Fried foods that have been cooked with vegetable oils and canola oils wreak havoc on the body's alkalinity. Try cooking with coconut oil or ghee butter at low temperatures, instead.

- **Avoid or limit your intake of dairy products** – Most dairy products are acid-forming. If you are to consume dairy, know that buttermilk, kefir and whey are alkalinizing dairy products.

- **Avoid drinking fluoridated and chlorinated tap water** – They not only add to the body's toxic load, but are also acid-forming.

- **Add alkalizing foods into your diet such as:**
  - alkalizing vegetables like broccoli, celery, cucumber, peppers and spinach
  - alkalizing fruits like apples, berries, melons, pears and pineapples
  - alkalizing nuts like almonds and coconuts
  - alkalizing meats like fish, chicken, turkey and duck
  - alkalizing miscellaneous foods like alfalfa, ginger, honey, kelp and mint

- **Consume low-acid coffee** – If you drink coffee, purchase coffee that has a lower acidity level. The acidity of a coffee is partly due to the growing region and partly influenced by the way the bean is processed and roasted. Look for organic, acid-free coffee at your local grocer.

- **Try to reduce your stress** – Stress and negative emotions have been shown to increase body acidity.

The following diagram shows examples of health habits with corresponding hack levels. To download the *Hack Your Health Habits Worksheet*, visit

www.hackyourhealthhabits.com/worksheets

READY #HEALTHHACKER?
EXAMPLES OF LEVEL 1, 2 AND 3 HACKS FOR THIS CHAPTER

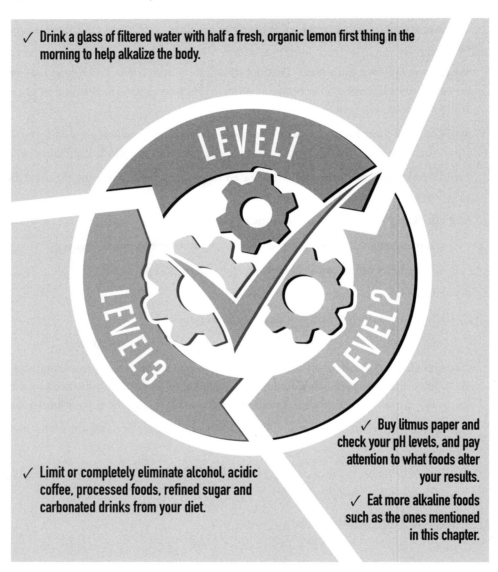

✓ Drink a glass of filtered water with half a fresh, organic lemon first thing in the morning to help alkalize the body.

✓ Buy litmus paper and check your pH levels, and pay attention to what foods alter your results.

✓ Eat more alkaline foods such as the ones mentioned in this chapter.

✓ Limit or completely eliminate alcohol, acidic coffee, processed foods, refined sugar and carbonated drinks from your diet.

HACK YOUR HEALTH PROGRESS

||||||||||||||||||||||||||||||||||||||||||||||||||||||||||||||

CHAPTER 15

SECTION 4

Get Rid of Toxins—The Key to Real Cellular Detox for Optimal Health

Do you know what harmful substances are hidden in our foods and self-care products? From personal products to household items, Section 4 emphasizes how to make better choices that reduce your daily toxic exposure. You will also learn simple lifestyle modifications to optimize your body's detoxification capabilities to combat today's increasing chemical burden.

TOXINS
What Are You Exposed To?

"Pay attention to your toxic load, be it food, products, or people."

— Dr. Nathalie Beauchamp

THINK IT OVER

- Do you know the toxic load of your body?

- Are the foods you eat, body products you use, and the furniture you have in your house contributing to your toxic load?

- Do you know the main chemicals that you should avoid?

From cleaning supplies to beauty products, and from our water supply to pesticide-ridden foods, our toxin exposure has increased exponentially in the last couple of decades. Whether we're aware of it or not, we are bombarded with synthetic substances each and every day. In fact, it is said that as many as 80,000 commercial and industrial chemicals are used in the United States. Additionally, approximately 2,000 new chemicals are registered for use in everyday items each year—including food, personal care products, prescription drugs, household cleaners and lawn-care products.[1] Talk about a "chemical soup!"

The accumulation of toxins is unavoidable in our modern world, but it should not be assumed that the current industry and governmental safeguards protect human health from the adverse effects of ordinary chemical exposures. We would like to think that most of the chemicals that we are exposed to have been tested for safety, but for most products, this is just not the case.

In 1976, the Toxic Substance Control Act (TSCA) was passed in the United States.[2] Its regulations grandfathered in a total of 62,000 "old" chemicals, with the assumption that the U.S. Environmental Protection Agency (EPA) would eventually assess the safety of these chemicals. It is said that, at the current rate, it would take 1,000 years to adequately document the health effects of the chemicals now on the market. In Canada, the department of health promised to re-assess 4,000 common chemicals in 2006, acknowledging that they may pose health risks. Despite this, these chemicals have yet to be barred from use.[3] Scary, isn't it?

> ✪ The more I read, the more I realize how little safeguards there are, in terms of the safety of our foods and products. We really need to take matters (and our health) into our own hands.

If one chemical can have a negative effect, imagine the damage several chemicals can have on the body. Unfortunately, testing is complex. Though it is known that chemicals combine in our bodies, they are rarely tested that way. Toxicity testing is typically done with individual compounds in highly controlled settings and almost never investigates the effects of complex mixtures. There is also very little safety monitoring that occurs after a new chemical is released.

PRECAUTIONARY PRINCIPLE ANYONE?

Did you know that, unlike drugs, which are assumed to be toxic and must be proven safe (by FDA standards) before they can be marketed, industrial chemicals are considered safe until proven hazardous? The 1998 Wingspread Conference's Statement on the Precautionary Principle states: "When an activity raises threats of harm to human health or the environment, precautionary measures should be taken even if some cause and effect relationships are not fully established scientifically. In this context, the proponent of an activity, rather than the public, should bear the burden of proof." Without implementation of this principle, we are basically guinea pigs in a huge science experiment.[4]

Thankfully, there are organizations like the Environmental Working Group (EWG), an American non-profit group, whose mandate is "to empower people to live healthier lives in a healthier environment." With breakthrough research and education, this group drives consumer choice and civic action. Unfortunately, this is not met without resistance. According to the EWG, *"We have an industry that has no legal obligation to conduct safety tests or monitor for the presence of its chemicals in the environment or the human population and a financial incentive not to do so."*

Before we dive in, here are definitions of some important concepts you will see throughout this section:

- **Toxic** – Capable of causing injury or death, especially by chemical means (poisonous).

- **Toxin** – A toxic substance that is produced by a living organism (e.g. plants, animals, fungi and bacteria).

- **Detoxification** – To rid a person of a poison or its effects.

- **Xenobiotic** – A chemical compound that is foreign to or not normally produced by the body. Examples of xenobiotics are pesticides, plasticizers, perfluorooctane, industrial pollutants (e.g. dioxins), pigments, paints and dyes, preservatives and flame retardants, petrochemical fuels (e.g. perchlorate) and solvents.

- **Chemical Body Burden** – The quantity of an exogenous substance (xenobiotic) or its metabolites that accumulates in an individual or a population.

- **Persistent Organic Pollutant (POP)** – A substance that persists in the environment, bio-accumulates through the food chain and poses a risk of adverse effects to humans and environmental health.

RISK ASSESSMENT FOR SYNTHETIC CHEMICALS – NOEL

For our French readers, NOEL does not have anything to do with Christmas. It stands for "No Observable Effect Level," and this rating is given when a chemical is assessed and said to not produce effects on the body. What is wrong with that? Well, for starters, it is based on short-term observations and assumes a linear dose-effect of toxins. It also assumes that individuals will have a similar reaction to the toxin, when, in reality, sensitivity and metabolism can vary greatly from person to person. In addition, it ignores windows of vulnerability like puberty, discounts the potentially cumulative effect of low-dose toxic exposures, and ignores the impact and synergistic effects of one's total toxic load and lifetime environmental exposure. It also fails to account for epigenetics and other transgenerational effects.

In order to truly evaluate a person's total toxic load and disease risk level, multiple components need to be taken into consideration. Total toxic load addresses not only what we are exposed to, but also our body's ability to transform and get rid of toxins. Moreover, disease risk addresses the toxins' potency, if they have accumulated in the body and whether or not we are predisposed genetically to developing the disease.

In addition, there exists certain predisposing factors that explain why some individuals are more sensitive to toxins or retain them in greater levels. These factors include:

- increased or ongoing exposure to toxins

- nutrient deficiencies (in B vitamins, antioxidants, magnesium, selenium, etc.)

- high-sugar, low-protein diet

- heavy metals

- stress or emotional trauma

- intestinal dysbiosis

- variations in detoxification genes

SOURCES OF ENVIRONMENTAL TOXICITY

- Ionizing radiation (i.e. UV light and radioactive elements)

- Oxidation (or free radicals)

- Animal, plant and fungal toxins

- Products of combustion (smoke, incineration)

- Heavy metals/metalloids

- Industrial chemicals

- Pharmaceuticals

- Food-preparation by-products

- Personal-care products

- Electromagnetic fields

As mentioned earlier, the biological effects of toxicants are not linear. Chemical sensitivities can vary considerably depending on age, biochemical individuality and compounding effects from multiple toxicants.

When discussing toxins and our environment, I often hear the following: *"We did not eat organic or 'detox' when we were growing up and are fine—what's the big deal?"* Well, considering that on average, we have 30,000 to 50,000 more toxic chemicals in our bodies than our grandparents did, we really are comparing apples to oranges. In fact, a 2005 study conducted by the EWG found an average of 200 industrial chemicals and pollutants in the umbilical cord blood of the 10 babies they tested. This a strong indicator that man-made toxins have infiltrated our environment and our bodies.[5]

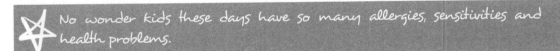

No wonder kids these days have so many allergies, sensitivities and health problems.

THE TOXIC BUNCH

According to Dr. T. R. Morris, N.D., there are nine major toxic chemicals that affect our health. He calls these the Toxic Bunch:

1. Heavy Metals (lead, mercury, arsenic and cadmium)

2. Polycyclic Aromatic Hydrocarbons (PAH)

3. Phthalates and Phenols

4. Organochlorine (OC) Pesticides

5. Organophosphate (OP) Pesticides

6. Polychlorinated Dibenzo-dioxin and Furans (PCDDs and PCDFs)

7. Polychlorinated Biphenyls (PCBs)

8. Polybrominated Diphenyl Ethers (PBDEs)

9. Polyfluorinated Compounds (PFCs)[6]

Trust me, I know, the names of these chemicals are hard to pronounce. Reading the list above might make you feel like you are in over your head, but don't be discouraged. The whole point of this chapter is to make things easier for you to understand and show you that there *are* things you can do. I am not saying it won't be challenging, but decreasing your toxic load is well worth it. Please don't put your head in the sand. The Toxic Bunch are, unfortunately, here to stay. Your health depends on taking action, and the first step is learning about them. So, let's get started! Below are the main sources and health effects of the Toxic Bunch, and how to avoid them.

1 – HEAVY METALS: LEAD, MERCURY, ARSENIC, CADMIUM AND ALUMINUM

Lead

Sources: A very small amount occurs naturally in the environment. Lead is often found in agricultural pesticides, cosmetics, batteries, pipes, mining and smelting.

Health effects: No safety threshold for lead has been established. Competes with calcium, iron and zinc. It causes neurological brain damage and cancer. Lead poisoning for a child is deemed, by the Centers for Disease Control (CDC), to be 50 parts per billion (ppb). The half-life of lead in blood is approximately 30 days, in soft tissues 40 days, and in bone, 20 years.

What to do: Beware of lead pipes, solder and fixtures (They were banned in 1998.). Beware of pre-1978 paint chips or dust. Vacuum often, using a HEPA filter vacuum. Beware of older imported toys, furniture, ceramics and leaded glassware. Be careful with water that may have been in contact with lead. Make sure to test and filter.

Mercury

Sources: Found in thermometers, batteries, pesticides, CFL fluorescent light bulbs, dental fillings and vaccines.

Health effects: Mercury is the most toxic element on the planet, especially in an organic form. It can cause symptoms from headaches or cognitive impairment to neurological brain damage.

What to do: Limit fish high in mercury. High Fructose Corn Syrup (HFCS) has been shown to contain mercury, so avoid this as well. Avoid amalgam dental fillings as they are 50 percent mercury. Filter water: The Environmental Protective Association suggests a maximum limit of 2 ppb.

Resources: www.ewg.org/safefishlist and http://www.ewg.org/tunacalculator

Arsenic

Sources: Arsenic is found in drinking water, in certain foods like chicken, eggs and rice products. Also found in treated wood and certain herbicides.

Health effects: Long-term exposure causes neurotoxicity, cancer, developmental issues, heart disease and diabetes. It can also cause cadmium-induced cell damage.

What to do: Remove or paint over treated wood. Avoid arsenic-containing herbicides. Check the arsenic level of your city water. Avoid foods high in arsenic such as rice syrup and non-organic poultry. The safe levels set by the EPA are .010 ppb.

Cadmium

Sources: Cadmium is found in batteries, cigarettes, some water sources and certain foods.
Health effects: In high doses, it can cause nausea, vomiting and severe gastroenteritis. The reference dose is 0.001 mg/kg/day.
What to do: Do not smoke or expose yourself to smoke. Have your water tested. Keep cadmium batteries away from kids. Beware of ceramic kilns.

Aluminum

Sources: Aluminum is found in pots and pans, soda cans, cosmetics, antacids, antiperspirant, sunscreen with nanoparticles, infant formulas, and vaccines and flu shots. The highest levels in foods are found in cocoa, baking powder, tea leaves, and herbs and spices.
Health effects: High amounts will settle in tissues and accumulate in the bones. Aluminum is able to cross the blood-brain barrier and cause Alzheimer's disease, Parkinson's and dementia.
What to do: Use aluminum-free beauty and personal products. Inform yourself on what is in vaccines and flu shots. Use aluminum-free baking powder and try to cook with herbs and spices that have low levels of aluminum.

2 – POLYCYLIC AROMATIC HYDROCARBONS (PAH)

Source: PAH come from the incomplete combustion of coal, oil, gas, wood, garbage, tobacco and conventional meat.
Health effects: Known for carcinogenicity and immune suppression, PAH can also cause reproductive issues and genetic damage.
What to do: Make sure to limit consuming grilled and charred meats. Avoid smoke and exhaust from cigarette, wood, vehicle, forest fires, or trash incineration.

3 – PHTHALATES AND PHENOLS (E.G. BPA AND TRICLOSAN)

Phthalates

Sources: Phthalates are found primarily in di(2-ethylhexyl) phthalate (DEHP) and mono(2-ethylhexyl) phthalate (MEHP). DEHP is a plasticizer found in flexible vinyl, like toys, flooring, car interiors, IV bags and tubing, dental composites, wallpaper, shower curtains, etc. Meanwhile, MEHP is a metabolite of phthalate used in paint, shampoos, lotions, nail polish, perfume, etc. Interestingly enough, phthalates can also be found in fast and processed foods, too, likely because of things like food-handling gloves, vinyl tubing at processing plants, etc.
Health effects: Phthalates are linked to asthma, attention-deficit disorder, obesity, breast cancer, type 2 diabetes, behavioral issues, autism spectrum disorder and fertility issues.
What to do: Use glass containers for food storage, do not microwave or store hot food in soft plastic

containers, avoid vinyl cling wraps. Use unscented fragrance-free personal-care products and remove vinyl shower curtains—choose cotton, polyester, or nylon instead.

Phenols/BPA

Source: A chemical with one of the highest production volumes—used in polycarbonate plastics and canned food lining. Also found in cash receipts.

Health effects: A known endocrine disruptor, it can affect the thyroid and also mimic estrogen, leading to estrogen dominance. It is also linked to cancer, diabetes, obesity, birth defects and brain development disorders.

What to do: Avoid plastic containers marked with #7, as they may contain BPA. Avoid hard plastics, and opt for glass, porcelain, or stainless steel—especially with hot foods or liquids. Don't eat from cans, or buy only BPA-free cans.

Phenols/Triclosan

Source: Found in synthetic antibacterial agents and used as a preservative in consumer products, including toothpastes, soaps, detergents, toys and surgical cleaning treatments.

Health effects: This is another known endocrine disruptor, as well as an immune system suppressor. Exposure in kids has been shown to increase the chance of developing asthma, allergies and eczema.

What do to: Products with a certified organic logo are triclosan-free. Opt for organic personal and beauty products.

4 – ORGANOCHLORINE (OC) PESTICIDES

Sources: The most common source is DDT. It is highly lipophilic, meaning it can persist in fatty tissues and cause issues during weight loss. It was banned in the early '70s in the United States and Canada. However, by 2004, the CDC still found DDE (a metabolite of DDT) in 99.7 percent of kids under the age of 12.

Health effects: OC is a neurotoxin that is known to cause cancer. It can also affect developmental and reproductive toxins. It is another suspected endocrine disruptor.

What to do: Avoid foods from countries where OCs are not banned. Choose organic, local, fresh products. Choose organic meats and low-fat products—not necessarily because fat is bad, but because of potential toxin accumulation in the fat. Cook meat where fats can drip away.

5 – ORGANOPHOSPHATE (OP) PESTICIDES

Sources: Currently, the most widely used group of pesticides, OP was developed from nerve gas research and is an acetylcholinesterase inhibitor.

Health effects: It is a known neurotoxin.

What to do: Choose organic, local products. Wash all fruits and vegetables. Monitor your municipal water levels for pesticides. Don't wear outdoor shoes in your home.

6 – POLYCHLORINATED DIBENZO-DIOXIN (PCDD)

Sources: This chemical loves fat and can be found in high-fat foods. It's also found in PVC production, paper bleaching and incineration.

Health effects: Known to cause cancer, it's also an endocrine and immune disruptor.

What to do: Choose low-fat or no-fat animal products as toxins tend to accumulate in fats. Avoid fish like catfish, trout, or carp as they tend to have higher dioxin levels. Remove the skins and fatty areas from fish fillets, and do not fry fish—bake or broil instead. Wash fruits and vegetables before eating. Avoid smoke and vapors from chemical factories.

7 – POLYCHLORINATED BIPHENYLS (PCBS)

Sources: PCBs were banned in 1979 due to extreme persistence, bioaccumulation and toxicity.

Health effects: They can cause cancer and birth defects. PCBs can also cause brain, nervous system, immune system and reproductive issues. They are another known endocrine disruptor.

What to do: Never eat farmed fish, often called 'Atlantic salmon'. Avoid fish high in PCBs like bluefish, striped bass, croaker, flounder and blue crab. Use low-fat conventional meats or full-fat organic meats and dairy products to avoid consuming toxins stored in animal fats.

8 – POLYBROMINATED DIPHENYL ETHERS (PBDES)

Sources: Used as flame retardants in furniture, foam, bedding, toys, electronics and plastics.

Health effects: PBDEs are lipophilic, meaning they, too, accumulate in our tissues and environment. They can cause cancer, liver damage, thyroid dysfunction, birth defects and neurotoxicity.

What to do: Avoid all foam items made before 2005, as they are likely to contain PBDE. Cover mattresses with an allergen barrier to reduce exposure from dust. Remove old carpets. Use a HEPA filter when vacuuming. Avoid farmed fish as PBDEs accumulate in fats. Use low-fat conventional meats or full-fat organic meats and dairy products to avoid consuming toxins stored in animal fats.

9 – POLYFLUORINATED COMPOUNDS (PFCS)

Sources: These are fluorine-containing chemicals that make material resistant to stains and adhesion. They are used to make packaged fast food grease-resistant. PFCs are also used in Scotch Gard, Teflon, shampoos and denture cleaners. There are two types—PFOA and PFOS. PFOA is not biodegradable, so it never breaks down.

Health effects: PFOAs affect the liver, pancreas and thyroid. They can also cause testicular and breast tumors. They are known to cause thyroid cancers and decrease thyroid production.

What to do: Don't eat fast foods—especially those that are packaged in PFC treated paper. Avoid microwave popcorn bags or treated pizza boxes. Avoid stain-resistant products and non-stick cookware. Don't use pots and pans that are scratched. Check personal-care products for ingredients starting with "fluoro" or "perfluoro." Be wary as PFCs may be found in dental floss and cosmetics.

KEY THINGS TO REMEMBER

You probably noticed that a lot of the suggestions above are quite similar. When it comes to chemicals, they mostly affect five main areas: personal beauty products, water, air quality, cookware and food. All of these will be discussed at length in the chapters to come. However, here is a general list of things to do in terms of minimizing your toxic load:

- Test and filter your water.

- Filter your home air. Don't wear outdoor shoes indoors and remove all carpets. Be careful with other highly-treated flooring materials as they can emit vapors.

- Avoid personal-care products with synthetic ingredients; look for an organic certification logo.

- Eat local and organic as much as you can. Better yet, grow your own food whenever possible.

- Eat grass-fed organic meats to decrease exposure to the toxins that can be stored in animal fats.

- Be careful if rapidly losing weight. Toxins are stored in fat cells so you need to make sure your liver, lymphatic system, kidneys, and gut can flush out toxins adequately before and during a weight-loss program.

- Store food in glass containers.

- Be aware of toxins in coffee. Make sure the beans are fresh and certified organic. Most coffee in the store is at least eight weeks old and can contain mold).

- Don't drink from plastic cups or containers—especially hot beverages.

- Beware of your furniture and the materials out of which it is made—is it time to upgrade?

- Consider getting tested for heavy metal and chemical toxicity. There are different tests that can be done to measure one's level of toxicity. More on this in **Chapter 17: Detox—Is Your Body Flushing Out Toxins Efficiently?**

Also, keep in mind that emotional trauma can be just as bad as physical toxicity. Stress puts us in sympathetic overload (i.e. fight-or-flight mode), while a calming state put us in parasympathetic (i.e. rest/digest/detoxify mode) where healing occurs. If we are in chronic stress all the time, we don't get into the rest/digest/detox stage, and we will accumulate toxins in our body.

The following diagram shows examples of health habits, with corresponding hack levels. To download the *Hack Your Health Habits Worksheet*, visit

www.hackyourhealthhabits.com/worksheets

READY #HEALTHHACKER?
EXAMPLES OF LEVEL 1, 2 AND 3 HACKS FOR THIS CHAPTER

✓ Next time you shop for beauty and cleaning products, pay attention to labels and start to make changes in the brands you buy.

✓ Instead of plastic containers, use glass containers to store food.

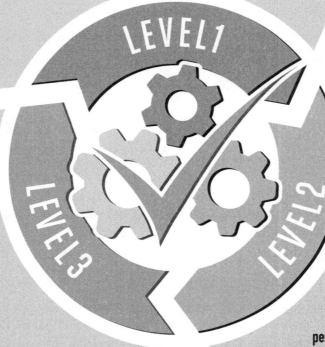

✓ When purchasing new furniture, research the materials used.

✓ Pick an afternoon or a weekend to go through your cosmetics and personal products. Ditch what is toxic, and make a list of things you need to replace. Go online and research organic makeup and less-toxic cleaning products.

✓ Eat unprocessed, organic foods most of the time.

✓ Install a water filtration device in your home to reduce fluoride and chlorine exposure.

HACK YOUR HEALTH PROGRESS

||||||||||||||||||||||||||||||||||||||||||||||||||||||||||||||||||||||||||||||||||||||||||||

CHAPTER 16

DETOXIFICATION

Is Your Body Flushing Out Toxins Efficiently?

"A healthy outside starts
from the inside."

— ROBERT URICH

THINK IT OVER

- What systems in the body are responsible for detoxification, and how do you know if they are functioning optimally?

- How do you find out if toxins are negatively affecting your health?

- What does a proper detox program consist of?

Although our bodies all function the same way, the toxins we encounter in our daily lives can have a different impact on each of us, depending on how much we are able to handle. Have you ever wondered why two people that seem to have similar lives—who work or live together—can have different responses to illness? Why does one person get sick, but not the other? To explain why this happens, let's use the analogy of a bucket.

Buckets come in all shapes and sizes and will hold a certain amount of liquid before they overflow. Imagine that there is a bucket in front of you. This bucket represents your body. It's filled with liquid that represents the toxins you have been exposed to, from your birth to now. Your bucket is half-full. On the other hand, your spouse's bucket is close to full. What do you think will happen if more liquid is added? Your bucket may be able to handle it, but your spouse's will likely overflow. This is exactly what happens in our bodies and is why some individuals get sick after a certain amount of toxin exposure, whereas others do not. We all carry a certain toxic load. Some of us are less toxic than others; it all depends on what we have been exposed to in the past.

Those who are less toxic are usually better-equipped to deal with chemical stressors. That's the reason why one family member may have environmental allergies and others don't. When it comes to being sick or feeling unwell, toxic load is often overlooked. Many do not think that they are exposed to huge amounts of toxins. Nor do they understand that symptoms can stay dormant for years until their "bucket" is full. In other words, people do not realize that the chemicals they are exposed to—no matter how big or small the dose—can build up in their body and can eventually wreak havoc on their health. For example, toxin exposure may be originating in the mouth from metals (from amalgams, crowns, implants and orthodontic appliances), BPA and phthalates (from some dental composites and night guards) and infections (from periodontal disease, root canals and jaw osteonecrosis). However, the above-mentioned are used by many, without realizing the amount of toxic exposure that comes with them.

Without getting too complex, here are the ways that toxins can create damage in the body:

- They can increase what are called Radical Oxygen Species (ROS) formation, also known as free radicals.

- They can damage DNA and cells by inhibiting enzyme function. Enzymes are catalysts that bring about a specific biochemical reaction.

- They can create endocrine disruption, resulting in hormone imbalances.

WHAT IS NEEDED FOR A PROPER DETOXIFICATION PROCESS?

The detoxification process is a complex one. When we think of detox, we mostly think of the liver, the lymphatic system, the kidneys and the gut. Yes, these organs and systems play an important role in the detoxification process; however, they remain downstream from the problem. When it comes to detoxification, the true problem can be found upstream at the cellular level. Every cell in our body needs to be able to get nutrients in and toxins out. If and when that mechanism is impaired, our toxicity levels will rise, and our detoxification process will be compromised.

To clarify, here is an analogy: Imagine that you are at the bottom of a river. The river has been dyed purple, and your job is to return the river to its natural color. From downstream, you start filtering the water. You're able to remove some of the color—turning the river from a dark purple to a lighter purple, but can't seem to be able to get it back to its natural color. Being the smart person that you are, you decide to venture upstream and stumble across the source, which is a big block of purple dye. You remove the source and make your way back downstream. After a few days, the river is no longer purple. The source was the real problem. You could have filtered the water downstream forever, and the water would never have returned to normal until you took away the source.

There are seven channels the body uses for elimination: the lungs, the liver, the kidneys, the skin, the blood, the gut and the lymphatic system. They all play a role in removing toxins from our body, but their roles, as important as they are, are secondary. If we want to have a permanent impact, we need to truly address the source—our cells.

The cell membrane plays a key role in cellular detoxification and health. Inflammation to the cell membrane can impede the cell's ability to get nutrients into the cell and toxins out. In addition, inflammation reduces the ability for hormones to reach the cell-receptor sites to be activated. Inflammation of the cell membrane can be caused by heavy metal toxicity, mycotoxins from molds, and a diet high in inflammatory sugar or pesticide-ridden foods.

Before we dig deeper into the cells, let's review some of the major players in the detoxification process.

LIVER AND DETOXIFICATION

The liver is a large, meaty organ that is located on the right side of the body, beneath the diaphragm and just above the stomach. Weighing approximately three pounds, it is one of the largest organs in your body. Along with the gallbladder, pancreas and intestines, it works to digest, absorb and process food. But, that is not your liver's only function.

Researchers have found that your liver is responsible for performing nearly five hundred vital functions, including:

- producing bile, which helps carry away waste and break down fats in the small intestine during digestion

- clearing the blood of drugs and other poisonous substances

- resisting infections by producing immune factors and removing bacteria from the bloodstream

- producing certain proteins for blood plasma

- producing cholesterol and special proteins that help carry fats through the body

- converting excess glucose into glycogen for storage

- regulating levels of amino acid in the blood, which form the building blocks of proteins

- processing of hemoglobin for use of its iron content

- conversion of poisonous ammonia to urea, which is excreted in the urine

To simplify, your liver is your body's processing plant, breaking down anything that you consume. It is your liver's job to distinguish between the nutrients you need to absorb (like vitamins and minerals), and the dangerous or unnecessary substances that must be filtered out of your bloodstream (like drugs or alcohol).

Without giving you a physiology course, let's talk briefly about the two major detoxification pathways inside the liver, which are called Phase 1 and Phase 2 detoxification pathways.

PHASE 1 LIVER DETOXIFICATION PATHWAY

Phase 1 detoxification consists of processes of oxidation, reduction, hydrolysis, hydration and dehalogenation. To put it simply, this pathway will convert a toxic chemical (that is nonpolar and lipid-soluble) into a less harmful chemical (more polar, less lipid-soluble). Nutrients used for this phase are vitamins B2-B3-B6-B12, folic acid, glutathione, branched chain amino acids, flavonoids and phospholipids. During this process, free radicals are produced, which, if excessive, can damage the liver cells. Antioxidants (such as vitamin C and E and natural carotenoids) reduce the damage caused by these free radicals. If antioxidants are lacking, and toxin exposure is high, toxic chemicals become far more dangerous.

PHASE 2 LIVER DETOXIFICATION PATHWAY

This is called the conjugation pathway. Phase 2 of detoxification consists of the processes of sulfation, glucuronidation, glutathione conjugation, acetylation, amino acid conjugation and methylation. The nutrients used in this process are glycine, taurine, glutamine, n-acetylcysteine, cysteine and methionine. The goal of the phase 2 detoxification process is to take the more polar, less lipid-soluble intermediary metabolites produced from phase 1 detoxification and make them polar and water-soluble so they can be excreted from the body via feces and urine.

In **Chapter 55: Know Your Numbers—Understanding Your Tests Results to Take Control of Your Health**, we will be discussing how to interpret the results of a liver-enzymes blood panel. However, in the meantime, symptoms and signs of liver biotransformation issues include acne, bloating, thinning hair, swelling, weight gain, hormonal imbalances, poor bowel function and foul-smelling sweat.

What about the gallbladder? The gallbladder is the organ that sits just beneath the liver. This small organ plays an important role in the digestion of our food. Its main purpose is to store bile that is produced by the liver. It stores the bile until it is needed for digesting fatty foods in the duodenum of the small intestine.

What does the gallbladder have to do with detoxification? If functioning properly, the liver will remove toxic substances from our blood and discard them via bile into the intestines. If the liver and gallbladder are *not* functioning properly, bile containing harmful chemicals can be recirculated throughout the body and reabsorbed into the liver. This can cause issues, not just for the liver, but also for the entire body.

THE KIDNEYS AND DETOXIFICATION

The kidneys play an important role in detoxification. They extract waste from our blood, help balance our bodily fluids, and form urine so we can excrete toxic waste. To support the kidneys, it is important to avoid excess protein, drink a lot of pure filtered water, and eat foods rich in potassium like avocados, spinach and coconuts. Lemon water in the morning not only helps you start your day on an alkaline note but also helps prevent kidney stones from forming. You can also drink unsweetened herbal teas like dandelion and ginger teas, but make sure to stay away from artificial sugars.

GUT AND DETOXIFICATION

We will discuss the gut at length in Section 8, but since it plays a crucial role in the detoxification process, it's important to address it here, as well. If the bowel has dysbiosis (i.e. imbalances in the microflora), increased permeability or inflammation, the liver is forced to work overtime. This means that good gut bacteria are not only important for gut health but for liver function, as well.

Heavy metals such as mercury, aluminum, and lead can damage the gut mucous membrane and tissues, causing it to become more permeable and allowing toxins to spread throughout the body. This is known to cause allergies, intolerances and potential immune reactions. Toxins found in the gut need to be bound properly for excretion, or they will be recirculated in the body. This condition is often referred to as Leaky Gut Syndrome, which you will learn all about in **Chapter 38: Your Gut—Understanding How It Works and What Could Go Wrong.**

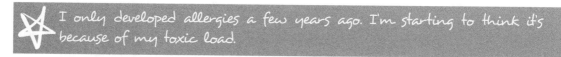
I only developed allergies a few years ago. I'm starting to think it's because of my toxic load.

Another key aspect of bowel detoxification is the portal vein, which carries blood from the gut and spleen and drains it into the liver. This is why enemas such as coffee enemas, are efficient to help detox the liver and increase glutathione production. Glutathione is used by every cell in the body, where it acts as an antioxidant to neutralize free radicals and prevent cellular damage.

THE LYMPHATIC SYSTEM AND DETOXIFICATION

Next on our list is the lymphatic system. What does the lymphatic system do? The lymphatic system is a vital part of the immune system. It consists of vessels and nodes that carry a fluid called lymph from tissues and organs to the bloodstream. There is approximately three to five times more lymph fluid in the body than there is blood. Lymph is meant to help the body filter and clean toxins, debris and pathogens that accumulate in our circulatory system as a result of toxic environments, medications and an unhealthy diet. Lymph fluid passes through lymph nodes in our organ tissues. The nodes act as filtering station that move the lymph fluid to the surface of our skin near the neck, abdomen, armpits and groin. These nodes are meant to remove waste products, damaged cells, infectious organisms and foreign particles to prevent blockages and protect against infection.

Think of the lymphatic system as a city waste-removal service; garbage is removed on a regular basis, and if not, the garbage will build up and eventually overwhelm a household. It is possible for our lymphatic system to become blocked and congested, causing stagnation in circulation and, therefore, having adverse effects on the body. Properly functioning kidneys are also key for a properly functioning lymphatic system.

TESTING FOR TOXICITY

There are several methods of testing for toxicity. Serum (blood), urine and fecal levels of toxins represent only acute exposure to toxins and do not necessarily reflect the toxicity of a toxin, per se. For example, 90 percent of the body's lead is stored in the bones, so a blood test on its own would not evaluate lead levels accurately. This is because the biological half-life of lead in blood is approximately 30 days, so the test would indicate only recent lead exposure.[1]

To determine toxicity levels, a very detailed health history analysis needs to be done. Has the person been exposed to metals? Do they have or have they had dental amalgams in the past? Do they eat tuna regularly? Are they taking low-quality herbal supplements that could have a high level of toxicity? Did they grow up near a chemical plant? Do they work with toxic fumes?

There are different ways to test for heavy metal exposure. One of them is a hair analysis. Some experts disagree with the validity of this testing method, but the idea is that hair permanently binds heavy metals in levels proportionate to those found in the body. However, there are limitations to hair analysis. For one, it reflects what the person has been exposed to only in recent months and does not reveal the inorganic type of toxins common in things like amalgam tooth fillings.

Another method is the provoked urine test, which is said to be one of the best tests to determine metal toxicity. In this method, a person is given a chelation agent before the collection of urine. This agent pushes any metals into the kidneys so that they can be excreted in the urine. The MELISA test is also another test that can detect hypersensitivity to metals; MELISA stands for Memory Lymphocyte Immunostimulation Assay. MELISA is said to be a scientifically proven and clinically validated blood test that detects delayed hypersensitivity to metals such as mercury, nickel and titanium. Lastly, a stool analysis can be another tool and is often best suited for kids and adults who are sensitive to the chelating agent.

In addition to all this, there also exists another useful tool that can measure the amount of cellular inflammation caused by toxins in the body. This test is called the Meta-Oxy Test. The Meta-Oxy Test measures malondialdehyde in the urine, which is a marker for oxidative stress and cell membrane damage due to free radicals. The level of malondialdehyde in the urine indicates the amount of oxidized fat; therefore, the more malondialdehyde measured in the urine, the greater the amount of cell membrane damage.

FOODS TO SUPPORT DETOXIFICATION

When it comes to food and the detoxification process, one could get very specific. In fact, different foods and nutrients are needed to support phase 1 and phase 2 of detoxification. In general, a plant-based diet high in phytonutrients is key for proper detoxification. Nutrients can help induce or inhibit specific enzymes, provide soluble and insoluble fibers, and ensure the consumption of antioxidants. Here are foods, in general, that can help the detoxification process:

- foods high in sulfur like garlic, legumes and onions
- good sources of water-soluble fiber like apples, oat bran and legumes

- cruciferous vegetables like Brussels sprouts, cabbage, cauliflower, kale and broccoli

- artichokes, beets, carrots and dandelion greens

- herbs and spices like turmeric, cinnamon and licorice

- green leafy vegetables, green tea, wheatgrass juice, chlorella and spirulina

Please note that if an extensive detox is required, it is best to work with a natural health practitioner who specializes in detoxification.

DETOXIFICATION—WHAT IS OUT THERE?

From teas, to cleanses, to exercise routines, there are many types of detox therapies on the market today. In their book, *Toxin Toxout*, authors Bruce Lourie and Rick Smith discuss some of the most popular methods. I've adapted their list below to tell you which methods are proven, which methods produce limited results, and which have no proof at all. [2]

PROVEN METHODS OF DETOX

- chelation—using the chelation agents I mentioned earlier to bind heavy metal toxins, allowing for excretion

- sauna therapy

LIMITED METHODS OF DETOX*

*These methods have some evidence supporting them; however, further research is needed before it is considered proven.

- fasting
- exercise

- probiotics and prebiotics
- herbal supplements

You may have encountered some other methods of detox such as:

- ionic foot baths

- colonic cleansing—there is some research showing benefits, but it mostly lacks empirical evidence. It might be good to flush encrusted fecal material, but be careful not to disturb normal flora

- food and drink cleanses—eating these foods can help keep the body in tip-top shape, but no evidence has been found that they can actually remove toxins

- leeching—some people believe that leeches will suck toxins from the blood; and

- hot springs

However, not much empirical evidence currently exists showing that these methods safely and effectively remove toxins from the body, although often promoted as such. If considering any of these methods, ensure to do your own research before beginning.

HEAVY METAL DETOXIFICATION

Chelation is often used to treat heavy metal toxicity with agents like EDTA, DMSA or DMPS, which are abbreviations for ridiculously long words that you probably don't need to know. Because of how powerful they are, chelators are available only with a prescription and should be used only when working with a qualified health-care professional. A health-care professional will ensure that, during the detox process, minerals that are being depleted are replaced, enough antioxidants are consumed, and that the detoxification of the liver and the gut is supported.

Adding to the complexity of these, it's important to note that heavy metals in the brain can affect the hypothalamus and pituitary glands, which play a crucial role in the HPA (hypothalamus-pituitary-adrenal) axis and can cause major dysregulations in many hormones.

Be aware that some supplements used for binding heavy metals may not actually eliminate toxins. Take, for instance, chlorella and cilantro. Neither are "true binders," meaning that while they may bind toxins, they do not necessarily eliminate them. When it comes down to it, chlorella is a great superfood but not great for heavy metal detoxification, and cilantro is a delicious garnish, but you need to watch how much you eat. Bound metals that are not eliminated remain in the body and seek refuge in other tissues and organs, causing more health problems.

Have you heard of zeolites? Zeolites are another known heavy metal detoxification agent that has been promoted as a more natural, more efficient, and less expensive alternative to chelation. That being said, there is some debate over its efficiency. Zeolites are not soluble, and while they are great binders, they are too big to cross the gut, which is a huge limitation. Dr. Nikolaos Tsirikos-Karapanos seems to have resolved that issue by creating a product called "CytoDetox," which is a clinptilolite form of zeolite that is hydrolyzed and able to cross not only the gut but also enter the cells and get into the brain.

DETOXIFICATION AT THE CELLULAR LEVEL

Earlier in this chapter, I talked about the importance of detoxification at a cellular level. Dr. Daniel Pompa, health expert and founder of *True Cellular Detox*, has conceived a program that focuses on detoxifying at the cellular level.[3] Empowered by his own struggles with severe heavy metal toxicity, Dr. Pompa developed a protocol focusing on the detoxification of heavy metals with safe and effective nutraceutical supplements. It's important to mention that his program is not a quick fix. Detoxifying the body after years of toxicity takes time, but it can be life-changing for those who have yet to find a solution to their health challenges. Dr. Pompa's program is based on what he calls the five Rs:

1 - REMOVE THE SOURCE

What kind of sources are we talking about? Things like:

- pathogens (bacteria, virus, mold or fungus, parasites)
- petrochemicals and toxins (herbicides, pesticides, fungicides)
- heavy metals (mercury, lead, aluminum, arsenic and cadmium)

Removing the source may sound like the obvious thing to do, but often people don't realize how exposed they are. Toxic stressors quickly shut down detox pathways and allow other toxins to bio-accumulate. This is where testing and an inventory of our food, water, air and personal products can be helpful.

2 - REGENERATE THE CELL MEMBRANE

According to stem-cell biologist Dr. Bruce H. Lipton, the cell membrane is so important that it should be considered the "brain" of the cell.[4] Simply put, the cell membrane holds the intelligence of the cell, allowing it to turn genes on and off and regulate hormones. A supple lipid bilayer membrane allows for things to be able to flow in and out of the cells. When a cell membrane becomes inflamed, it loses its ability to move good things *in* such as hormones and nutrients, and bad things such as toxins and debris *out*—which can lead to abnormal cellular function and disease.

3 - RESTORE CELL ENERGY—ADENOSINE TRIPHOSPHATE (ATP)

The body can't heal properly without its mitochondria working properly, in order to produce energy. Mitochondria are the cell powerhouses which create ATP, or energy. Think of how having gasoline in a car makes it run. Cellular energy is the gasoline of the cell and nothing runs or functions without it. As nutrients flow into the cell, they feed the mitochondria. Without adequate production of ATP, cells are unable to detoxify or regenerate properly. What's more, the lower your ATP, the more inflammation occurs at the cellular level. The lack of ATP production has almost become an epidemic in the modern world; and individuals suffer from symptoms like fatigue, brain fog, digestive problems and hormone issues.

4 - REDUCE INFLAMMATION AND FREE RADICAL DAMAGE

Reducing inflammation and damages caused by free radicals created by the detoxification pathways are key elements in improving cell function.

Cellular inflammation is driving the epidemic of pervasive chronic diseases and hormone disruption in our culture today—specifically, inflammation of the cell membrane affects the way the cell communicates and detoxes, which ultimately can change gene expression. Understanding how to downregulate inflammation is essential to improve almost any health condition and maintain good health.

5 – RE-ESTABLISH METHYLATION

Methylation, as mentioned earlier, is one of the steps in phase 2 of liver detoxification. Methyl groups (CH3) are applied to countless critical functions in the body such as repairing DNA, turning genes on and off, fighting infections, and getting rid of environmental toxins. When methyl groups are not available, the body becomes vulnerable to inflammation and toxins.

The "methylation priority principle" states that the body prioritizes where methyl groups go, sending them where they are most needed. Prioritization is based on the immediate adaptation to stress. In a sense, methyl groups turn our stress receptors on and off. People under high stress can deplete their methyl groups, resulting in heightened levels of anxiety and an inability to sleep. In cases where depletion is severe, their stress response is affected, and DNA goes unprotected. Known methyl depleters are the birth control pill, antidepressants, some diabetic medications, antacids and cigarette smoke.

To make matters even more complex, some people can have what are called single nucleotide polymorphisms (SNPs, pronounced "snips"), or "copying errors" in one of their methylation genes (e.g. MTHFR). This means that they have a genetic mutation that may decrease DNA methylation (which acts to repress gene expression).

How do these copying errors happen? In order for new cells to be made, an existing cell must divide itself into two. During this process, it makes a copy of its DNA so the new cell will have a complete set of genetic instructions. Sometimes a mistake is made in the copying—kind of like a typo—and these typos lead to a variation in the DNA sequence at a particular location, called SNPs.

There are specific SNPs that can affect the detoxification pathways. Knowing this information can be helpful to optimize and support a person's detoxification process. For example, I myself have the genotype (+/-) for the MTHFR gene SNP C677T, which makes me a poor methylator. Therefore, in order to support my overall methylation, I've started making some lifestyle changes and taking specific supplements.

TIPS AND STRATEGIES FOR BETTER DETOXIFICATION

- **Water** – Drinking plenty of water (2-3L per day) will aid greatly in liver detoxification by flushing out toxins more easily.

- **Eat a phytonutrient-dense diet** – Nutrients are needed to help the detoxification process. Therefore, it is important to not be nutrient-depleted before and during a detox.

- **Fiber** – If we don't eat enough soluble fiber, our bile, instead of being ushered out of the body and then replaced with fresh bile produced by the liver, is repeatedly re-circulated within our system. In the process, it becomes more concentrated with toxins, which, in turn, can lead to all sorts of inflammatory diseases such as gallbladder disease, intestinal inflammation, and even skin conditions like acne, eczema and psoriasis. Ultimately, a low-fiber diet can contribute to elevated levels of toxicity throughout the body.

- **Eat organic** – Stay away from GMOs and eat organic as much as you can to reduce your exposure to pesticides, herbicides and fungicide. Remember, Roundup is one of the most toxic herbicides and products containing glyphosate.

- **Avoid drugs and alcohol** – Drugs and alcohol can be very taxing on the liver, which is the primary organ of detoxification. Try to limit your alcohol intake even more if you are a woman, as it can also affect hormonal balance.

- **Use organic beauty, skin care and cleaning products** – Try to eliminate exposure to harmful toxins by using products that are void of known carcinogenic substances. Yes, they may smell good, but, at what cost? More brands now offer products made with organic or non-toxic ingredients. Let's not only read labels for things we eat but also for what we put on our body.

- **Mattress and beds** – Get 100 percent wool, organic cotton, or rubber pillows and natural mattresses free of flame retardants and harmful chemicals.

- **Remove dental amalgams** – Silver amalgam fillings are 50 percent mercury. Mercury vaporizes over time, crossing into the brain and bio-accumulating over time. The scientific journal, FACETS, published a study that found that the number of fillings in your mouth is proportional to how much mercury is found in your brain and pituitary glands, which control your endocrine system. Removal is strongly suggested but has to be done correctly in order to avoid toxicity and long-term health effects. The mercury vapors that come off the filling when drilling can go up the nose and to the brain. Therefore, seek out a biological dentist that is trained to remove the amalgams properly and safely. After the removal of your fillings, make sure to detoxify your body with a proven detoxification program such as True Cellular Detox. For more information, check out the International Academy of Oral Medicine and Technology website: www.iaomt.org. The academy is an advocate for safer dentistry.

- **Regular use of infrared saunas** – Infrared saunas have been shown to restore lymph function by causing the body to sweat. Sweat detoxifies the body, cleaning and draining your system. It's important to note that use of the sauna is not suggested if you have amalgams since breathing in their vapors can raise toxicity levels.

- **Dry brushing** – Brushing your skin with a dry brush, especially after exercise or an infrared sauna, can help to not only remove dead skin cells but can also help to improve blood flow and lymph circulation.

- **Exercise and rebounders** – Rebounders that resemble mini trampolines are a great way to help activate your lymphatic system and help move toxins out of your body. Physical activity also promotes healthy circulation, which prevents lymph from becoming stagnant. Better blood circulation also helps with nutrient and oxygen distribution. In addition, sweating will also help eliminate toxins through your skin.

- **Cleanse using herbs and spices** – Herbs and spices such as dandelion root, milk thistle, burdock, turmeric, cinnamon and licorice—along with green and white teas—can help your body cleanse itself more efficiently, *but* be careful that the herbs and spices you are using do not have high levels of toxicity or molds!

- **Supplements to support your liver** – Glutathione, B vitamins, N-acetyl cysteine and alpha-lipoic acid are all supplements to be considered. L-glutamine and probiotics can also help the gut.

- **Get your Zs!** – Restful sleep helps facilitate clearance of metabolites from the brain. Without proper sleep, you aren't detoxifying right.

It is important to realize that detoxification is not a thing you do once in a while. Steps to proper detoxification should be ongoing. Remember that our environments are pivotal. We can treat a condition, but if the environment stays the same, our symptoms will return. Our cells respond to our environment, so if you don't change the environment, you won't get rid of your health issues.

The following diagram shows examples of health habits, with corresponding hack levels. To download the *Hack Your Health Habits Worksheet*, visit

www.hackyourhealthhabits.com/worksheets

READY #HEALTHHACKER?
EXAMPLES OF LEVEL 1, 2 AND 3 HACKS FOR THIS CHAPTER

✓ Ensure you are well hydrated, as water helps flush out toxins.

✓ Assess your environment to see how much exposure to toxins you may have in your everyday life.

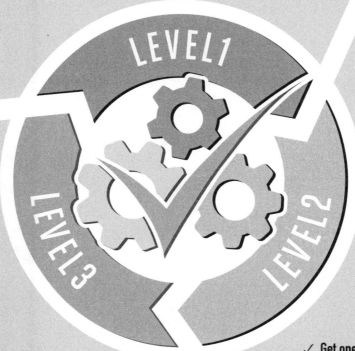

✓ Detox your cells with the True Cellular Detox Complete Program.

✓ Safely remove dental amalgams.

✓ Get one out of the three tests done to assess your levels of toxicity. How did you score? What can you do to improve that score?

HACK YOUR HEALTH PROGRESS

|||||||||||||||||||

CHAPTER 17

YOUR SKIN
What Are You Soaking Up?

"We're the guinea pigs
when it comes to testing
the long-term chronic
health impacts of all the
chemical substances in our
shine-boosting shampoos,
wrinkle-retardant clothes,
and pain-killing pills."

— ADRIA VASIL,
ECOHOLIC BODY

THINK IT OVER

- Do you know what ingredients are in your favorite beauty products?

- Could the chemicals found in your cosmetic and hygiene products be negatively impacting your overall health?

- What are some safe alternatives to conventional, store-bought personal-care products?

For more than a decade, I have been organizing an annual Health and Wellness Expo in my hometown. A few years ago, I invited Adria Vasil to speak. Vasil is known as Canada's "straight shooting, green living expert." Her series of books (*Ecoholic, Ecoholic Home and Ecoholic Body*) discuss pretty much everything you need to know about becoming environmentally friendly. At the time of the expo, Adria was promoting *Ecoholic Body*. I remember picking her up from the train station and being asked if we could make a quick stop at the drugstore. She needed to buy some products for an article she was working on.

At this point in time, I had already started making greener and healthier product choices. I was trying natural shampoos, shopping for natural cosmetics, and using natural deodorants and toothpastes. With that said, while going through the aisles with Adria, I couldn't help but feel a bit overwhelmed. Cosmetic shopping at a drugstore with the "Queen of Green" was like shopping at a butcher shop with a vegan. For almost every item on the shelf, Adria could name off several reasons why it should be avoided. Even some of the products I thought were good, natural options were on the "no-no list!"

While I've learned much more since first meeting Adria, I'm not going to pretend that I am a green expert. My primary concern is health. I choose products based on whether or not they contain harmful toxins that could negatively impact my well-being. To this day, I still reference Adria's book and the Environmental Working Group's (EWG) website when searching for new products. As a journalist, Adria stays unbiased and impartial when making recommendations, and I appreciate that.

The point of this chapter isn't to go through every single cosmetic or skin product on the shelves. If you are looking to switch over to natural body care, I strongly suggest that you research products on an individual basis. Adria's books and the EWG website can be great resources. Buyer beware: Just because a company makes one stellar all-natural, organic product, doesn't mean that all their products will be as good. You really need to be mindful when shopping.

My goal for this chapter is to shine a light on why natural is better, and provide some concrete examples regarding cosmetics, women's sanitary products, deodorants and sunscreens. It's true that swapping your go-to products for their natural alternatives might be easier said than done. But when it comes down to it, being healthy is more important to me than the perfect shade of lipstick. Finding the best products can be difficult, but there are good resources out there, and the hassle is definitely worth it in the long term.

THE NOT-SO-PRETTY SIDE OF COSMETICS

"The term 'cosmetic' means: (1) articles intended to be rubbed, poured, sprinkled, or sprayed on, introduced into, or otherwise applied to the human body or any part thereof for cleansing, beautifying, promoting attractiveness, or altering the appearance, and (2) articles intended for use as a component of any such articles; except that such term shall not include soap."

— Federal Food, Drug & Cosmetic Act (U.S.), Sec. 201 (I)

The primary role of your skin is to act as a barrier. That being said, pretty much everything you slather onto your skin—from body products to makeup—is absorbed into your bloodstream. According to research, the average person absorbs about five pounds of cosmetic chemicals every year. What's more, nine out of 10 women use makeup past its best-before date, thereby increasing the risk of irritation or contamination.[1] Ultimately, we really shouldn't put anything on our skin that we wouldn't want to eat!

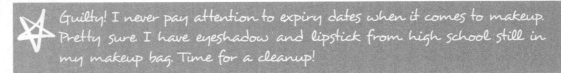

Guilty! I never pay attention to expiry dates when it comes to makeup. Pretty sure I have eyeshadow and lipstick from high school still in my makeup bag. Time for a cleanup!

Take note of how many personal products and cosmetics you use every day. If you're a "typical" female, your daily routine might look something like this: The alarm goes off in the morning, you jump in the shower, use shampoo, conditioner, body soap... then you get out of the shower and perhaps put on body and face cream, then comes the foundation, bronzer, eyeshadow, eyeliner, mascara, lipstick, followed by deodorant and maybe some perfume. Throughout the day, you may re-apply some lipstick, moisturize your hands, etc. Before you go to bed, you use a makeup remover and moisturizer, and, of course, you brush your teeth with toothpaste and rinse with a mouthwash. That's a total of 16 products used in a day! See my point?

The chemicals in your cosmetics can seep into your bloodstream in a variety of ways. Take note that powders are absorbed the least, while those that are oil-based or designed to moisturize will be absorbed more. Eye makeup most certainly affects the health of the eye—which is a very sensitive mucous membrane. Lipstick is often ingested. And, hairspray and perfumes can irritate your lungs when inhaled.

Unfortunately, cosmetics in the U.S. and Canada are not currently regulated by an overseeing body. The cosmetics industry is, in fact, a self-regulated one, which means your safety isn't going to be a priority—sales are.

> ✴ *Wow, that's not terrifying at all!*

This means that you're not only what you eat, you're also what you absorb! Shockingly, more than one-third of our personal-care products contain ingredients that have been linked in some way to cancer. And, according to the Environmental Working Group, only 11 percent of the 10,500 ingredients used in cosmetics, creams, deodorants, and antiperspirants, have ever been tested for safety. This is because neither the U.S. nor Canada have a mandate to safeguard the cosmetics industry. With nearly 4,000,000 synthetic chemicals out there, it seems too daunting a task.

As mentioned in the previous chapter on toxins, many of the chemical compounds created before 1970 have been grandfathered in and do not require testing for safety—it's assumed that time has been a good enough test. While some chemicals have been lightly tested and deemed to be substances "Generally Recognized as Safe" (GRAS), even those chemicals have not been studied adequately, and their long-term effects haven't been determined, nor what kind of consequences they could have when mixed with other synthetic products. Of course, not all of the ingredients used are harmful. However, many are known carcinogens (cancer-causers); neurotoxins (disrupters of the nervous system and brain), and reproductive-disrupting toxins (disrupters of fertility). Even babies are being born pre-polluted, due to the amount of toxin exposure around us!

Studies have shown that marketing may be even more important for some of the cosmetics companies than new product development. In a $50-billion-dollar industry, many companies spend just as much, if not more, on advertising and promotion as they do on research and development. Most consumers will choose a product based on branding or advertising promises rather than on scientific evidence.

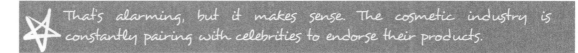

COSMETIC HAZARDS

There are some chemicals in cosmetics of which you need to stay clear. These are known to be hazardous to human health. Similar to Adria Vasil's recommendations in *Ecoholic Body*, the Environmental Working Group (EWG), a non-profit organization, has created a cosmetic safety database that will help you find out the safety rating of makeup:

www.cosmeticsdatabase.com

In this database, products are ranked from one (low hazard) to 10 (high hazard), and the site will tell you whether a product has been linked to cancer, causes allergies, is hazardous to your organs, could affect an unborn baby, and more.

If you haven't found a certain product on the cosmetics database, and the ingredients aren't included on your product's label, try looking up the ingredients online or even calling the cosmetics company to find out. You need to know what your body is absorbing. Campaigns by organizations like the EWG are pushing for changes in the legislation of cosmetics to help better protect you.

In *Ecoholic Body*, Adria lists the "Mean 15"—a list of chemicals used in cosmetics that should be avoided or, at the very least, limited:

1. **BHA (Beta Hydroxy Acid) and BHT (Butylated Hydroxytoluene)** – These are preservatives with links to cancer. BHA is the worst of the two and has to come with a cancer warning in California.

2. **DEA/MEA/TEA (diethanolamine)** – These can create carcinogenic nitrosamines when mixed with preservatives. At the time of writing, California now demands that cocamide DEA (found in shampoos, etc.) come with a cancer warning.

3. **Formaldehyde-releasing preservatives** – These include DMDM hydantoin, diazolidinyl urea, imidazolidinyl urea, methenamine, quaternium-15 and Bronopol. These are all known carcinogens, with links to allergies.

4. **Oxybenzone (BP-3/benzophenone) and octinoxate (octyl methoxycinnamate)** – These two sunscreen chemicals may disrupt your hormone system and can trigger allergic reactions.

5. **Palm oil** – This includes anything with "palm" or "palmate" in its name, like sodium palmate. Palm oil is not necessarily bad for the skin but is very bad for the earth. So much forest has been clear-cut for palm oil monocultures that it has threatened endangered species. Avoid unless it's fair trade and organic.

6. **Parabens** – These are commonly found in shampoos and deodorants to extend their shelf life. Parabens are stored in your body fat and can mimic the hormone estrogen. Parabens have also been linked to cancers, particularly breast cancer.

7. **Partum/fragrance** – When you see this word on a label, it can indicate the presence of up to 4,000 separate ingredients. These are potentially laced with phthalates and other hormone disruptors and sensitizers.

8. **PEGs** (polyethylene glycol compounds, and anything with '-eth' in its name) – These are often contaminated with the carcinogenic 1,4-dioxane.

9. **Petrolatum/paraffin/mineral oil/petroleum distillates** – These are by-products of petroleum, the same stuff you put in your car! These ingredients sit on your skin and block pores by forming an oil film, creating a buildup of toxins, which may aggravate acne and promote premature aging.

10. **PPD** – PPD is in all permanent hair dyes and is linked to some cancers. It can also be called p-Aminoaniline; 1,4-benzenediamine; p-benzenediamine CI 76060; p-Diaminobenzene; 1,4-phenylenediamine; 1,4-diaminobenzene.

11. **Phthalates** – This hormone-disrupting family of chemicals hides behind the word 'fragrance,' but you can look for the phrase "phthalate free." It is also used as a plastic softener, common in vinyl and PVC. Several phthalates have been banned from children's toys and child-care items in North America, but not from children's body care. These chemicals can be harmful to your liver and kidneys—and can even harm a developing fetus.

12. **Retinyl palmitate** – Keep this one out of the sun as it seems to speed up the carcinogenic effect of UV rays in mice.

13. **Siloxanes** – Pass on anything with the prefix "cyclo-" or the suffix "-methicone." Cyclotetrasiloxane (D4) and cyclopentasiloxane (D5) are eco-toxic siloxanes, silicone based polymers. Cyclomethicone is a mix of D4, D5 and D6 siloxanes.

14. **Sodium laureth sulphate** – Used as a foaming agent in soaps and shampoos, this chemical is actually a harsh skin irritant that is potentially carcinogenic.

15. **Triclosan and triclocarban** – These are suspected thyroid disruptors. Health Canada was poised to declare triclosan officially toxic to the environment, but did not deliver. Instead, they are asking companies to voluntarily reduce their use. This is pretty weak, considering the U.S. FDA just told soap makers they would have to stop using triclosan—along with 18 other antibacterial chemicals—in their products.[2]

Other Chemicals to Avoid:

- **Lead** – Lipstick can contain lead, which is a neurotoxin and can cause health problems, including learning, language and behavior problems.

- **Aluminum** – Occurring in some eyeshadows, aluminum has been linked to Alzheimer's disease.

- **Coal Tar** – Used to color products, this chemical has been linked to cancer.

- **Talc** – Found in some powders, this has been shown to cause cancer in animals.

- **Propylene Glycol** – This is found in thousands of cosmetic products to help moisturize. It is also an ingredient used in antifreeze and brake fluid…no surprise that it may cause liver abnormalities and kidney damage.

"NATURAL," "ORGANIC" OR "MINERAL" MAKEUP

Beware of cosmetic products claiming to be "Natural," "Organic," or "Mineral-based." They still need scrutiny. Since the terms "organic" and "natural" aren't regulated in the cosmetic industry, it's hard to tell whether cosmetics making such claims are going to be any better for you. Look, when possible, for a third-party-certified organic logo and/or eco-certification.

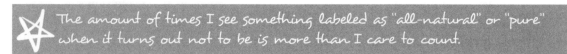

The amount of times I see something labeled as "all-natural" or "pure" when it turns out not to be is more than I care to count.

True natural makeup will use base products such as jojoba oil or candelilla wax instead of the petrochemicals such as mineral oil, which is not recommended because it will clog pores and leave an oily residue on your skin. It is also absorbed very rapidly and goes into your bloodstream.

Mineral-based makeup—not to be confused with mineral oil—is gaining popularity. Minerals in cosmetics are not new; they are already in most of the cosmetics you own—there are minerals and tons of other added chemicals. What's new, however, is that the demand for pure mineral cosmetics is growing. This kind of makeup is free of chemicals, preservatives and dyes. Since they are more granular powders, mineral-based cosmetics are minimally absorbed by the body. Dermatologists and health-care practitioners also like them because they don't cause many allergic reactions; they're highly recommended to those who suffer from acne, dermatitis and other skin diseases. Mineral makeup typically includes inorganic dyes and minerals such as mica, titanium dioxide, zinc oxide and iron oxide.

The price of mineral cosmetics isn't that much higher than conventional ones. If you traditionally buy high-end cosmetics, you'll notice that the price is about the same or even less. Knowing, however, that you're putting something on your body that isn't hazardous to your health is priceless.

A word of warning, though: To make application smoother and less noticeable, titanium dioxide and zinc oxide are sometimes broken down into tiny particles called nano minerals. If breathed in, these particles can cause long-term lung inflammation and oxidative stress. Generally, anything higher than 100 nanometers is considered safe. Unfortunately, companies are not required to declare the presence of nanoparticles on their labels. To find out, you'll have to call the company's hotline.

The following sources can help you determine whether your current cosmetics are safe and also recommend product lines for you to try:

- *Ecoholic Body: Your Ultimate Earth-Friendly Guide to Living Healthy & Looking Good*, by Adria Vasil

- Environmental Working Group, www.ewg.org

- Skin Deep: Cosmetic Safety database, www.cosmeticsdatabase.com

- Cosmetic Ingredient Review panel, www.cir-safety.org

- Campaign for Safe Cosmetics, www.safecosmetics.org. You can download a *"healthy cosmetic party kit,"* where you will find tons of useful information, resources for campaigns, contacts and even homemade recipes for face scrubs, masks, etc.

WOMEN'S SANITARY PRODUCTS—BEWARE!

Did you know that sanitary products—including pads and tampons—can be similarly hazardous to your health? The average woman who menstruates until menopause uses an average of 16,000 tampons in her lifetime, not including pads and liners. That's a whole lot synthetic chemicals being directly inserted inside the vagina month after month!

Most common brands of tampons are made from genetically engineered cotton, rayon and synthetic fibers—all bleached in harsh chemicals to achieve the look we are used to seeing. It's scary to think, but there are a lot of issues with the ingredients that go into making a tampon.

> To be honest, I never thought twice about the kind of tampons I was using until period cups started to become more popular a few years ago. I had no idea that they could have such negative effects.

To start off, studies show the effects of inserting genetically engineered cotton directly into the body is no different than ingesting GMO food, due to the walls of the vagina being highly permeable and allowing direct access into the bloodstream. In fact, it is believed that substances absorbed through the vagina actually reach other parts of the body quicker than when ingested orally.

In addition to the cotton being genetically engineered, this also runs the risk of the pesticide contamination. We all know to avoid those in our food, so why have them in our sanitary products? Also, cancer-causing chemicals such as phthalates, styrene, pyridine, methyl eugenol, chlorine and artificial fragrances are added that give the tampon and the tampon applicator the look, color and feel that they have. Now, most of these chemicals such as chlorine create harmful by-products like dioxin, which are linked to:

- abnormal tissue growth in the abdomen and reproductive organs
- abnormal cell growth throughout the body
- immune system suppression
- hormonal and endocrine system disruption

Another rare but important issue regarding tampon use is Toxic Shock Syndrome (TSS). You have probably seen the warning signs on the boxes and labels, but never really given it a second thought. Toxic Shock Syndrome is the result of a bacterial infection inside the vagina, typically with staph or strep bacteria. Although its occurrence is rare, it can have serious effects on the body. Symptoms include fever, vomiting, diarrhea, dizziness, seizures, rashes and muscle aches that result from keeping the tampon in for prolonged periods of time. There are a few precautions you can take to prevent TSS:

- Avoid super-absorbent tampons and opt for the lowest absorbency.

- Only use pads overnight—never leave a tampon inside while you sleep.

- Be careful to not scratch your vaginal lining when using plastic applicators.

- Change tampons at least every four to six hours.

There are, however, safer alternatives to the commercial tampons that you can pick up at your local store. There are 100 percent certified organic cotton tampons available, which are processed without chlorine, which avoids toxic by-products such as dioxin; they are free of synthetic fibers and plastics, hypoallergenic and scent-free. You still get the benefit of stopping flow without the harmful side effects of traditional commercial tampons.

Want a greener option, but not into the idea of cloth pads? Period cups are becoming more and more popular. They are usually made of silicon, are reusable, so they're good for the environment and the wallet, need to be emptied every 6-18 hours, depending on your flow. Inserting and removing them may be a little daunting at first, but most women get used to them in no time and end up loving them.

THE STINKY TRUTH ABOUT DEODORANT

We all sweat, so it's not surprising that 90 percent of us regularly use antiperspirants and deodorants. In fact, sales of these products are exceeded by only one other bathroom staple—toothpaste. You likely use deodorant to mask underarm odor or use antiperspirants to reduce sweating. Unfortunately, health concerns over both are growing. If you have to use one, go with a deodorant. Antiperspirants clog and close your pores, inhibiting you from sweating; this is not a normal or healthy thing.

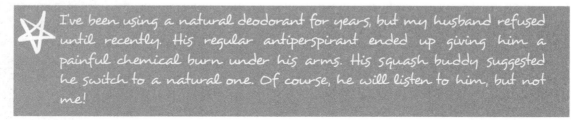

I've been using a natural deodorant for years, but my husband refused until recently. His regular antiperspirant ended up giving him a painful chemical burn under his arms. His squash buddy suggested he switch to a natural one. Of course, he will listen to him, but not me!

While deodorant is a better choice than antiperspirant, there is some evidence that the chemicals used in both products may be contributing to a higher incidence of breast cancer. Unfortunately, the priority of most companies that sell skin products is their financial bottom line, not your long-term health. Ultimately, we can't ignore the fact that all the chemicals we use on our body may increase our risk of developing cancer. Knowledge is power, but you have to act on that knowledge.

To protect yourself, here are a few things you can do:

- Don't apply deodorant right after shaving your underarms.

- Avoid application if there are open cuts.

- Read labels, and look for a more natural deodorant.

- Keep your body alkaline. Oral chlorophyll tablets can help reduce body odor and can eliminate the need for deodorants.

HEALTHIER ALTERNATIVES TO DEODORANT

- **Baking soda** – Take a pinch of baking soda powder in one hand. Drop several drops of water on it, blend and then rub underarms. You'll be amazed how effective it is!

- **Natural Mineral salts** – A natural mineral-salt deodorant stick will improve your skin's pH level while protecting against odor-causing bacteria.

- **Natural deodorant** – Natural health-food stores will carry deodorants that don't have harmful chemicals.

- **Au Natural** – Consider not using any deodorant! If you feed your body the right food and keep your body alkaline, you may not actually need it. Give it a try. Why add more to your daily toxic load if you don't have to?

SUNSCREEN SAFETY

How do sunscreens work? Chemical agents in sunscreens absorb the sun's UV rays and convert them into harmless thermal energy or reflect it off the body. While this product may help protect you from sunburns, you need to be aware of the chemicals in your sunscreen and whether they might pose more of a health risk than the sun itself. Sunscreen may protect you from the sun, but, if you think the lotion is harmless, think again.

Don't forget—your skin is the largest organ in your body, and everything that you put on it is absorbed into your bloodstream. Look at nicotine and hormone patches, for example, to see how effectively your skin absorbs whatever you put on it. As mentioned at the beginning of this chapter, you shouldn't put anything on your skin that you wouldn't eat. Now, go read the ingredient list on a bottle of sunscreen: Would you willingly eat any of that?

It is important to note that The Environmental Working Group, in a 2011 report, claimed that nearly half of the 500 most popular sunscreen products may actually increase the rate at which malignant cells develop and spread skin cancer.[3]

Sunscreens have also been shown to:

- act like estrogen and disrupt hormones

- cause allergic reactions

- accumulate in the body[4]

 For the longest time, I thought I was allergic to the sun. Anytime I would go out for long periods, I would develop a rash all over my

body. It turns out I was actually allergic to the chemicals in the
sunscreen I was using. Since switching to natural sunscreens, I have
yet to break out.

Sunscreen can actually block the absorption of vitamin D, and studies have shown that vitamin D can prevent up to 16 types of cancers.[5]

So, all that said, sunscreens are effective in reducing sunburns, but may not reduce the risk of cancer. The debate over sunscreen, however, is still ongoing and, in the meantime, you need to educate yourself about sunscreen.

The first question that needs to be answered concerning SPF is—what does it mean? SPF stands for Sun Protection Factor and is actually a test designed to measure how much a product protects against UVB rays. It does not test the protection against UVA rays (the effects of UVA and UVB will be discussed in greater detail in **Chapter 25: Vitamin D—Are You Operating on Low?**) For this reason, it gives many a false sense of protection against the sun, and many may stay out longer because of it. There are, however, products on the market that provide protection against both UVA and UVB rays; they contain zinc oxide. Unfortunately, regulatory bodies have not yet established proper standards for the efficacy or the safety of sunscreen ingredients. In fact, sunscreen manufacturers are free to market products that haven't actually been proven to protect from the sun.

HOW TO BE SAFE IN THE SUN

- **Use a natural, non-toxic, full-spectrum sunscreen that contains zinc oxide** – Zinc oxide offers broad-spectrum protection, meaning it decreases the risk for cancer and sunburns. You may be surprised to learn that chemical sunscreens aren't physical reflectors, meaning they allow the sun's wavelengths to enter the skin, where they can cause genetic damage. The ideal sunscreen is both kid- and adult-friendly, while being highly effective at blocking UVA and UVB rays, and doesn't have ingredients that break down in the sun. When buying natural sunscreen, be wary of the nanoparticles we discussed earlier. They can be found in some mineral sunscreens.

- **Beware of bug repellent** – Also, make sure you don't combine sunscreen with bug repellent. The ingredients in the repellent will make you absorb a higher amount of the chemicals present in the sunscreen.

- **Use UV-resistant clothing** – One other option to protect yourself from the sun—if you have to be outside for some time—is to buy some UV-resistant clothing. These items come with protective factors as high as 40.

- **Go gradually** – To avoid being burnt, limit your sun exposure to 10 minutes a day. Gradually increase your time spent in the sun as the summer season continues; in a few weeks, you will be able to have normal sun exposure without risk of a burn or cancer.

- **Balance your omega-6 to omega-3 ratio** – In 2001, the National Academy of Sciences published a comprehensive review showing that a proper omega-6:3 ratio is key in preventing skin cancer.

- **Don't be fooled by super high SPF** – They protect against UVB rays, which cause sunburns, but can leave your skin exposed to damaging UVA rays. They also give you a false sense of security; 60 SPF is just 2 percent more effective than 30 SPF at blocking UVB rays.

 That's it?!

A FINAL WORD

There are toxins in pretty much every body-care item you can imagine. This chapter touched on only a few items. Start with these, and move onto other items as time progresses. Making gradual changes can help ensure you stick with your new natural approach. It will also ensure that you don't break the bank. As mentioned above, there are plenty of resources available to you. Adria Vasil's books and articles are a great starting point. So is the Environmental Working Group website. You may have to try different products before you find something you really like, but it's worth taking the time to do it. Read ingredient lists and keep the "Mean 15" in mind when making choices—your body will thank you for your efforts.

The following diagram shows examples of health habits, with corresponding hack levels. To download the *Hack Your Health Habits Worksheet*, visit

www.hackyourhealthhabits.com/worksheets

READY #HEALTHHACKER?
EXAMPLES OF LEVEL 1, 2 AND 3 HACKS FOR THIS CHAPTER

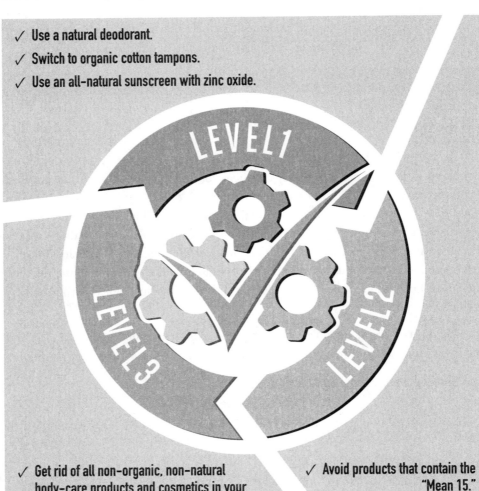

✓ Use a natural deodorant.
✓ Switch to organic cotton tampons.
✓ Use an all-natural sunscreen with zinc oxide.

✓ Get rid of all non-organic, non-natural body-care products and cosmetics in your household and switch to well-rated organic, natural products, instead.

✓ Avoid products that contain the "Mean 15."

HACK YOUR HEALTH PROGRESS

CHAPTER 18

10
COOKWARE
Is Yours Safe or Toxic?

"Safety is more important
than convenience."

— Don Hambidge

THINK IT OVER

- Are your pots and pans exposing you to unwanted toxins?

- Are you using plastics in microwaves?

- Do you know which cooking methods are the healthiest for you?

You try to buy organic food as much as you can, cook your meals at home, and try to eat as healthy as possible. But, did you know that even the healthiest foods can become toxic when prepared in unsafe cookware? How you prepare your food is just as important as the food itself.

UNSAFE COOKWARE?

When it comes to pots, pans, and other cookware, there are many options available. From non-stick to glass, it's hard to know which option is safest for you and your family.

What's the big issue? If you are using poor-quality cookware, particles can leach into your food and get absorbed by your body when consumed. Depending on what kind of cookware you use, this can cause problems, as food ions react with plastic, synthetic, and even metallic ions from cookware that are toxic to the body. These toxins can cause a multitude of health problems—cancer being one of the biggest.

In general, temperature affects reactivity, so hot food will react with a container more quickly than cool food. In other words, heating food will produce more toxins.

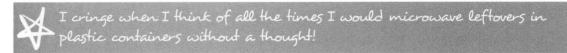

I cringe when I think of all the times I would microwave leftovers in plastic containers without a thought!

Though refrigeration deters the uptake of metal or plastic ions, some materials can still be absorbed even in colder temperatures. Ever notice a funky taste after storing your leftovers in plastic overnight?

All of this means that we need to be careful with the containers in which we cook or store our food. Though Teflon and plastic may be easy to clean, the fact of the matter is that they leave a mess in the body.

When playing chef, try to avoid the following types of cookware:

NON-STICK COOKWARE

Non-stick cookware is one of the most popular kinds of cookware on the market as—just like the name says—it allows us to cook food without it sticking to the pan due to its non-stick-coated surface. Unfortunately, this type of cookware can chip off and get into our food. It also contains perfluorooctanoic acid (PFOA), a synthetic chemical with major health risks linked to it. As convenient as they are, stay clear to stay safe!

ALUMINUM COOKWARE

Aluminum is a lightweight product that conducts heat well and is fairly inexpensive, but it's also a suspected factor in Alzheimer's disease. The World Health Organization estimates that you can consume 50 milligrams of aluminum a day without enduring harm, but it's probably almost impossible to measure the quantities you ingest from the products you use—and the longer food is cooked or stored in aluminum, the more it gets into your food.[1] Green leafy vegetables and acidic foods like tomatoes will absorb the most aluminum.

PLASTIC COOKWARE

As noted previously, plastics are also a concern. The softer the plastic, the more apt it is to react with food and beverages. Microwaving increases the reactivity of plastics and food. And, since we are often in a hurry and just want to "nuke, grab and go," we are regularly exposing ourselves to dioxins—often present in plastic—which are known carcinogens. It is best to microwave your food in glass or ceramic containers. So, even if the instructions say it's safe to microwave in the plastic store-bought container, take the extra few seconds and switch your meal to a dinner plate.

WHAT'S SAFER TO USE?

STAINLESS STEEL

Stainless steel is a better cookware choice, but it still contains iron, nickel and chromium, which can be harmful to your health. Contrary to popular belief, stainless steel may not be a completely inert metal. It's not recommended to store foods that are highly acidic in such containers. Once a stainless-steel container has been scratched—even through normal scouring—the leaching of metals is higher. If buying stainless steel, look for a high-quality, heavy-duty one.

SILICONE

Silicone is a synthetic rubber that contains bonded silicon—a natural element that is abundant in sand, rock and oxygen. Silicone cookware is non-stick and stain-resistant, inert and safe up to 428 degrees Fahrenheit (220 degrees Celsius). If heated above its safe range, silicone melts but does not give off toxic vapors. There are no known health hazards associated with silicone cookware at this time, and it does not react with food or beverages.

CAST IRON

Cast iron is also a good choice of cookware because it reacts very little when heated and is less harmful to your health. It is, nevertheless, important to consider that cast-iron cookware can leach iron into food, impacting our health. One disadvantage of this type of cookware is its heaviness.

GLASS ENAMEL

There's good reason why glass beakers are used in chemistry labs—it's because glass is non-reactive. Enamel-based cookware has a fused-glass surface. With proper care, an enamel pot can last a lifetime, but inexpensive enamel cookware will have only a thin enamel layer. Cheap enamel cookware will chip easily, and the fragments will find their way into your food.

 Glassware is also great in the oven. So much easier to clean!

CERAMIC

Ceramic-based cookware is non-reactive and offers the most effective heat for cooking. With ceramic cookware, the subtlest flavors emerge because there is no leaching from the container. Be aware, however, that antique ceramic may contain lead—better to buy new.

Bottom line: It can be frustrating to cook without non-stick cookware as food will stick more. Cook on low to minimize sticking, and remember all the negative health impacts you're avoiding. It's worth the small inconvenience.

FOOD CAN ALSO BE REACTIVE

Fat, acidic ingredients and water absorb more from containers than proteins and carbohydrates do. This explains why high-quality oils, vinegars and wines are sold exclusively in non-reactive glass containers. Not to mention, some fats become 'bad' when heated and should not be used to cook with. As mentioned in the chapter on fats, when you're cooking with high heat, you want to use oils that do not oxidize or go rancid easily.

Once again, the best sources of saturated fat to cook with are:

- coconut oil
- ghee
- grass-fed animal fats such as lard
- grass-fed butter
- avocado oil

REVAMP YOUR COOKING METHODS

Not only do we have to be cautious of what we use to cook, we also need to be cautious of *how* we cook. Heat can break down and destroy 15 percent to 20 percent of some vitamins in vegetables—especially vitamin C, folate and potassium. To be fair, that's not the case for every vegetable; some actually become more nutritious when cooked. It all depends on the cooking method used.

BBQ/GRILLING

Studies show that eating meat cooked under high heat to the point of burning or charring may increase the risk of pancreatic or breast cancer.[2] This appears to be true for meats cooked by frying, grilling and barbecuing. Grilling can also make meats harder for the body to digest, causing stomach problems. Why? Anytime you cook meat at high temperatures, nasty chemicals are created. These are some of the worst:

- **Heterocyclic Amines (HCAs):** These form when food is cooked at high temperatures, and they're linked to cancer. They worsen when food is blackened or charred.
- **Polycyclic Aromatic Hydrocarbons (PAHs):** Cooking fats causes smoke to surround your food and transfer cancer-causing PAHs to the meat.
- **Advanced Glycation End Products (AGEs):** When food is cooked at high temperatures, it increases the formation of AGEs in your food. AGEs build up in your body over time, leading to inflammation and an increased risk of heart disease, diabetes and kidney disease.

If you're a BBQ lover, don't fret. There are things you can do to make grilling a little healthier. Studies show that marinating your meat in red wine or beer will drastically reduce the number of HCAs transferred. What's more, including something acidic like citrus or vinegar in your marinade can reduce the amount of AGEs. Always opt for organic, free-range meat. Lastly, consider cooking your meat on a cedar plank or a higher rack.

FRYING

Fried foods also contain AGEs, which have been linked to an increased risk of developing age-related diseases such as high blood pressure and stroke. If you are looking to fry your food, opt to stir-fry.

BAKING

Again, any cooking method that involves high temperatures can strip foods of nutrients and also increase the risk of carcinogens as the food browns. To avoid this, try lower roasting temperatures, even if this will increase the cooking time.

STEAMING

Steaming is one of the healthiest ways to prepare foods. Allowing fresh vegetables or fish fillets to stew in their own juices ensures that they retain all their nutrients.

BOILING

Boiling is quick and easy. However, high temperatures can dissolve and wash away water-soluble vitamins and a high percentage of minerals. Opt for steaming vegetables—except in the case of broccoli and carrots—where boiling is the best way to preserve their nutrients.

Healthy cooking is about more than just the ingredients you use. Ditch the non-stick cookware, get rid of the plastic, and try steaming your vegetables for a change. Your body will appreciate the extra effort.

The following diagram shows examples of health habits, with corresponding hack levels. To download the *Hack Your Health Habits Worksheet*, visit

www.hackyourhealthhabits.com/worksheets

READY #HEALTHHACKER?
EXAMPLES OF LEVEL 1, 2 AND 3 HACKS FOR THIS CHAPTER

✓ Never microwave food in a plastic container.

✓ Avoid charring or blackening foods.

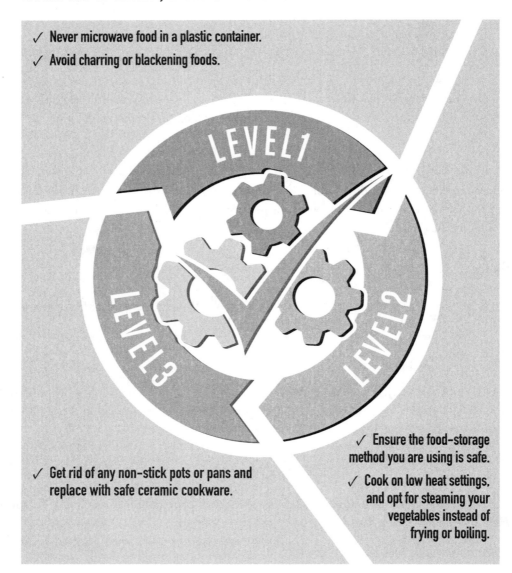

✓ Get rid of any non-stick pots or pans and replace with safe ceramic cookware.

✓ Ensure the food-storage method you are using is safe.

✓ Cook on low heat settings, and opt for steaming your vegetables instead of frying or boiling.

HACK YOUR HEALTH PROGRESS

|||||||||||||||||||||||||

CHAPTER 19

AIR QUALITY
What Are You Breathing?

> "We are so busy doing the urgent that we don't have time to do the important."
>
> — CONFUCIUS

Our bodies process hundreds, if not thousands, of substances. Food, water and oxygen are three crucial substances our body requires. While the body can store food and liquid, it cannot store oxygen. Our cells require a continuous supply of oxygen to survive. This is why breathing problems pose serious health risks, and why the quality of our air should be taken seriously.

CHEMICALS, NATURAL ALLERGENS AND POLLUTANTS

You can't control pollution when you step outside, but you can definitely have some control over the quality of air you breathe inside your home. North Americans spend an average of 90 percent of their time inside.[1] Astonishingly, research shows that exposure to contaminants indoors can be two to one hundred times higher than the contaminants outside.[2] You might be thinking that your house is clean and not polluted, but, in all likelihood, it is. The following list of pollutants are hazardous to your health:

- construction materials like lead, formaldehyde and paint
- solvents, insecticides, herbicides and disinfectants from household products
- dust, dander and chemicals on carpets, clothes and bedding
- food waste, cooking odors and vapors in the kitchen
- pollen, mold, hair and skin in air vents
- sewer gas and mildew in the bathroom

All these contaminants can have an effect on your health, if present in high enough quantities, and if you are exposed to them day in and day out.

MAJOR HEALTH PROBLEMS RELATED TO INDOOR AIR POLLUTION

- **Asthma** – Symptoms of Asthma can be triggered or aggravated by indoor air pollution.
- **Sick Building Syndrome (SBS)** – This may take time to notice because the symptoms usually resolve themselves once you leave the area. SBS can involve health problems with multiple systems of the body, including headaches, nausea, and eye, throat, and skin irritation.
- **Multiple Chemical Sensitivity (MCS)** – This is when your body negatively responds to low levels of chemicals that are commonly found in indoor environments. Symptoms are similar to SBS, and usually fade when you leave the environment that's making you ill, although, for some people, symptoms persist outside the environment.
- **Hypersensitivity Pneumonitis** – This is caused by bacteria, fungi and molds that contaminate home humidifiers, heating, ventilation and air-conditioning systems. The symptoms are flu-like and include chills, fever, fatigue, cough, chest tightness and shortness of breath. This is usually reversible when regular exposure to the harmful environment is halted.

Possible symptoms of SBS, MCS and general indoor air pollution are:

- headache
- chest tightness
- fatigue
- skin irritation
- eye and throat irritation
- shortness of breath
- nausea

HOW CLEAN ARE YOUR CLEANING PRODUCTS?

Have you ever wondered if any of your cleaning products are contributing to an increase in your body's toxic load? From antibacterial wipes to hand sanitizers, there are a range of long-term health consequences these products may cause that are being overlooked. Scented sprays and plug-ins have gained popularity for home perfuming and are marketed as having a "cleansing effect" on your home, and certain brands even claim to "eliminate odor-causing bacteria." However, research is showing that these products can include an array of hazardous substances as ingredients. These, in turn, can cause lung damage, changes in blood flow, tumors, hormone interferences, and life-long problems such as asthma and migraines.[3]

The Consumer Product Safety Commission, which regulates the safety of cleaning supplies, air fresheners, and laundry products, currently does not require manufacturers to disclose any ingredients on the label, including fragrances in these products. Before WWII, household cleaning products were just that, household products that were combined to clean your house. A combination of vinegar, baking soda and lemon juice were really all that was required.

☆ *My grandmother always had a jar of this made up in her cupboard.*

Since the war, more than 80,000 synthetic chemicals have been created.[4] The majority of these were made from coal and petroleum, many originally for the purposes of chemical warfare. Since their creation, these products have been added to cleaning products, often without testing their safety. The reason so many companies use harmful chemicals in their cleaning products is because petroleum-based cleaners are cheaper and faster to manufacture, and chemical compounds are ready-made cleansers.

Here is an interesting quote from the U.S. National Research Council:

> "No toxic information is available for more than 80 percent of the chemicals in everyday-use products. Less than 20 percent have been tested for acute effects and less than 10 percent have been tested for chronic, reproductive or mutagenic effects."[5]

This means that less than 20 percent of chemicals found in everyday-use products have been tested for safety before they are put on the shelves. Would you fly with an airline that inspects only 20 percent of its planes? So, why is it that we are OK with not knowing what is in our everyday-use products? Of course, not all of the ingredients used are harmful; however, many are known carcinogens, neurotoxins and reproductive-disruptive toxins.

☆ *I would definitely want to know if those are in any of my products!*

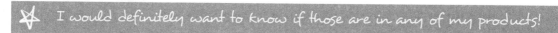

PERFUME: A STINKY SUBJECT?

Many synthetic fragrances are also known respiratory irritants, which essentially means that they cause inflammation in the lungs. This can possibly lead to increased mucus production, and a greater vulnerability to other chemicals, allergens and infections. Ninety-five percent of synthetic fragrances are derived from petroleum.[6] They include benzene and aldehydes, which are known to cause cancers, reproductive effects, and problems with the central nervous system. These effects on the nervous system result in increased cases of Alzheimer's disease, multiple sclerosis, Parkinson's disease and more. Most scented candles even produce formaldehyde, which is a known carcinogen and the culprit for sore throats, coughs, scratchy eyes and nosebleeds.

You know, I never put two and two together, but I do get a scratchy throat whenever I'm in a room with a heavily scented candle. As an alternative, pure beeswax candles are eco-friendly, have a lovely, gentle scent, and clean the air.

Even products that claim to be scent-free or "all natural" often contain phthalates. If you remember, phthalates are a toxic ingredient used in plastics, especially PVC. According to the Environmental Working Group, phthalates can accumulate in the liver and cause serious health problems.[7]

Chemicals such as these are emitted from air fresheners, gel plug-ins, laundry detergents and other toxic household products. They accumulate in the fatty tissues over time, increasing risk as they build up inside a body. Since the human body uses fat to store certain materials that are too toxic for it to process, breaking down the fat would mean releasing those toxins—so such a body must resist its fat loss for self-defense. Thus, fat-loss resistance can sometimes be the result of an immune system properly responding to a danger.

DO FLAME RETARDANTS CAUSE MORE HARM THAN GOOD?

From couch cushions to carpeting, flame-retardant chemicals can be found in just about everything these days. Though created to keep us "safe" by inhibiting or delaying the spread of fire, these chemicals have been linked to a variety of health problems, including cancer, birth defects and neurological disorders.

Interestingly, flame retardants were developed in the 1970s, when 40 percent of Americans smoked and cigarettes were a major cause of house fires. At this time, pressure was placed on the tobacco company to create "fire-safe" cigarettes that would self-extinguish. Refusing to make the change, the tobacco industry created a front group called the National Association of State Fire Marshals that pushed for the creation of federal standards regarding fire-retardant furniture, instead.

Though flame retardants have been linked to several serious health problems, many outdated regulations are still in place today. Due to their continued use, it is reported that nearly 90 percent of Americans have some level of flame-retardant chemicals in their system.[8] To keep yourself and your family safe, it's important to act with due diligence. Most exposure to these chemicals comes from household dust. So, if you dust, wash your hands and vacuum often; then you can minimize your exposure to the flame retardants lurking in your home. Try to pay attention to the furniture and products you buy, ask questions about the material used, and stay away from items laced with flame retardant when possible.

TIPS FOR BETTER INDOOR AIR

There are several things you can do to ensure better indoor air. Consider implementing the following:

- Use a high-efficiency filter in your central heating/cooling system with at least a 60 percent efficiency grade. This will help remove harmful airborne particles.

- Minimize the humidity in your home by letting more outdoor air in and ensuring sufficient ventilation. By doing this, you'll prevent moisture from building up on walls and windows, reducing the possible growth of bacteria. You may need to buy a ceiling fan to optimize airflow in highly humid areas.

- Measure the humidity in your home by using a hygrometer – you can get an inexpensive one at a hardware store. The relative humidity in your home should be below 50 percent in the summer and below 30 percent in the winter. If your home doesn't achieve this on its own, you should invest in a dehumidifier.

- Repair leaky roofs, walls and foundations.

- Clean frequently and thoroughly to prevent dust and mold build-up.

- Regularly clean and disinfect filters of furnaces, humidifiers, dehumidifiers and air conditioners.

- Keep aerosol product use to a minimum.

- Restrict smoking to outdoor areas, or better yet, just quit!

- Use exhaust fans that vent to the outdoors when cooking.

- When purchasing building materials and furniture, choose products that do not emit formaldehyde; ask a salesperson or the manufacturer when in doubt.

- Carefully follow safety instructions on consumer products such as cleaning agents, paints and glues.

- Consider using chemical-free cleaning products. There are several on the market now. They're better for you and the environment.

- Use microfiber cleaning cloths, which have a great ability to pick up and trap dirt, coupled with superior absorbency and scrubbing power.

- Limit the use of candles and incense indoors, as they can elevate indoor particle levels. Essential-oil diffusers are a great alternative to candles.

- Use plenty of ventilation.

A WORD ON AIR FILTERS

Air-cleaning devices are either central filtration systems, often called in-duct systems, which are placed into the heating, ventilation and air-conditioning system of a home, or portable units with an attached fan. Portable units help clean the air in a single room, while central-air units can improve the air throughout the whole home.

Here is a list of different air filters and cleaners and their attributes:

HEPA (High-Efficiency Particulate Air) Mechanical Air Filters – These are the most efficient mechanical filters for removing small particles, which can be breathed deep into the lungs. The highest efficiency mechanical filters available today are up to 99.97 percent effective and can remove particles just 0.3 microns in size.[9] **Electronic Air Cleaners** – There are four general types of electronic air-cleaning technologies:

1. **Ozone Generator Technology:** These air cleaners work by producing ozone. But, be aware that ozone can have its challenge for our health. Ozone in the upper atmosphere protects us from the sun's ultraviolet rays, but ground-level ozone is an irritant that can aggravate asthma and hinder lung function. Ozone, at this level, is a harmful air pollutant and will affect the respiratory system of children, the elderly, asthmatics and those with respiratory problems. Long-term ozone exposure can also reduce the average person's breathing ability. Some health experts argue that ozone can be safe and effective if levels are properly controlled. The FDA has established that 50 ppb should be your maximum allowable ozone emission for medical devices. If you opt for an ozone generator, ensure that the machine allows you to adjust the amount of ozone being released.

2. **Electrostatic Precipitator Technology:** Electrostatic precipitator technology uses a small electrical charge to collect particles from air that is pulled through the device—a charged-plate electrical system. A major drawback of this technology is that because there is no fan, air doesn't circulate as much, making it less efficient. This process produces some ozone as a by-product of the ion-generating technology.

3. **Ionizers or Negative Ion Generator Technology:** Both of these technologies work by generating negative ions. Now, the word "negative" might make you think they're not healthy. In this case, "negative" is simply referring to atomic charge; electrons carry a negative charge, and a negative ion is simply a molecule with an extra electron. Negative ions are found in natural environments like forests and waterfalls. They also create a soothing, relaxing atmosphere—as if you were surrounded by nature. Household air conditioners reduce the number of negative ions present in an indoor environment, so a negative-ion generator can help correct this imbalance. Having negative ions in our air is good! Now, let's talk about the technology. Ionizers work by causing particles to stick to materials near the ionizer (e.g. the carpet and wall), taking them out of the air we breathe. Not only does this process produce ozone as a by-product, it does not necessarily clean the air of the particles created, which could easily become loose again and re-circulate. A better and safer type of negative-ion technology is called a clean-ion generator. This adds negative ions after mechanical filtering, not as part of the filtering process.

4. **Photocatalytic Oxidation Technology:** Another type of electronic air cleaner technology is called photocatalytic oxidation (PCO). PCO technology uses ultraviolet light to help clean

the air. If you decide to choose PCO technology, be aware that they can also produce a small amount of ozone and can create chemical by-products like formaldehyde.

OTHER AIR PURIFIER TOOLS

You may have seen large salt lamps being sold at your local health-food store and wondered: "What do those do?" Himalayan Salt Lamps are essentially a large piece of Himalayan salt with a light bulb inside. Himalayan salt lamps purify the air through the power of hygroscopy. To put it simply, the lamp attracts water molecules, and the toxins trapped in these molecules and absorbs them into salt crystals. As the salt heats from the bulb inside, the water molecules evaporate back into the air while the trapped particles of dust, pollen, smoke, etc., remain locked in the salt. Salt lamps have been shown to reduce coughing and allergy symptoms, neutralize electromagnetic radiation, purify the air and much more.

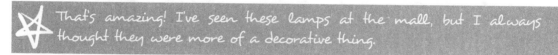

That's amazing! I've seen these lamps at the mall, but I always thought they were more of a decorative thing.

Essential-oil diffusers have also gained popularity in recent years. Diffusers help purify the air, killing the bacteria and fungus present in air particles. Research has shown that oregano, cinnamon bark, thyme and clove bud are the most effective for this purpose.[10] When it comes to essential oils, quality does matter. Ensure you are buying oils that are 100 percent natural.

As with anything else, do your research before choosing an air-purifying system; they are often a significant investment, and you want the highest quality for the best price.

The following diagram shows examples of health habits, with corresponding hack levels. To download the *Hack Your Health Habits Worksheet*, visit

www.hackyourhealthhabits.com/worksheets

✓ Dust and vacuum your home often.

✓ In the warmer months, open windows to air out the house.

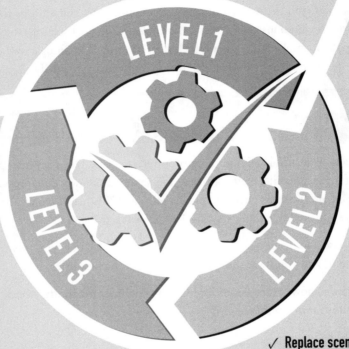

✓ Determine which air filter will work best for you and your space. Purchase one or more for the spaces in which you spend the most time.

✓ Replace scented candles and home fragrances with essential oils.

✓ Replace your cleaning products with safer and less toxic ones.

HACK YOUR HEALTH PROGRESS

||||||||||||||||||||||||||||||||||||||||||||||||||||||||||||||||||

CHAPTER 20

MOLDS
Are They Making You Sick?

"What you don't see, can hurt you."

— DR. NATHALIE BEAUCHAMP

THINK IT OVER

- Do you know if you are exposed to toxic molds in your environment?

- Do you know what the common symptoms of exposure to toxic mold are?

- Should you test your environment for mold?

Beyond tossing out moldy food or repairing a leak in the basement, most people don't give mold much thought. However, after watching *moldy* by Dave Asprey, you may think twice. The film exposes the dirty truth about how mold and mycotoxins are affecting the health of hundreds of thousands—if not, millions—of people. In his documentary, Asprey tells the stories of several mold toxicity sufferers. Viewers quickly learn that, while mold itself is not necessarily dangerous, the mycotoxins that it produces can be extremely detrimental to overall health.

SYMPTOMS THAT DON'T FIT ANY "MOLD"

Mold toxins are unique and can affect the body and mind in different ways, causing a variety of symptoms. This, in itself, makes it very difficult for a doctor to correctly diagnose these symptoms.

According to Dr. Ritchie Shoemaker, mold expert and author of the book *Surviving mold*, mold toxins are even more toxic than pesticides and heavy metals and affect a greater number of body systems.[1] Mold mycotoxins can affect all of the body's systems—from respiratory to immune to digestive to neurological, just to name a few. Common symptoms include headaches, migraines, insomnia, coughing and phlegm build-up, depression, skin irritations or rashes, infertility and brain issues.

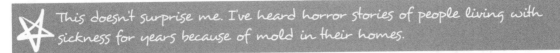
This doesn't surprise me. I've heard horror stories of people living with sickness for years because of mold in their homes.

Biotoxins from mold also affect leptins receptors. Leptin is the hormone that regulates hunger. When leptin is disrupted, people will generally feel hungrier. This can cause weight gain and hormonal imbalances. Symptoms of mold toxicity may mimic fibromyalgia, Chronic Fatigue Syndrome, Irritable Bowel Syndrome, Attention Deficit Disorder, Multiple Sclerosis and other autoimmune disorders. Mold toxicity can also affect the brain. We think that it is "normal" to be forgetful as we get older, but the truth is that any brain issue, regardless of your age, should be investigated. According to Dr. Daniel Amen, author of the book, *Change Your Brain, Change Your Life*, it does not matter whether you are 40, 50, or 70—brain symptoms are a clear indication of trouble.[2]

What's more, when it comes to mold, some might be more affected than others. Different people can be subject to the same amount of mold, for the same amount of time, and experience different symptoms. According to Dr. Shoemaker, up to 24 percent of people are considered "genetic canaries in the coal mine" and have a genetic susceptibility to chronic mold illness based on their immune response genes (or HLA–DR). HLA-DR stands for Human Leukocyte Antigens – antigen D Related. They are found on the surface of nearly every cell in the human body. They help the immune system tell the difference between body tissue and foreign substances.

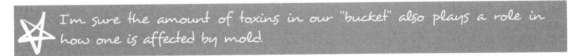
I'm sure the amount of toxins in our "bucket" also plays a role in how one is affected by mold.

TOXIC MOLD IN OUR ENVIRONMENTS AND FOOD

Mycotoxins have not always been a problem. In fact, they've been used for years in the fermentation and preservation of food. What's changed? The introduction of herbicides like Roundup have had a serious implication on the quality of our soil. As we learned in the chapter on organic foods, Roundup acts as a chelator, binding essential nutrients in the soil and plants. This disturbs the natural balance of the soil, destroying nutrients and affecting the nutrient density of plants. In addition, Roundup increases the toxicity level of mycotoxins, contributing to harmful effects on the body.

Ironically, the widespread use of a fungicide on crops and in our paints—to stop the growth of mold in our buildings and homes—has contributed to the growth of highly toxic and dangerous molds similar to superbugs. It's scary to think about, but mold has invaded a large number of the buildings we spend time in. If your home or place of work has had water damage, it is likely hiding toxic mold. Even if the visible mold has been removed, it can remain embedded in your carpets, furniture, bed, clothing and other belongings, causing unwanted health problems.

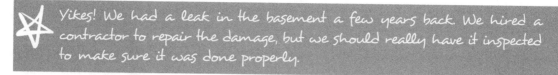

Yikes! We had a leak in the basement a few years back. We hired a contractor to repair the damage, but we should really have it inspected to make sure it was done properly.

Let's not forget about food. Not all food turns green when going bad. Peanuts, coffee, some cheeses, corn, wheat, alcohol and melons often contain molds invisible to the human eye. And, if you are part of the "canary in the coal mine" population, you may be reacting to these foods without even realizing it. If someone is sensitive, mold-ridden foods can cause headaches, coughs, phlegm and a host of other symptoms that mimic typical allergy symptoms.

WHAT'S A MOLD SUFFERER TO DO?

Chronic fatigue and other unexplained health conditions may be due to toxic mold exposure. While it may be difficult to diagnose mold toxicity, you should consult a health-care practitioner, who specializes in environmental issues, to explore the possibility. There are numerous blood tests that can be done to confirm your diagnosis. In addition, if you suspect that your home or workplace contains mold, have it inspected by a specialist who will take air and carpet samples. If you start feeling ill when you walk into a building, get out of that building and stay out—your health is not worth the risk.

Like carbon monoxide, toxic mold can go unnoticed before symptoms appear. Because you can't see or smell it, testing is needed to determine whether there is mold in your environment. Unfortunately, many standard tests only test for mold spores, despite mycotoxins being to blame for most health problems. Oftentimes, test results will come back negative for mold even though harmful mycotoxins are present. This is why it is important to hire a professional to properly test for mycotoxins and deal with proper removal of mold, as well. Keep in mind that cleaning your house is not always enough; mold spores can remain in your carpets, furniture and clothes for months.

ERMI is the Environmental Relative moldiness Index. Based of leading scientific technology, ERMI is an objective, standardized DNA-based method of testing, which can identify and quantify molds. It uses the analysis of settled dust in homes and buildings to determine different species of molds. According to Dr. King-Teh Lin and Dr. Shoemaker, "the automated analysis provides for rapid, reproducible results that can be reliably interpreted. For patients, prospective home-buyers, industrial hygienists and remediators alike, ERMI shows great promise for the future."[3]

GET TESTED!

There are different ways to test for mold toxicity. The Visual Contrast Sensitivity (VCS) test is considered a good screening tool. You can find the tool online at www.survivingmold.com or find a qualified health professional who has a handheld VSC test in their office.

If you are tested and a mold illness is indicated, find a health-care practitioner who specializes in chronic mold illnesses to aid you in your recovery. Avoid foods that are known to grow mold. This includes coffee—yes, you might be drinking moldy coffee—peanuts, wheat, corn, dairy, wine, beer, etc. Eat fruit while it is still fresh; melons, in particular, have a tendency to grow mold quickly. Boost your immune system with vitamin C and glutathione, and follow an anti-inflammatory food plan to help reduce the inflammation in your body caused by mold toxicity. Finally, if you know that you have been exposed to molds, consider doing the True Cellular Detox Program described in the detoxification chapter to help rid your body of mold toxins.

Your health is dependent on the air that you breathe, the water that you drink and the food that you eat. So, make sure that your air, water and food are as healthy, pure and clean as can be.

The following diagram shows examples of health habits, with corresponding hack levels. To download the *Hack Your Health Habits Worksheet*, visit

www.hackyourhealthhabits.com/worksheets

READY #HEALTHHACKER?
EXAMPLES OF LEVEL 1, 2 AND 3 HACKS FOR THIS CHAPTER

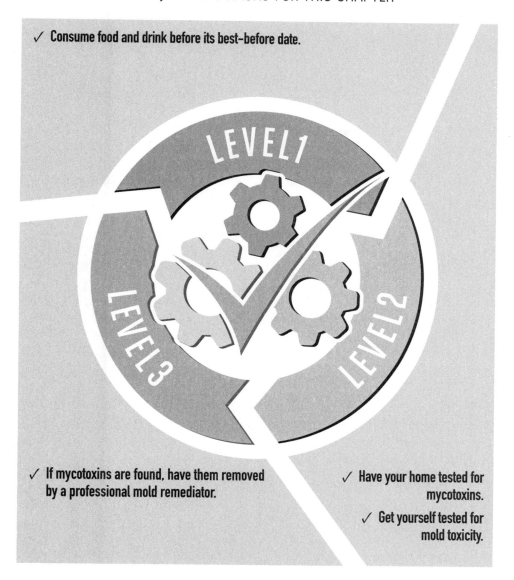

✓ Consume food and drink before its best-before date.

✓ If mycotoxins are found, have them removed by a professional mold remediator.

✓ Have your home tested for mycotoxins.

✓ Get yourself tested for mold toxicity.

HACK YOUR HEALTH PROGRESS

||||||||||||||||||||||||||||||||||||||||||||||||||||||||||||||||||||||||||||

CHAPTER 21

WATER

What Should You Be Concerned About?

"Water is the only drink for a
wise man."

— Henry David Thoreau

THINK IT OVER

- **Can you recognize symptoms of dehydration?**

- **Is tap water safe to drink?**

- **Do plastic water bottles really have negative implications on our health?**

Pop Quiz! How many glasses of water should you drink per day? It's kind of a trick question. Many may say drink eight glasses, which is a great starting point, but there are many factors that can affect this number, like how much exercise you get, your age and your weight. Considering that water is often free and readily accessible, drinking eight glasses shouldn't be a problem. Just find a tap, pour a glass and drink, right? Not so fast! By now, you've probably come to the realization that the easiest options aren't always the healthiest. Unfortunately, tap water is no different. Where you get your water from really does matter.

To be honest, I never fully realized the impact that different sources of water can have on our health and well-being until I started doing research for my first book, *Wellness On The Go*, many years ago. It was a serious eye-opener and led me to make changes in my own life. To this day, there is a great deal of controversy surrounding the safety of tap and bottled water. In this chapter,

I will explain the benefits of staying hydrated and outline the pros and cons of the different types of water available to us. To get started, let's discuss the role and importance of water.

WHY IS WATER SO IMPORTANT?

Water is integral to humans. We need it to survive. Being well-hydrated will:

- relieve fatigue
- improve mood
- treat headaches and migraines
- help in digestion and constipation
- aid weight loss
- flush out toxins
- regulate body temperature
- promote healthy skin
- beat bad breath
- keep muscles and joints hydrated

At birth, our bodies are made up of approximately 90 percent water, which decreases to 75 percent by the age of three. Then, as we grow older, water levels can dip to as low as 65 percent—even though our bodies are healthiest when they are well-hydrated. For most adults, the body is composed of about 70 percent water, which is recycled approximately every 15 days. Notice that it's not 70 percent coffee, tea, pop, or juice!

I don't know how many times I get this answer from my patients when I ask about their daily water intake: "I drink a lot of water—I have at least five coffees per day—that's water, right?"

Wrong! Caffeinated beverages are actually diuretics and will dehydrate your body. Therefore, they actually increase your need to consume more water. What about juice? Be wary—take into consideration the sugar content and the additional water your body needs to dilute sugars in order for them to be digested. Also, beware of flavoured waters with artificial sweeteners; these chemical sweeteners have been shown to be toxic and detrimental to our health.

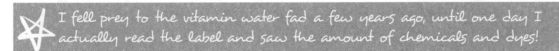

I fell prey to the vitamin water fad a few years ago, until one day I actually read the label and saw the amount of chemicals and dyes!

A QUICK WORD ON SODIUM

I think everyone had the experience of eating a meal with too much salt at some point—leaving you in desperate need of water for hours afterward. That is because sodium and water are closely linked when it comes to hydration. The Mayo Clinic explains that sodium is needed for bodily functions like proper fluid balance, nerve conduction, and the contraction and relaxation of muscles. Your kidneys work to maintain an optimal salt balance in your body. However, with excessive salt intake, balance can be difficult to maintain, leading to chronic diseases and other health issues. High blood pressure, strokes, and heart and kidney disease may result from overconsumption of salt.

Beware: Your table salt is actually 97.5 percent sodium chloride and 2.5 percent chemicals, such as moisture absorbents and iodine. Dried at over 1,200 degrees Fahrenheit, the excessive heat alters the natural structure of the salt. Opt for Himalayan sea salts as opposed to table salt, as they are much healthier for you.

RESULTS OF SLIGHT DEHYDRATION

- Premature aging
- Sunken eyes
- Kidney problems
- Migraines
- Indigestion and heartburn
- High cholesteral
- Joint and back pain
- Muscle and nerve pain
- Excess body weight
- Asthma

- Dry skin
- Slowed urine production
- Dizziness
- Fatigue
- High blood pressure
- Arthritis
- Osteoporosis
- Muscle cramping
- Diabetes
- Allergies

Keep in mind that you can lose up to 2,500 ml of water every day through urine, stool, lungs and skin. If you add other dehydrating factors such as a hot climate, exercise and dehydrating or sugary foods and beverages, your need for water increases dramatically. Apart from oxygen, water is the only other constant bodily requirement; without it, we can survive only a few days, further reinforcing the importance of water.

If you're not one who likes to guzzle lots of water, keep in mind that fruits and vegetables are very good sources of water. Cantaloupe and melons contain more than 90 percent water, as do leafy vegetables such as lettuce. Kiwis are another great source of water, and they also contain essential electrolytes such as potassium and magnesium. Be proactive in giving your body the water it needs, and it will reward you in countless ways!

WHAT'S THE PROBLEM WITH TAP WATER?

We all know that there are chemicals used in our tap water to help ensure it is free of harmful bacteria, such as E. coli. This is good; we wouldn't want to fall ill from untreated water. We also know that, in many cities, fluoride is added to our drinking water. This is done because years ago, the dental association told us that fluoride was good for our teeth.

Why is it so great for our teeth? Well, the theory is that fluoride helps strengthen teeth. Teeth, like bones, are made up of calcium. Fluoride reinforces the calcium in our body. Sounds good, right? For the most part, it is, but here is where it becomes a concern: Calcium is partly to blame for this hardening of the arteries. So, if we ingest more calcium and fluoride than our bodies are able to use and flush out, then we are at risk of artery hardening. In addition, some research shows that fluoridation of water does not really have much impact on the prevention of tooth decay, but has also been shown to cause bone fluorosis, meaning that it causes damage to bone cells.[1]

To make matters worse, fluoride has now officially been listed as a neurotoxin, with direct effects on the nervous system. A lifetime of excessive fluoride ingestion will undoubtedly have detrimental effects on a number of biological systems in the body. Some published studies point to fluoride's interference with the reproductive system, the pineal gland and the thyroid.[2] Does this sound like a substance you want to be ingesting on a regular basis?

MORE THINGS TO CONSIDER ABOUT TAP WATER:

- **Tap water acidity** – Tap water can be more acidic than pure water, which has a pH of 7. When consumed regularly, it can increase the body's acidity and cause an imbalance in our pH levels, potentially increasing the risks of disease.

- **The source of tap water** – Tap water quality varies depending on where you get it. For example, in some industrialized cities, municipal drinking water can have traces of lead, arsenic, asbestos, benzene, mercury, nitrites, radium, sulphate, PCBs, Coliform bacteria, and more than 70 other contaminants. Chlorine is added to this water to kill bacteria, but the dead bacteria and the chlorine still remain in the water. Chlorine has been linked to cancer, heart disease and strokes. Some people say they can also taste the chlorine in tap water due to its very distinct taste and smell. I know I have travelled to other cities, and, when I drank the tap water, I could smell and taste the chlorine right away.

- **Possible agricultural runoff** – There are concerns that agricultural runoff adds pesticides and fertilizers to the water system.

- **Decaying pipes and reservoirs** – Tap water is stored in potentially decaying or rotting pipes and reservoirs before getting to your sink. Ask yourself if you're comfortable knowing this every time you reach for the tap.

- **Prescription drug contamination** – The Environmental Working Group (EWG) did a study in 2008 that showed that at least 40 million Americans drink water that contains detectable levels of prescription drugs, such as antibiotics, hormones and drugs that treat epilepsy and depression.[3]

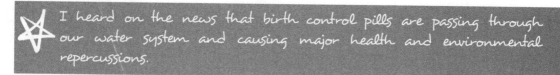

For information on your local drinking water, go online and enter your city's name in your search engine. All cities have water-quality information listed on their websites.

BOTTLED WATER VS. TAP WATER

Is one better than the other? The bottled water industry claims that bottled water is better for you than tap water, although governmental agencies such as Health Canada claim there is no evidence to support that theory.

In the United States, tap water is regulated by the Environmental Protection Agency (EPA) for hazardous chemicals, pesticides and bacteria, and is tested almost daily. In Canada, tap water is regulated by Health Canada and the provinces and territories. Municipalities test their water sources constantly. Bottled water is not subject to the same guidelines because it is classified as a food and falls under the Food and Drug Act.

BOTTLED WATER—SPRING, MINERAL, TAP OR DISTILLED WATER

Spring water does not contain fluoride naturally, so if the water is truly sourced from a spring, it could be a good option. Of course, if the bottling company chooses to add fluoride, this would no longer be true.

Non-spring water is typically just municipal tap water that has been purified by the bottling company and then packaged to sell to the consumer. Since most of the purification systems these companies use do not eliminate all minerals—in order to allow the good ones to remain—they tend to still have fluoride in them. The exception would be water that has been treated through reverse osmosis. However, again, the company may then choose to add fluoride to the finished product. You can easily find the amounts of fluoride (measured in parts per million, or ppm) by reading the labels. For comparison's sake, in Ottawa at the time of writing, the city I live in, tap water usually contains 0.70 mg/L (ppm) of fluoride.[4]

Here are some other facts about bottled water:

- It is expensive—carrying a markup of up to 3,000 percent.

- It creates a landfill problem.

- It may still contain bacteria.

- The plastic container leaches toxic chemicals into the water.

- A lot of bottled water sold in North America is municipal-filtered and treated tap water—bringing the concerns of tap water into play.

- Bottled water tends to have a pH lower than 7.

More and more evidence shows adverse health effects associated with the use of bottled water. A major concern is the significant leaching of toxic chemicals antimony and Bisphenol-A (BPA) from certain plastic bottles. There is also a concern that washing plastic water bottles and re-using them increases the chemical leaching process. BPA may be capable of altering the normal function of genes. It has also been shown to mimic the hormone estrogen and can disrupt reproductive functions. While the precise adverse health effects associated with the leaching of chemicals are uncertain at this time, it is recommended that you do not refill a plastic single-use water bottle. Also, be aware that while most beverage companies issue a two-year expiry date for unopened water bottles. It is recommended that you keep them for no more than six months.[5]

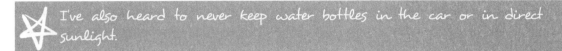

I've also heard to never keep water bottles in the car or in direct sunlight.

Independent researchers and the plastic industry do not see eye to eye when it comes to the health impact of BPA leaching from bottled water, as the plastic industry continues to claim the effects are minimal. Industry studies show no harmful effects, while independently funded research contradicts these studies. Who to believe? Why take the chance? Why not try to minimize the risk?

WHAT IS PLASTIC?

Plastic is a moldable material made from petroleum. Each plastic item, including water bottles, is marked with an identification number that identifies which particular type of plastic was used. The code is typically found on the bottom of a container and is often displayed inside a three-arrow symbol: like this <<< 3 >>>. While the codes help identify different plastics for recycling, there is still some controversy over whether they provide guidance on the safety of the plastic product being authorized for use.

Here are the categories of plastic and helpful guidelines:

Safer Plastics

- #2 High-Density Polyethylene (HDP) – Found in milk and detergent bottles, freezer bags.

- #4 Low-Density Polyethylene (LDPE) – Found in sandwich bags and bread bags.

- #5 Polypropylene (PP) – Found in medicine bottles and cereal liners.

Questionable or Harmful Plastics

- #1 Polyethylene Terephthalate (PET or PETE) – Found to leach antimony and BPA. Found in single-use water bottles, pop and juice bottles.

- #3 Polyvinyl Chloride (PVC) – Found to leach 2-ethylhexyl phthalate (DEHP) and Bisphenol-A (BPA), both endocrine and hormone disruptors. Found in shower curtains and meat wrap.

- #6 Polystyrene (PS) – May leach styrene—a possible endocrine disruptor and human carcinogen—into water and food. Found in take-out containers and foam packaging.

- #7 Polycarbonate (PC/PLA) – This plastic is made with BPA. Leaching is a huge concern. Found in baby bottles, food-can liners and nylon.

ENVIRONMENTAL CONCERNS

For years, for years, environmentalists have spoken against the environmental evils of bottled water—the pollution generated, the energy expended in their production and the shipping is tragic. Despite being recyclable, plastic bottles often make their way to landfills. Since plastic breaks down at a very slow rate, those plastic bottles will remain in landfills for hundreds of years to come.

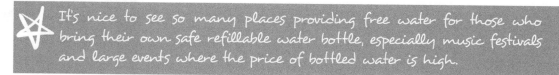

It's nice to see so many places providing free water for those who bring their own safe refillable water bottle, especially music festivals and large events where the price of bottled water is high.

Just the processing of plastics can cause serious pollution, affecting both the environment and our health. The production of one kilogram of PET plastic, which is often used for water bottles, requires 17.5 kilograms of water, which is significantly more than what those bottles themselves will contain! There is also concern related to the petroleum waste from the manufacturing of plastics.

Not only is water being wasted to create bottled water, but did you know that a large percentage of the water produced worldwide every year is consumed outside of the country in which it was produced? That means we should also be concerned about the carbon dioxide emissions caused by transporting bottled water, as this contributes to the global problem of climate change. Forgoing bottled water could greatly reduce our carbon footprint!

WATER FILTRATION

Clearly, the health values of these two types of water sources—tap and bottled—are questionable, so where should you get your water? I recommend finding a source you can control yourself; your own home-filtration system. Filtering out the contaminants with a quality home water-filtration system at the point of source, just prior to consumption, is the best way to be certain that you are consuming healthy water!

The choices when it comes to water-treatment devices are anything but simple: There are carbon filters, mechanical filters, distillation units, reverse osmosis units, water softeners, iron filters and neutralizers. Out of these, the three most common are distillation, reverse osmosis and common filtration devices. It is worth the time to do your own research on filtration methods. There is a great deal of information and opinions out there to explore, but here are the basics.

DISTILLATION

Process: Distillation units boil water to create steam, which is then condensed, leaving pure water behind. Distilled water may not have fluoride in it, but it's lacking in important minerals. It is water in its truest form. This sounds like a great thing, but is it really? Water, by nature, contains natural minerals. Distilled or demineralized water will attempt to replenish its missing minerals to get back into balance. So, if you use it for cooking or steaming your vegetables, it will absorb their minerals, leaving you with food that may be devoid of these important minerals that benefit the body. Drinking and using distilled water is OK, as long as is not used 100 percent of the time.

Some important facts about distillation are:

- it reduces chlorine, heavy metals, viruses and bacteria
- it removes minerals such as nitrate, sodium, sulphate and many organic chemicals
- contaminants such as chloroform, a known carcinogen, will remain in the end product
- the heating chamber must be cleaned regularly
- it is time-consuming
- it is noisy
- distilled water is depleted of minerals, and long-term consumption may lead to the leaching of minerals from your body
- it creates acidic water

REVERSE OSMOSIS

Process: Contaminants are removed by forcing water through a semipermeable membrane to filter out contaminants. Different membrane materials will be more or less effective on different chemicals. The variety of materials for membrane will impact effectiveness on different chemicals. Like with distillation, reverse osmosis depletes water of essential minerals, and it creates a more acidic water.

Reverse osmosis is also:

- expensive
- slow
- wasteful—it takes at least four gallons of unprocessed water to produce one drinkable gallon of water

ACTIVATED CARBON FILTERS

Process: Water flows through a carbon filter as contaminants are attracted to the positively charged and highly absorbent carbon particles.

- Activated carbon filters reduce general taste and odour problems, as well as chlorine residue.

- Activated carbon filters do not remove nitrate, bacteria, or metals.

- The design of the filters greatly influences individual efficiency.

- They filter a high percentage of contaminants.

- The filters need to be replaced regularly.

- The process is cost-efficient.

- Water may be depleted of essential minerals.*

- Water may be on the more acidic side due to the depleted minerals.

*Some activated carbon filters come with mineral rocks to place in the system to put back minerals in the water, and to make the water more alkaline.

CHOOSING THE RIGHT FILTRATION SYSTEM

One sure way to take the guesswork out of a filtration device is to check if it's certified by the National Sanitation Foundation (NSF). Certification by the NSF International signifies that the manufacturer's performance claims have been validated and that the materials used in the construction of the device are safe and up to standard.

Do your research when choosing a water system. Having a home-filtration system gives you control over what you are drinking and is a step toward decreasing your plastic use. Portable water bottles with integrated filters are also now available. Do your research on the efficiency of the filter, and remember to use a safe plastic or a glass bottle. These filter bottles are great when you don't have access to your home-filtering system and are on the go. You can refill with tap water, and the filter does the job!

Filtration systems aren't just great for drinking water. The chemicals found in regular tap water, like chlorine, can be harsh on the skin, hair and bodily systems. Consider installing a filter in your showers and bathroom sinks, as well.

My daughters and I suffer with some skin problems. The water we bathe in seems to have a big effect on our outbreaks. We've installed a shower filter in our home, which has helped significantly.

A quick note—though the pitcher-style filter is one of the most popular filtration systems on the market, it is the *least* effective. Designed primarily for taste and odour, most pitchers are certified to remove only five substances and can actually add heavy metals into the water. What's more, though the carafe is cost-efficient at first, replacing the cartridge every 30 gallons can add up quickly. It's best to invest more at the start, and buy a filtration system that will actually work.

It is true that our bodies are designed to filter out some of the impurities that we ingest, and it is difficult to always have access to pure filtered water. However, if we focus on using the best option most of the time, it takes the burden off the body of having to continuously process and eliminate toxins. So, raise a glass of water to your health and drink up!

The following diagram shows examples of health habits, with corresponding hack levels. To download the *Hack Your Health Habits Worksheet*, visit

www.hackyourhealthhabits.com/worksheets

READY #HEALTHHACKER?
EXAMPLES OF LEVEL 1, 2 AND 3 HACKS FOR THIS CHAPTER

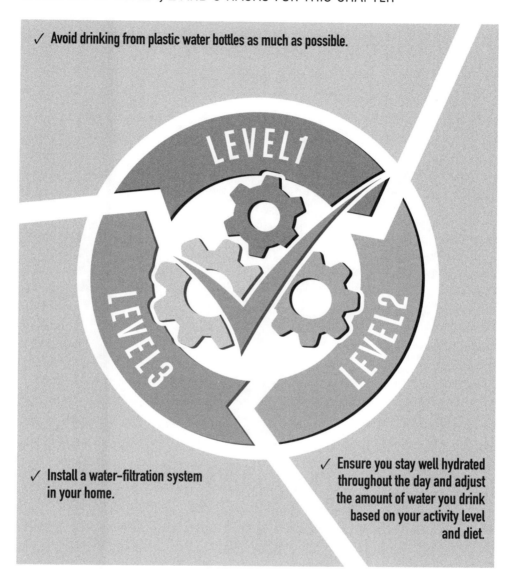

✓ Avoid drinking from plastic water bottles as much as possible.

LEVEL 1

LEVEL 2

LEVEL 3

✓ Install a water-filtration system in your home.

✓ Ensure you stay well hydrated throughout the day and adjust the amount of water you drink based on your activity level and diet.

HACK YOUR HEALTH PROGRESS

|||||||||||||||||||||||||||||||||||||||||||||||||||||||||||||||||||||

CHAPTER 22

SECTION 5

Get the Right Vitamins to Help Your Body Perform at its Best

Should you be taking supplements? Your body relies on vitamins, minerals and essential nutrients to function optimally, and unfortunately in today's world, we are often not getting what we need from our food. In Section 5, you will learn the roles different vitamins play in your body and which supplements would contribute to your overall health and wellbeing.

23

THE LOW-DOWN ON VITAMINS
Do We Need Them, and Are They All Created Equal?

> "So many people spend their health gaining wealth, and then have to spend their wealth to regain their health."
>
> — A. J. REB MATERI

THINK IT OVER

- What are the signs and symptoms of vitamin deficiencies?

- Does quality matter when it comes to vitamin supplementation?

- How are vitamins regulated?

To be honest, I could write an entire book on vitamins and supplements. There is so much information out there that it can get quite confusing. What supplements do you need? Are you taking the right ones?

According to the 2015 Council for Responsible Nutrition consumer survey, 68 percent of Americans take supplements. This equates to a 37-billion-dollar-a-year industry.[1] And, according to the National Institutes of Health, multivitamins are the most commonly used dietary supplements, accounting for $5.7 billion in annual sales.[2] Based on these statistics, it's quite clear that people recognize the benefits of vitamins. But, how important are vitamins, really?

IS VITAMIN SUPPLEMENTATION NECESSARY?

As previously mentioned, our diet should be our main source of vitamins and nutrients. I know it sounds cliché, but, we really are what we eat. Focusing on a whole food diet is paramount. Eating organic is also very important. As discussed in earlier chapters, eating organic decreases our toxic load and increases our nutrient intake. In a perfect world, we shouldn't have to rely on supplements to get the nutrients we could be getting through food. But sadly, as discussed in the previous section, today's food supply does not provide us with the nutrients it once did.

In recent years, there has been a lot of controversy over whether or not supplements are needed. Critics claim that supplements are a waste of money because we can get all of what we need from our diet. I agree that quality does matter when it comes to vitamins and supplements. But, to deny that industrial farming and the reliance on synthetic fertilizer have negatively impacted valuable micronutrients in our soils is plain silly. This soil depletion has real consequences, in terms of the nutrients available to us in food.

To top it off, most clinical studies on vitamins use flawed methodology, often reaching negative conclusions. Researchers study the effects of nutrients like they would evaluate the effects of a prescription drug. Most clinical studies do not identify the baseline nutritional inadequacies of a person's diet; without this information, it becomes almost impossible to make accurate clinical conclusions.

One of the biggest questions asked in regards to vitamins is: Are they safe? Over the past 30 years or so, since data has been available, there have been *zero* deaths as a result of vitamin consumption and more than *3 million deaths* related to the use of prescription drugs.[3] Considering that the average drug label contains well over 70 side effects, one has to ask which of the two—the vitamins or drugs—we should be treating warily.

WHY ARE VITAMINS IMPORTANT?

As we have learned, our bodies are bombarded every day by biochemical stresses such as pesticides, herbicides, preservatives, genetically modified and fast foods. While we know fast food isn't great for us, we sometimes eat it anyway because we're on the run. As a consequence, we may end up eating not enough nutrient-dense foods. The problem with fast food is not only what they contain, but also what they are lacking. One way to make sure our bodies are getting the nutrients they need is to complement our diet with high-quality vitamin and mineral supplements.

Vitamins are organic compounds vital to our bodies' basic functions. They play an important role in numerous enzyme reactions in our body. Since our bodies can't manufacture vitamins, they need to be ingested through diet or supplements. This comes with the exception of Vitamin D, which can be synthesized by the body from the sun. Vitamins help regulate our metabolism, fight infection, repair and grow body tissues, give us energy and make us fertile. They even make us look good by making our hair shiny and thick, our nails strong, our teeth healthy and our skin youthful.

> I really do feel like I have more energy when I take my vitamins regularly.

VITAMINS 101

The following information is designed to give you an overview on why vitamins are important, and what to look for when buying them. It is not a prescription. We are all different and all have different needs. Your natural health-care provider can recommend which specific vitamins and supplements are suited to you. Note that what you eat will have a tremendous impact on the vitamins recommended for you. When it comes down to it, food should always come first as our source of nutrients.

In an ideal world, it would be best to get all the nutrients we need from high-quality, wholesome foods, but how realistic is that? With our busy lifestyles, we often don't take the time to plan and prepare well-balanced, nutritional meals. If I were to ask you how much manganese you took in yesterday, you would be at a loss to answer. Some may not know that manganese is a trace mineral, let alone what foods contain it and how much they've had!

Unfortunately, even if you think you eat fairly well, it's hard to know if you're covering all of your nutritional needs on a daily basis. Taking a broad-spectrum nutritional supplement can ensure that you are getting all the right nutrients. Each vitamin and mineral plays an important role in maintaining your body's normal functions, repairing cellular and tissue damage, and promoting optimal wellness.

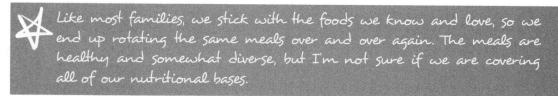

Like most families, we stick with the foods we know and love, so we end up rotating the same meals over and over again. The meals are healthy and somewhat diverse, but I'm not sure if we are covering all of our nutritional bases.

Another reason we don't get necessary nutrients from our everyday foods is due to the depletion of nutrients in our earth's soil. As I've stated before, our agriculture is not what it used to be: from genetically modified organisms to herbicides, pesticides, erosion and increased radiation, the quality of our soil and agriculture has decreased significantly. Nitrogen, phosphorus and potassium fertilizers have played a big role in depleting our soil of essential nutrients, and when nutrients aren't in our soil, they won't be found in our food.[4] This is why eating organic as much as possible is highly recommended to avoid dealing with the side effects of these chemicals and to provide ourselves with a healthier nutrition.

The message surrounding vitamins, specifically multivitamins, has changed dramatically over the years. Twenty years ago, experts told us not to take multivitamins if we ate a healthy diet, as they were considered a waste of money. However, in a 2015 report, the Centers for Disease Control and Prevention (CDC) stated that only one in every ten Americans eat enough fruit and vegetables, making the rest deficient in many essential vitamins and minerals.[5]

FAT-SOLUBLE AND WATER-SOLUBLE VITAMINS

Without getting into all the details of the vitamins' individual roles—as it will be discussed in the next chapter—know that there are 13 essential vitamins:

- thiamine (B1)
- riboflavin (B2—which gives your urine the fluorescent yellow color)
- niacin/niacinamide (B3)
- pantothenic acid (B5)
- pyridoxal/pyridoxamine/pyridoxine (B6—often deficient in people who consume excessive alcohol)
- biotin (B7)
- cobalamin (B12)
- folic acid
- ascorbic acid (vitamin C)
- retinol/retinal/retinoic acid (vitamin A)
- calcitriol (active vitamin D form)
- tocopherols/tocotrienols (vitamin E family)
- menaquinone (vitamin K active form)

Vitamins are categorized as either water soluble or fat soluble. Fat-soluble vitamins (i.e., A, D, E and K), are stored in the fat tissues in your body and your liver until your body needs them. They can be stored for a few days—or sometimes even months. Water-soluble vitamins, like C and B, are easily excreted and are, therefore, hard to consume in toxic amounts. This also means they must be replenished daily.

MINERALS

Minerals also perform essential functions. They are divided in two groups: major minerals and trace minerals. Major minerals are sodium, potassium, calcium, phosphorus, magnesium, chloride and sulfur. These minerals are generally required in amounts greater than 100 mg per day. Trace minerals are iron, zinc, manganese, fluoride, iodine, selenium, copper, molybdenum and chromium. These minerals are needed in only microgram (mcg) amounts.

DANGERS OF VITAMIN AND MINERAL DEFICIENCIES

Deficiencies can also occur if you have a pre-existing disease that prevents the food in your intestines from being absorbed properly. Alcoholism, multiple pregnancies and lactation can also deplete vitamins from your body. When the body is deficient in the vitamins it needs, serious health issues can occur.

Some of the dangers of ongoing deficiencies are:

- cancer susceptibility

- the development of allergies

- impaired growth, especially in children and teens

- decreased immune system function

- the development of nervous system disorders

- muscle degeneration

- depression

- anxiety

HOW DO I KNOW IF I AM VITAMIN DEFICIENT?

Many people suffer from micro-deficiencies, which may not display drastic symptoms. However, such deficiencies may eventually manifest themselves as:

- difficulty concentrating
- headaches
- loss of hair
- sinus trouble
- unpleasant body odor

- lack of energy
- loss of appetite
- dry skin
- memory loss
- digestive problems

If you start taking vitamin supplements after suspecting you're deficient, don't expect to see instant results. Depending on how deficient your body has become, it could take time before you are healthy again.

Your annual regular bloodwork is most likely not comprehensive enough to test for specific vitamin and mineral deficiencies. Luckily, there are ways to find out before you start supplementing. An example of such a test is NutrEval by Genova, which assesses for core nutrients in five key areas: antioxidants, B vitamins, digestive support, essential fatty acids and minerals.[6] By knowing exactly which nutrients you are deficient in, you no longer have to guess. You can determine what your body is in need of and supplement accordingly. This allows the patient to have great insight on their individual needs and make decisions for their health, based on their own results. Unfortunately, not many people are aware that these tests do, in fact, exist. And, they do come at an extra cost. But, personalized nutrition is truly the way of the future in health.

NOT ALL VITAMINS ARE CREATED EQUAL

When buying supplements, it is important to do your research. Good supplements should be whole-food based—without chemicals, dyes, binders, or fillers. Thankfully, there are companies specializing in nutrition and health research that focus primarily on vitamin and mineral supplementation. One such company is NutriSearch Corporation, and one of their main products is the *NutriSearch Comparative Guide to Nutritional Supplements*, which examines current research on the health benefits of supplementation for the prevention of degenerative disease. The guide also includes comparisons of a wide variety of supplements offered in various markets around the world—including Canada and the U.S.

As stated in the *NutriSearch Comparative Guide to Nutritional Supplements*:

"Each supplement is given a Health Support Profile based on 18 criteria— completeness, potency, mineral forms, vitamin E forms, immune support, antioxidant support, bone health, heart health, liver health, metabolic health, ocular health, methylation support, lipotropic factors, inflammation control, glycation control, bioflavonoid prole, phenolic compound profile, and potential toxicities. Each product is then given a score based on a star system (zero stars to five stars)."[7]

It is important to note that the guide is a non-sponsored publication.

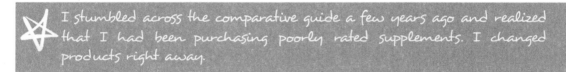

I stumbled across the comparative guide a few years ago and realized that I had been purchasing poorly rated supplements. I changed products right away.

A good-quality multivitamin may not be as simple as a "one-a-day" supplement, as quality supplements are not stuffed with fillers and binders—which help to "bind" the contents together to make it fit in one pill. This is why, with quality supplements, you will often have to take more than one tablet or capsule per day as they often have less fillers present. But remember, convenience shouldn't win over quality. Since nutrients do not work in isolation, a good supplement regime will ensure proper ratios to help you absorb the most nutrients.

Take note, as well, that regulations for vitamins made in Canada are more stringent than those in the U.S.—not to say that the U.S. doesn't have great vitamins. Canadian regulations fall under pharmaceutical guidelines, and therefore have a higher standard than those in the U.S., which fall under more lenient food regulation guidelines. Food-grade supplements may contain a wide array of unhealthy binders and fillers, including petroleum products, coal tar derivatives, shampoos, sands—the list goes on.

In addition, because they are considered foods and not drugs, the American Food and Drug Administration (FDA) does not monitor the content of the supplements or the source of the nutritional ingredient(s). In Canada, purity and potency of supplements are more stringent. The drawback, however, is that it can take seemingly forever to get a great supplement approved for sale due to these stricter regulations. Safety and performance should always be the bottom line, so get the proper information on the vitamins you are taking to ensure you're getting the highest of quality!

It's important to know the following:

- The two certifying bodies are the International Organization for Standardization (ISO) and the National Sanitation Foundation (NSF). These organizations ensure that products are made using the highest standards available. [8]

- Look for vitamins certified GMP (Good Manufacturing Practice) to ensure that what is said on the label is actually in the bottle—nothing more, nothing less. [9]

It is important to note that taking multivitamins, or acidic vitamins such as vitamin C (ascorbic acid), on an empty stomach can sometimes cause nausea and upset stomach for some. Minerals such as copper, iron and zinc can often cause such ill effects, as well. Take these vitamins and minerals with food to help avoid these side effects.

MY TWO CENTS ON VITAMIN REGULATION

Taking a poor-quality supplement can be worse than taking no supplement at all. Not only do you get a false sense of security about getting adequate nutrition, but—depending on the supplement's fillers— you can also be ingesting toxic substances.

I believe that regulations surrounding vitamins and supplements need to be reviewed. We need to create better worldwide evaluation systems and communications around vitamins and supplements. This has the potential to extend the human lifespan, which could save our health-care system millions of dollars, if not billions.

To sum up, vitamins and minerals play an important role in maintaining your body's normal functions, repairing cellular and tissue damage, and maintaining your optimal wellness. Are you getting enough from your diet? Why not make sure by supplementing with high-quality vitamins? It is that important!

The following diagram shows examples of health habits with corresponding hack levels. To download the *Hack Your Health Habits Worksheet*, visit

www.hackyourhealthhabits.com/worksheets

READY #HEALTHHACKER?
EXAMPLES OF LEVEL 1, 2 AND 3 HACKS FOR THIS CHAPTER

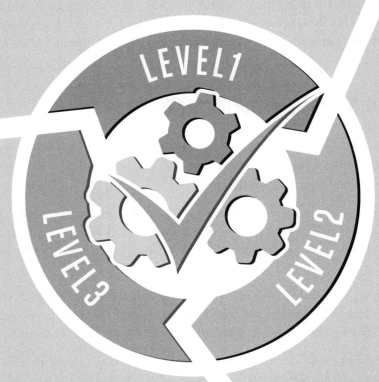

✓ Use the <u>NutriSearch Comparative Guide to Nutritional Supplements</u> to rate your current supplements.

✓ Establish the habit of taking a high-quality multivitamin daily.

✓ Find a health-food store or natural health-care provider that carries higher-quality supplements.

HACK YOUR HEALTH PROGRESS

||||||||||||||||||||||||||||||||||||||||||||||||||||||||||||||||||||

CHAPTER 23

24
VITAMINS AND MINERALS
Understanding Their Specific Roles

"Nutritional supplements
are not a substitute for a
nutritionally balanced diet."

— Deepak Chopra

THINK IT OVER

- Do you know the main functions of each essential vitamin and mineral?

- Do you know what foods have what vitamins or minerals?

- Do you know if you are getting your 13 essential vitamins and your major and minor minerals?

Remember the Flintstones tablets your parents made you take as a child? Maybe they weren't the ideal vitamin choice, but your parents definitely had the right idea. Many of us assume that by eating a nutritious diet we get all the required daily nutrients our body needs to function properly. But, as we learned in the previous chapter, though a healthy diet is key to getting our nutrients, many of us are still deficient in certain vitamins and minerals.

In the perfect world, one would get a full panel of vitamin and mineral tests to determine whether he or she is deficient and then supplement accordingly. People may not be aware that such tests do actually exist.

When I started writing this chapter, I told myself that I would focus only on the main and most popular supplements out there, vitamins and minerals included. It did not take me long to realize that the chapter would have been an encyclopedia on its own, if I had gone that route, so I decided to keep it to the basics and focus solely on vitamins and minerals, what they do, where to find them in the food we eat, and what symptoms can be associated with their deficiencies.

THE 13 ESSENTIAL VITAMINS

As you recall from the previous chapter, vitamins are categorized as either water soluble or fat soluble. So, let's dig in!

FAT-SOLUBLE VITAMINS

The following list of vitamins need adequate fat to be absorbed properly by the body.

VITAMIN A (A.K.A. RETINOL AND BETA-CAROTENE)

Functions: The primary functions of vitamin A are related to vision, bone development, immune function, cell differentiation, growth and reproduction.[1]

Food Sources: Vitamin A is found in two primary forms: active vitamin A and beta-carotene. Active vitamin A comes from animal-derived foods and is called retinol. It can be used directly by the body. The other type of vitamin A is in the form of carotenoids, which needs to be converted to retinol by the body after the food is ingested. Sources for active vitamin A include liver, eggs yolks, whole milk and butter. Sources for carotenoids include yellow and orange vegetables, such as carrots, pumpkins, sweet potatoes and squashes—and some leafy green vegetables.

Toxicity Effects: Bone fractures, joint pain, headaches, dry skin and brittle hair, nausea, fatigue, liver failure and hemorrhaging.[2]

Deficiency Effects: Poor night vision, decreased protection against infectious agents, a reduction in cellular immunity and antibody production.[3]

Pairs Well With: Zinc, vitamin E and vitamin C.

VITAMIN D (WHICH IS CONSIDERED MORE LIKE A HORMONE THAN A VITAMIN)

Functions: Vitamin D increases the absorption of calcium and phosphorus, which leads to stronger bones and teeth.

Food Sources: Fish liver oils, fatty fish, fortified milk, cheese and egg yolks.

Toxic Effects: Unknown – high vitamin D dosage in adults is now being researched at a much higher level.

Deficiency Effects: Since vitamin D is absorbed in the small intestine, people with gut-related issues may have decreased absorption. Health conditions like kidney disease, Crohn's disease, hyperparathyroidism, osteoporosis, osteopenia, osteomalacia and adolescent rickets may develop with a vitamin D deficiency. Other signs include tooth decay, muscle cramps and hair loss.[4]

Pairs Well With: Vitamins A, C and E.

VITAMIN E

Functions: Vitamin E acts as an antioxidant, helps prevent free radical damage to specific fats and helps prevent diseases of the heart and blood vessels.

Food Sources: Salmon, sunflower seed, almond, wheat germ, mango, avocado, butternut squash, broccoli and spinach.[5]

Toxic Effects: Too much can interfere with anti-clotting medications such as Warfarin (a.k.a. Coumadin). Taken in high doses, it can cause nausea, flatulence, diarrhea, muscle weakness, fatigue and double vision.[6]

Deficiency Effects: Possible signs of deficiency are lack of sex drive, decrease in muscle tissue, slowed growth, decreased red blood count and poor bone calcification. Other deficiency effects are faulty absorption of fats and soluble vitamins, inflammation of the pancreas, developmental issues in children and worsened PMS.[7]

Note: Vitamin E exists in different forms (alpha-, beta-, gamma-, and delta-tocopherols, and tocotrienols) each of which has slightly different activity in the body. Even though there are eight forms of vitamin E, the most biologically active form of the vitamin is alpha-tocopherol.

Pairs Well With: Vitamin C and selenium.

VITAMIN K

Functions: This is one of the main vitamins involved in bone mineralization and blood clotting. It helps to maintain brain function, a healthy metabolism and to protect against cancer.[8]

Food Sources: Vitamin K1 is found in plants, especially green vegetables. Examples include cauliflower, cabbage, Brussel sprouts and broccoli. Vitamin K2 is produced by the bacteria that line the gastrointestinal tract. Increases in K2 can be achieved by eating fermented foods.

Toxic Effects: The effects of vitamin K toxicity can include jaundice in newborns, hemolytic anemia and hyperbilirubinemia.

Deficiency Effects: Rare, but can lead to heart disease, weakened bones, tooth decay and cancer. A warning sign of a vitamin K deficiency is bleeding and bruising easily.[9]

Pairs Well With: Probiotics.

WATER-SOLUBLE VITAMINS

This section looks at the vitamins that do not need fat in order to be absorbed. Note that all B vitamins help the body convert carbohydrates into fuel (glucose), which the body uses as energy.

VITAMIN B1 (THIAMINE)

Functions: Vitamin B1 is important for producing energy and for proper neuronal and neurocognitive function. It also helps the body make use of protein.

Food Sources: Brewer's yeast, sunflower seeds, pine nuts, beans, millet, oatmeal, wild rice, squash, asparagus, mushrooms, peas and cauliflower.

Toxic Effects: Very rare.

Deficiency Effects: Severe deficiency may result in anorexia, weight loss, GI disorders, poor memory, irritability, neurological and cardiovascular problems.[10]

Pairs Well With: Magnesium and manganese.

VITAMIN B2 (RIBOFLAVIN)

Functions: Vitamin B2 is responsible for maintaining healthy blood cells, helping to boost energy levels, facilitating a healthy metabolism, preventing free radical damage, contributing to growth, and protecting skin and eye health.

Food Sources: Food and beverages that provide riboflavin without fortification are organ meats, brewer's yeast, almonds, wild rice, mushrooms, egg yolks, collards and kale.

Toxic Effects: Vitamin B2 riboflavin deficiency is not very common in Western diets.

Deficiency Effects: Anemia, fatigue, anxiety, depression, nerve damage, sluggish metabolism, mouth or lip sores and cracks, skin inflammation and disorders, inflamed mouth and tongue, sore throat, and swelling of mucous membranes.[11]

Pairs Well With: Selenium.

VITAMIN B3 (NIACIN)

Functions: Vitamin B3 is important for the skin and digestive tract, tissue oxygenation, and circulation. It is vital to the activity of the nervous system.[12]

Food Sources: Brewer's yeast, organ meats, salmon, wild rice, sunflower seeds, asparagus, tomatoes, cauliflower and almonds.

Toxic Effects: Can cause flushing of the skin through dilatation of blood vessels.

Deficiency Effects: Chronic lack of niacin is called Pellagra.

Pairs Well With: Chromium.

VITAMIN B5 (PANTOTHENIC ACID)

Function: B5 is necessary to make Coenzyme A, which activates some enzymes and proteins that promote important chemical reactions within the body. It has a direct effect on the adrenal glands and is an important nutrient during stressful conditions.

Food Sources: Beef, pork, chicken, organ meats, brewer's yeast, lentils, oatmeal and hazelnuts.

Toxic Effects: None known.

Deficiency Effects: Fatigue, muscle cramps, tenderness in feet or heels, and reduced production of red blood cell and hormones.[13]

Pairs Well With: Biotin and folate.

VITAMIN B6 (PYRIDOXINE)

Functions: B6 helps the body make red blood cells, contributes to immune and nervous system function, and metabolizes proteins and fats. It also helps balance sex hormones and acts as a natural antidepressant.

Food Sources: Turkey breast, beef, tuna, asparagus, cauliflower, pinto beans, avocados, sunflower seeds, chickpeas and amaranth grains.

Toxic Effects: Taking very high doses for months or years can induce neuropathy.

Deficiency Effects: Rare, but chronic deficiency could lead to muscle pains, low energy, fatigue, irritability, anxiety and depression. Deficiency can also be caused by alcoholism, asthma, birth control pills, Crohn's disease and suppression of the immune system.[14]

Pairs Well With: Zinc and magnesium.

VITAMIN B7 (BIOTIN)

Functions: B7 contributes to energy production and the metabolism of proteins, fats and carbohydrates.

Food Sources: Brewer's yeast, liver, egg yolks, peanuts, walnuts and oatmeal.

Toxic Effects: Rarely occurs.

Deficiency Effects: Although deficiency is rare, symptoms can include sore tongue, dry skin, low energy, loss of appetite, depression and insomnia.[15]

Pairs Well With: Magnesium and manganese.

VITAMIN B9 (FOLATE OR ALSO CALLED FOLIC ACID)

Functions: B9 is critical for all cell functions since folate helps make DNA and RNA. It may protect against heart disease by lowering homocysteine levels. In pregnant women, it lowers the risk of neural tube defects in the baby.

Food Sources: Leafy green vegetables (especially spinach and turnip greens), legumes, broccoli, asparagus, citrus fruits, avocados, seeds and nuts.

Toxic Effects: The risk of toxicity from folic acid is low because folate is water-soluble.

Deficiency Effects: To prevent spina bifida and other neural tubal disorders in babies, pregnant women and women who have the potential to become pregnant should be on folate supplements. For all adults, too little folate can result in anemia, irritability, anorexia and headaches.[16]

Note: Folic acid is the synthetic form of folate, found in supplements and also added to processed or "fortified" foods. The term folate is often used to describe both natural and synthetic versions. The best active form is methyltetrahydrofolate, which does not need to be converted from the basic form of folic acid to be used by the body.

VITAMIN B12 (COBALAMIN)

Functions: B12 is important for proper nerve function. It works with folate, converting it to an active form. B12 also helps make red blood cells and metabolize proteins and fats. It is also essential for memory and is needed for the synthesis of DNA.
Food Sources: Meats, fish, poultry, milk, cheese and eggs.
Toxic Effects: None have been reported to date.
Deficiency Effects: May result in anemia, nerve damage and hypersensitive skin. Serious lasting side effects include soreness and tingling of the extremities, sore tongue, weakness, brain damage, shooting pains, mental deterioration and paralysis.
Note: In order to absorb B12, one needs a healthy gut, so when people are low in this vitamin, it should be the first thing to look at—before jumping to injections that may not be well-absorbed or short lived.
Note: B12's inactive form is cyanocobalamin, and its active forms are methylcobalamin and hydroxocobalamin. Most people are not able to convert the inactive form, and unfortunately, store-bought supplements are often the inactive form. [17]

VITAMIN C (ASCORBIC ACID)

Functions: Vitamin C is important for immune function, and acts as an antioxidant to keep the body healthy. It strengthens blood vessels and capillary walls. It also makes collagen and the connective tissue that hold muscles and bones together. It keeps gums healthy and helps the body absorb iron from foods.
Food Sources: Citrus fruits, dark green vegetables, strawberries, papaya, cantaloupe, peppers, broccoli, Brussel sprouts, cauliflower and red cabbage.
Toxic Effects: Very high doses of vitamin C supplements (i.e., more than 1,000 milligrams) can cause diarrhea and may cause kidney stones.
Deficiency Effects: Smokers and those with inflammatory bowel disease are at risk of deficiency. Deficiency can cause skin bruising, bleeding gums, impaired digestion, joint pain and excessive hair loss. Extreme deficiency causes scurvy. [18]
Pairs Well With: Bioflavonoids and vitamin E.

MAJOR MINERALS AND MINOR MINERALS

Now, how about minerals? Let's have a deeper look at the major minerals—and some of the trace minerals that are popular as supplements.

MINERAL: CALCIUM

Functions: The body needs calcium to build strong bones and teeth. Calcium also plays a role in nerve transmissions, cardiovascular health, muscle function and hormone production.
Food Sources: Kale, sardines, yogurt or kefir, broccoli, watercress, cheese, bok choy, okra and almonds.
Toxic Effects: May include fatigue, constipation, depression, muscle weakness, arteriosclerosis, arthritis, kidney stones and gallstones.

Deficiency Effects: Osteopenia, osteoporosis, tooth decay, muscle cramps and twitches and hypertension (i.e. dizziness and headaches). [19]

Pairs Well With: Magnesium and vitamin D.

MINERAL: MAGNESIUM

Functions: Magnesium supports more than 300 biochemical reactions in the body. It supports nerve function, a regular heartbeat, strong bones and immunity.

Food Sources: Kelp, almonds, cashews, buckwheat, spinach, dates, brown rice, avocados and bananas.

Toxic Effects: Diarrhea, drowsiness, lethargy and weakness.

Deficiency Effects: Symptoms include leg cramps, insomnia, muscle pain, fibromyalgia, anxiety, constipation, depression, high blood pressure, type 2 diabetes, fatigue and migraine headaches. [20]

Note: Currently, statistics show that 42.7 percent of Canadians and 68 percent of Americans are deficient in magnesium, though the number is widely believed to be much higher. [21]

Pairs Well With: Vitamins B1, B6, C, D, phosphorus and zinc.

MINERAL: PHOSPHORUS

Functions: Phosphorus plays an important role in building strong bones and teeth, balancing body pH, helping to detoxify through urination, and helping to maintain the energy needed for growth and cognitive functions. It is also a component of DNA and RNA.

Food Sources: Sunflower seeds, white beans, tuna, turkey breast, beef, almonds, brown rice, potatoes and broccoli.

Toxic Effects: None reported—although a diet high in sodas and fast food can lead to excess phosphorus in the phosphorus-to-calcium ratio.

Deficiency Effects: Weak bones and fractures, osteoporosis, joint and muscle aches, numbness and tingling, anxiety, trouble concentrating and weight loss or gain. [22]

Pairs Well With: Calcium and vitamin D.

MINERAL: CHLORIDE

Functions: Sodium chloride (a.k.a. table salt) helps balance the fluids in the body and plays an essential role in the production of digestive juices in the stomach.

Food Sources: With the high salt content of Western food, most people meet the daily recommended intake.

Toxic Effects: When in the form of salt, chloride can lead to symptoms such as pH imbalance, fluid retention and high blood pressure.

Deficiency Effects: Rare, known as hypochloremia and can occur with heavy sweating, excessive fluid loss, over-hydration, burns, congestive heart failure, or certain kidney disorders.

Note: Table salts have been "chemically cleaned" and reduced to be actually 97.5 percent sodium chloride and 2.5 percent chemicals. Dried at over 1,200 degrees Fahrenheit, the excessive heat alters the natural structure of the salt. Himalayan salt or sea salt is a much better choice.[23]

MINERAL: SODIUM

Functions: Too much sodium can increase risks for developing high blood pressure. The body needs sodium to stimulate nerve and muscle function, maintain the correct balance of fluid in the cells (preventing dehydration) and support the absorption of other nutrients including chloride, amino acids and glucose.[24]

Food Sources: Table salt is the major source of sodium. There is also kelp, green olives, dill pickles, sauerkraut, cheddar cheese and Swiss chards.

Toxic Effects: May lead to symptoms such as pH imbalance, fluid retention and high blood pressure.

Deficiency Effects: Rare, but can occur in cases of starvation, where it leads to dizziness, low blood pressure, mental apathy, headaches, diarrhea and vomiting.

Pairs Well With: Vitamin D.

MINERAL: POTASSIUM

Functions: Potassium plays an important role in nerve transmission, muscle contractions, glycogen and glucose metabolism, and the maintenance of cellular integrity.

Food Sources: Kelp, almonds, dates, avocados, spinach, broccoli, banana, chicken, carrots, cantaloupe and tomatoes.

Toxic Effects: High doses are safe—except for people with kidney diseases and those on a potassium-sparing diuretic or ACE (angiotensin-converting enzyme) inhibitors.

Deficiency Effects: Can impact the central nervous system, and lead to muscle weakness, bradycardia and bone fragility.[25]

Pairs Well With: Magnesium.

TRACE MINERAL: IRON

Functions: Iron is necessary to produce the proteins hemoglobin (found in red blood cells) and myoglobin (found in muscle cells). It also supports brain development, immune function and temperature regulation.[26]

Food Sources: There are two kinds of iron. Heme iron is found in animal tissues, while non-heme iron is found in plants, but is not absorbed as well as heme iron. Sources for non-heme iron include kelp, pumpkins seeds, brewer's yeast, almonds, Jerusalem artichokes and dates.

Toxic Effects: Excess iron is stored, mostly in the liver, as ferritin and hemosiderin. Excess can lead to hemochromatosis.

Deficiency Effects: Symptoms can be fatigue, lack of energy, shortness of breath, chronic infections, hair loss, paleness and brittle nails. Vegetarian diets and low stomach acid can be a cause of deficiency.

Pairs Well With: Vitamin C.

TRACE MINERAL: ZINC

Functions: As a component of more than 200 enzymes in the body, zinc promotes enzyme and nervous system activity, supports immune function, and aids in wound healing, DNA synthesis and cell division.

Food Sources: Oysters, pumpkin seeds, beef, cashews, chickpeas, mushrooms, spinach, chicken and cocoa powder.

Toxic Effects: Excessive intake for prolonged periods can lead to fatigue, fever, stomach pain, coughing and even increased chances of prostate cancer—as well as affecting blood iron levels.

Deficiency Effects: Poor neurological function, weak immunity, white marks on fingernails, diarrhea, allergies, leaky gut, acne and thinning hair. [27]

Pairs Well With: Vitamin A, E, B6, magnesium and calcium.

TRACE MINERAL: IODINE

Functions: Iodine is needed for many biochemical processes, including fat metabolism, mental development, muscle function, the production of sex hormones and thyroid function.

Food Sources: Clams, shrimp, salmon, sardines, kelp, seaweed, pineapple, eggs, asparagus, artichokes and dark green vegetables.

Toxic Effects: Excess iodine can negatively impact thyroid hormone production.

Deficiency Effects: Deficiencies are rare as most people get enough iodine from their iodized table salt unless they restrict their salt or use Himalayan salts. Low levels can affect thyroid function. [28]

TRACE MINERAL: SELENIUM

Functions: Acts as an antioxidant, helps defend against cancer, boosts immunity, improves blood flow, helps regulate thyroid function, helps decrease asthma symptoms and may boost fertility.

Food Sources: Brazil nuts, sunflower seeds, cabbage, tuna, chicken, salmon, chia seeds and mushrooms.

Toxic Effects: These are rare, but excess can cause reactions like fever, nausea and (potentially) liver and kidney problems. May be fatal in toxic amounts.

Deficiency Effects: Increased risk of mortality, poor immune function and cognitive decline. Also, an increased risk of chronic diseases like heart disease and cancer. [29]

Pairs Well With: Vitamins A, E and C.

TRACE MINERAL: CHROMIUM

Functions: Chromium enhances the action of insulin, a hormone produced by the pancreas to regulate the breakdown of carbohydrates, fats and protein. Also helps protect DNA and RNA, and is essential for heart function.

Food Sources: Broccoli, grapes, potatoes, garlic, beef, oranges, green beans, red wine, apples and bananas.

Toxic Effects: Possible links to digestive issues, low blood sugar; very high levels can potentially cause damage to vital organs.

Deficiency Effects: Poor blood glucose control, weak bones, fatigue, higher risk for heart complications, low concentration, poor memory, mood changes, anxiety, change in weight and appetite, and delayed time in healing wounds or recovering from surgery.[30]

Pairs Well With: Vitamin B3 and amino acids.

TO CONCLUDE

Vitamins and minerals play essential roles in most metabolic processes in the body. Complex interactions between vitamins and minerals play important roles in functions of the body like digestion, absorption and synthesis. As North Americans, we live in a fortified food bubble—meaning our foods are enriched with synthetic vitamins and minerals—which can keep us out of touch with global health issues. But, just because we eat fortified foods, does not mean our bodies are properly absorbing these fortified nutrients.

Another important issue to consider is gastrointestinal dysfunction or imbalances in the gut microbiome. They can negatively affect the absorption of vitamins, which can lead to deficiencies. Getting the daily recommended intake of vitamins through food or supplements cannot rule out the possibility that a person's signs and symptoms are not related to vitamin insufficiency. An extensive clinical nutritional evaluation needs to be done in conjunction with proper nutritional diagnostic tests. This is yet another reason to eat as many colors as possible! Remember, color equals phytonutrients.

The following diagram shows examples of health habits, with corresponding hack levels. To download the *Hack Your Health Habits Worksheet*, visit

www.hackyourhealthhabits.com/worksheets

READY #HEALTHHACKER?
EXAMPLES OF LEVEL 1, 2 AND 3 HACKS FOR THIS CHAPTER

✓ Evaluate which symptoms of mineral deficiencies you might be currently experiencing.

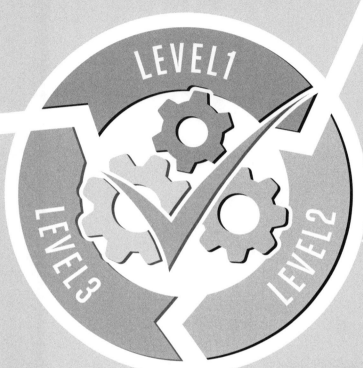

✓ Take a test (such as the NutrEval by Genova) to determine whether you are vitamin and mineral deficient, and supplement accordingly.

✓ Make a list of the foods that are high in the vitamins or minerals that you are deficient in, and make sure to add them to your grocery list.

HACK YOUR HEALTH PROGRESS

||||||||||||||||||||||||||||||||||||||||||||||||||

CHAPTER 24

VITAMIN D
Are You Operating on Low?

> "Your body is your most priceless possession; you go take care of it!"
>
> — Jack LaLanne

THINK IT OVER

- What are the signs and symptoms of vitamin D deficiency?

- Is sun exposure a safe form of vitamin D?

- How much vitamin D do you need to take?

You may be surprised to learn that vitamin D is different from most other vitamins. It is actually a hormone, a steroid that is produced out of cholesterol when your skin is exposed to the sun. For this reason, vitamin D is often referred to as the "sunshine vitamin." However, sun exposure is often inadequate (depending on where you live), making it necessary for people to get more of it from the foods they eat or from vitamin D supplements as vitamin D is absolutely essential for optimal health. Unfortunately, only a handful of foods contain significant amounts of this vitamin, therefore, deficiency is extremely common.

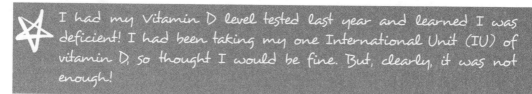
I had my Vitamin D level tested last year and learned I was deficient! I had been taking my one International Unit (IU) of vitamin D, so thought I would be fine. But, clearly, it was not enough!

Vitamin D is one of the fat-soluble vitamins, meaning that it dissolves in fat or oil and can be stored in the body for a long time.

There are actually two main forms of vitamin D found in the diet:

- vitamin D3 (a.k.a. cholecalciferol) – found in some animal foods, like fatty fish and egg yolks
- vitamin D2 (a.k.a. ergocalciferol) – found in some mushrooms

Of the two, D3 (cholecalciferol) is the one we're interested in, because it is almost twice as effective as the D2 form at increasing blood levels of vitamin D. Its benefits include:

- stronger bones and less risk for osteoporosis
- improved muscle function
- better hormone production
- protection from cardiovascular disease
- a reduced risk of type 2 diabetes
- a reduced risk of cancer
- prevention of cognitive decline
- a boost for immunity
- aid in weight loss
- help fighting depression
- improvements in the symptoms of autoimmune illnesses[1]

Now that we know the benefits of vitamin D, the signs of deficiency become a little clearer. Individuals experiencing deficiency may suffer from:

- increased calcium and mineral loss from their bones, osteoporosis and possible tooth decay
- poor wound healing
- increased muscle pain
- increased joint and back pain
- a greater risk of depression
- blood sugar imbalances
- an increased risk for schizophrenia
- increased migraines
- increased symptoms of autoimmune disease (e.g., lupus, scleroderma)
- increased allergy symptoms
- increased inflammation throughout the body[2]

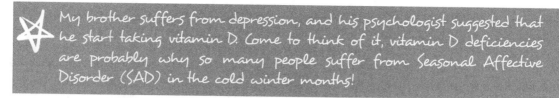

VITAMIN D AND THE SUN

The risks associated with sunlight exposure have been widely discussed in recent years. Health professionals and the media encourage people to stay out of the sun or apply sunscreen when going outdoors, citing a risk of a skin cancer. Unfortunately, little has been said about the benefits of sun exposure, nor the harmful effects of sunscreen application. As we learned in the chapter on skin, most sunscreens are made with toxic chemicals that make their way into the bloodstream via skin absorption. The harmful effects of these toxins actually rival those of sun overexposure, so be sure to opt for natural sunscreens when outside for long periods of time.

When it comes to sun exposure, the biggest fear is skin cancer. Skin cancer is very real, but you don't want to avoid the sun altogether. Did you know that tens of thousands of North Americans die of cancer and other illnesses every year due to an *inadequate* amount of sun exposure, and did you know the inadequate levels of vitamin D this causes? In fact, the annual cost for treating illnesses due to a lack of sun exposure far outweighs the amount spent on treating illnesses due to an overexposure to sunlight.[3]

These facts aren't meant to undermine the risks associated with overexposure to the sun. Sunshine is still the best source of vitamin D and a proven player in cancer-fighting. In fact, the closer to the equator you live, the easier it is for you to synthesize vitamin D from the sun all year round. However, since many of us in North America spend many months without sun exposure, we become deficient.[4] So, limit over-exposure by wearing a natural sunscreen if needed, but don't stay in the dark!

SUN EXPOSURE AND UV RAYS

In order to be sun-safe, it's important to be UV-knowledgeable. So, here's a little "Ultraviolet (UV) radiation 101" beyond what we learned in the skin chapter. To start, the sun emits ultraviolet radiation in UVA, UVB and UVC rays. The stratosphere filters out UVC rays, so they are of little concern to our health. We get the most benefit from UVB rays, which are responsible for vitamin D production. Unfortunately, UVB rays also pose the most risk. They are responsible for sunburn and damage to the surface of the skin. They are what cause moles, skin aging and some types of skin cancer. That being said, UVB rays make up only a fraction of UV light.

UVA rays make up the majority of UV light. They are what give us that bronzed glow in the summertime. When UVAs penetrate the skin, our skin produces melanocytes. These melanocytes produce melanin—a brown pigment that causes us to appear tan. UVAs do not produce sunburns and are less likely to cause skin cancer. However, they are linked with the most dangerous form of skin cancer: melanoma. What's more, UVAs contribute to rapid aging and DNA damage and are often less-effectively blocked by sunscreens.

It's impossible to avoid UV rays, and you don't have to! The UV Index—which is now included in most weather forecasts and websites—is a useful tool when it comes to sun protection. It tells you the strength of the sun's daily UV rays. The higher the number, the stronger the sun's rays, and the more important it is to protect yourself. On higher UV days, or any day when you need to be outside for long periods of time, limit sun exposure, or take some precautions. Wear a hat, use natural sunscreen containing zinc oxide, wear a long-sleeved shirt and pants and spend time in the shade.

YOUR DIET, SKIN CANCER AND VITAMIN D

Our main source of vitamin D is from sun exposure. Very few foods actually contain the recommended daily amount of vitamin D, which is why adequate sun exposure is highly recommended. If you are looking to add more vitamin D to your diet, consider adding the following foods to your weekly menu:

- mackerel
- salmon
- sardines
- cheese

- herring
- oysters
- beef liver
- eggs

Notice how most of these sources are fish? Skin cancers have been linked to a disproportion in the ratio of omega-6 to omega-3 in the body. Our North American diets are often much higher in omega-6, so this may place us at a greater risk of developing skin cancer. Increasing your intake of omega-3 by adding mackerel, herring, salmon, oysters and sardines to your diet will not only give you healthy omega-3s but will also provide you with some vitamin D.

It's important to note that food choices and sun exposure might not cut it. Older individuals and people with darker skin produce less vitamin D, and therefore, may need to supplement. Similarly, those of us living in cooler climates, with little sun exposure in the winter months, may also need to supplement.

It's also important to keep in mind that hormones and nutrients usually don't work in isolation. Many of them depend on one another, so an increased intake of one nutrient may increase your need for another. Some claim that fat-soluble vitamins (i.e., A, D, E and K) work together and that it is crucial to optimize Vitamin A and Vitamin K2 intake at the same time as supplementing with vitamin D3.

When trying to do this, vitamin K2 MK-7 is said to be the best form of Vitamin K2.[5] The foods richest in K2 are animal products like butter, cream, cheese, meat (especially organ meats), cultured yogurt and fermented foods.

HOW MUCH VITAMIN D DO YOU NEED?

I often get asked by patients, "How much vitamin D should I take?" Unfortunately, there is no one answer to this question. The best way to find out is to get tested. A simple blood test will tell you whether you are deficient or not. I suggest getting tested at the end of the winter when your levels are likely at their lowest. Knowing your levels will allow you to gauge how much Vitamin D you should be taking. As a baseline, it is recommended that everyone take 1,000 IU (25 mcg) daily. However, if you are deficient, 1,000 IU will not be enough to replenish your reserve. Vitamin D plays an important role in many of your body's functions, so you want to make sure that your levels are in the optimal range at all times.

Here are the range levels of vitamin D:

- less than 25 nmol/L or 10 ng/ml = deficient
- 25-80 nmol/L or 10 to 32 ng/ml = mild to moderately deficient
- 80-200 nmol/L or 32 to 80 ng/ml = optimal
- 200-250 nmol/L or 80 to 100 ng/ml = high
- more than 250 nmol/L or 100 ng/ml = possible toxicity[6]

Once you know your number, you can go online to determine how much vitamin D you should be taking. There are many online calculators available. Take the recommended dosage, and get tested again to see if you have achieved the optimal range.

> To my surprise, after reviewing my vitamin D test results, my naturopath suggested taking 7,000 IU for a month to boost my levels.

The bottom line is, vitamin D is important. We need it to be healthy. Play outside, get some sun but avoid getting burned. For those of us stuck inside during the cold winter months, eat vitamin D-rich foods and take a supplement if you don't think you are getting enough exposure (or buy that condo in Florida you've been eyeing; becoming a snowbird would certainly help your vitamin D levels!).

The following diagram shows examples of health habits with corresponding hack levels. To download the *Hack Your Health Habits Worksheet*, visit

www.hackyourhealthhabits.com/worksheets

READY #HEALTHHACKER?
EXAMPLES OF LEVEL 1, 2 AND 3 HACKS FOR THIS CHAPTER

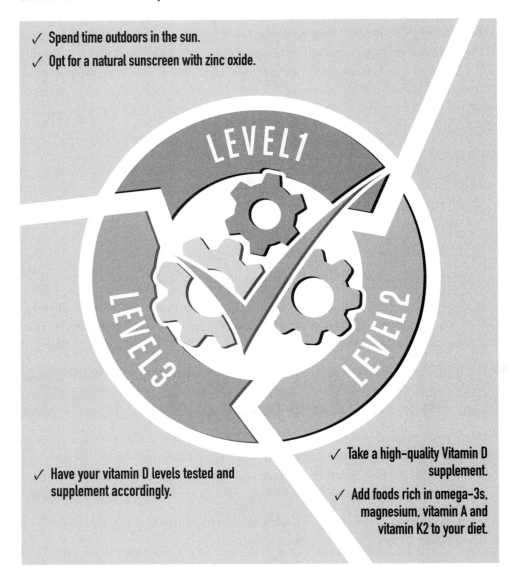

✓ Spend time outdoors in the sun.
✓ Opt for a natural sunscreen with zinc oxide.

✓ Have your vitamin D levels tested and supplement accordingly.

✓ Take a high-quality Vitamin D supplement.
✓ Add foods rich in omega-3s, magnesium, vitamin A and vitamin K2 to your diet.

HACK YOUR HEALTH PROGRESS

|||||||||||||||||||||||||||||||||||||||||||||||||

CHAPTER 25

ESSENTIAL FATTY ACIDS
Their Roles In Your Overall Health

"An ounce of prevention is
worth a pound of cure."

— BENJAMIN FRANKLIN

THINK IT OVER

- Do you understand the different types of Essential Fatty Acids (EFAs) and what foods are rich in them?

- Should you be supplementing with EFAs?

- Should you consider getting your EFA levels tested?

I did not think that this chapter would be so difficult to write, but the more I read on Essential Fatty Acids (EFAs), the more I realized the topic is far more complex than what it's made out to be. There has been a lot of research conducted on EFAs—more specifically on omega-3s and their effects on health conditions like cardiovascular diseases, cancer, diabetes and Alzheimer's disease. While some researchers argue that omega-3 supplements are of great benefit to our health, others claim that their health effects are not clear-cut. My goal with this chapter is to provide you with some basic EFA facts, and then address what the issues and concerns surrounding them might be.

ESSENTIAL FATTY ACIDS

Essential fatty acids are called *essential* since they need to be consumed in our diet. As discussed in the fat chapter, they are omega-3s and omega-6s. Omega-9s are not considered *essential* because they don't need to be consumed in the diet, as they can be produced by the body. Omega-3s and omega-6s are called polyunsaturated fatty acids (PUFA) while omega-9s are called mostly monounsaturated fatty acid (MUFA).

OMEGA-3s

There are three forms of omega-3 fatty acids. The primary one, ALA (alpha-linolenic acid) is found in flax, walnut, canola, soy, chia and hemp. The second one, EPA (eicosapentaenoic acid), is found in cold water fish, wild game and enriched eggs. The third one, DHA (docosahexaenoic acid), is also found in cold water fish, wild game and enriched eggs, as well as algaes.

OMEGA-6s

The primary omega-6 fatty acid is Linoleic Acid (LA). LA is found in seeds, nuts, grains and vegetable oils like: corn oil, soybean oil and sunflower oil. The second omega-6 fatty acid is Gamma-Linolenic Acid (GLA) and is found in borage, black currant seeds and evening primrose oil. The third one is called Arachidonic Acid (AA) and is present in animal fat, dairy and shellfish.

EFAs are important for proper functioning of our cell membrane (the outer layer of our cell). Our cell membrane has a double layer of lipids and proteins. When the cell membranes are healthy, they allow fluid and nutrients to pass through the membrane and support the metabolic needs of our cells. The lipid portion of the membrane is made of both saturated fats, meaning it is chemically non-reactive—does not react with oxygen or other substances—and of unsaturated fats—which does react with oxygen. The function of the saturated fat is to act as a barrier to help protect this delicate layer of unsaturated, oxygen-reacting fat in the membrane.

Essential fatty acids are important for various functions of the body, such as:

- improvement of blood vessel health
- dampening of inflammation
- support of healthy skin
- support of healthy brain and nervous system function

OMEGA-6 TO OMEGA-3 RATIO

The ratio of omega-6 to omega-3 is important for proper cellular function and optimal health. It is said that most people in North America consume a much higher amount of omega-6 than omega-3—as high as 25:1 with the average being 11:1.[1] This is in great part due to sunflower, cotton seeds, soybeans and canola oils found in our processed foods. The imbalance in omega-6 and omega-3 can create an inflammatory environment which can play a role in chronic conditions like heart disease, autoimmune disease, diabetes and brain degeneration. In order to minimize this inflammation, research suggests an omega-6:omega-3 ratio of 1:1 to 4:1 for disease prevention and optimal health.[2]

Most of the scientific community agrees that we don't usually need to supplement with omega-6, as we already get enough from our diet. But, to make things complex, others have raised concerns regarding omega-6 fats claiming that it is not just the fats themselves but rather what has been done to them that has caused the decrease in quality. For example, if the source of omega-6 is non-organic, we risk the presence of pesticides, herbicides, fungicides, GMO pesticides-inducing genes, chemical colorings, unnatural coatings and waxes. Also, many sources of omega-6 are adulterated (made inferior) by how they are processed using harsh chemical solvents and manipulated at high temperatures creating harmful free radicals when they are subjected to heat. Routinely eating processed oils or partially hydrogenated oils found in packaged foods, can cause the cell membrane to lose its flexibility. It is therefore important to consume organic and non-adulterated omega-6 as much as possible.

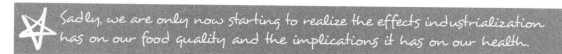

Sadly, we are only now starting to realize the effects industrialization has on our food quality and the implications it has on our health.

Another important note on this is that wild animals, wild fish and grass-fed cows naturally have a high amount of omega-3 fats in their flesh. The problem is, for human consumption, most of these animals are fed wheat, corn and soy, instead of grass, therefore the amount of omega-3 fats drop significantly and omega-6 fats increase, becoming yet another reason why our EFA ratios have become so imbalanced.

EFAs SUPPLEMENTATION

Before we start talking about *if* we should supplement with EFAs and *how much* and *which* ones we should supplement with, I suggest getting your fatty acid levels tested. Many labs offer a Fatty Acids Profile that can measure in detail the levels of the different omega-3s and omega-6s, fatty acid ratios like omega-6:omega-3 and AA:EPA ratios, monounsaturated fatty acids and saturated fatty acids levels. These tests are not usually part of your regular blood tests, so you may have to specifically request them from your healthcare practitioner. They are also not to be confused with a blood lipoprotein profile which measures LDL and HDL cholesterol and triglycerides. These tests can be well worth doing as they can give you a good "snapshot" of your fatty acid levels and can help guide you in adjusting your diet and supplementation to aim for a healthy levels of fatty acids.

There exists a variety of EFA supplementation from flaxseed oils to primrose oils to fish oils. Fish oil is usually the main one researched and discussed. A large number of studies show many benefits of omega-3 supplementation, however, there also exists some research showing that the consumption of omega-3 fish oil supplements may not be as beneficial as once thought, as there are many factors which have to be taken in consideration when it comes to EFAs.

The premise behind omega-3 fish oil supplementation is based on the fact that most people have high ratios of omega-6:omega-3, and that supplementing with EPA and DHA from fish oil will help balance that ratio. Why are the average ratios so high? As mentioned earlier, the high consumption of highly processed omega-6s in our industrialized diet combined with the fact that only about 5 percent to 10 percent of ALA can actually be converted to EPA and only about 2 percent to 5 percent converted to DHA.[3]

Most fish oil has a 1 to 1 ratio of EPA to DHA, which has shown to be beneficial in decreasing inflammation and supporting brain health. According to studies, EPA provides more on general anti-inflammation effects while DHA focuses more on brain support. From a therapeutic point of view, use of EPA and DHA will depend on what one is trying to support—i.e. for brain support the ratio can be 10:1 to 20:1 DHA to EPA whereas the ratio for reducing inflammation can be much lower.[4]

So what is the debate about? As mentioned earlier, the importance of EFA supplementation is not black and white—meaning much research has shown evidence for the benefits of their consumption, whereas other studies don't seem to support this standpoint. Here are some of the topics that are being challenged when it comes to EFAs supplementation:

- Some sources state that we don't need EPA and DHA in supplement form, as the body can make them from the ALA we get in our diet and that we also don't need as much EPA and DHA as it has been assumed. Therefore, supplementing can gives us *supraphysiological* doses of EPA and DHA. While other sources say that we need to consume long-chained EFAs as we can't make enough from the short chains EFA alpha-linolenic acid.

- Some sources are pointing to the fact that increasing PUFAs can lead to an increase in lipid peroxidation—the oxidative degradation of lipids which results in cell damage. Given that omega-3s susceptibility of oxidation is higher than omega-6, it may be just wiser to decrease omega-6s intake to prevent development of chronic diseases rather then supplementing with omega-3s.

- Some sources say that there it is practically impossible for fish oil companies to protect their oils from spontaneous oxidation, or perhaps worse, polymerization (cross-linking) of unsaturated bonds, once ingested, even despite companies adding antioxidants such as vitamin E to their fish oil products.

INDIVIDUAL DIFFERENCES IN EFA METABOLISM AND IMPORTANCE OF TESTING

You will hear me say it time and time again through this book—everyone is unique, therefore supplements, like diets, are not a one-size-fits-all approach. When it comes to EFAs metabolism, many factors have to be taken into consideration. For instance, delta-6 desaturase—an enzyme that converts between types of fatty acids—is down-regulated when one is insulin resistant (more on insulin resistance in Chapter 37). This results in less anti-inflammatory prostaglandins and leukotrienes which are involved in numerous homeostatic biological functions and inflammation. Moreover, when one is insulin resistant, this will at the same time up-regulate delta-5 desaturase—which shifts GLA to the pro-inflammatory Arachidonic Acid (AA). Consumption of the standard American diet (rightfully named the S.A.D. diet), which consists of high consumption of simple sugars and unhealthy fats, will lower the cellular insulin response and increase extracellular insulin. This alters fatty acid metabolism, resulting in elevated inflammatory end products and poor cellular communication. Therefore, those with a history of metabolic syndrome or pre-diabetes will more likely experience an increase in inflammation with increased omega-6 consumption since the blood sugar hormone, insulin, can increase conversion to the pro-inflammatory AA rather than anti-inflammatory prostaglandins.

> *Wow, I knew when I picked up this book that I'd have to put my science cap on for certain sections. This is one of those sections...let me re-read that again!*

Therefore, to see exactly *if* and *how much* EFA supplementation you may need, it is thus important to get your blood sugar levels tested to ensure you don't have any metabolic issues, and also test levels of omega-3 and omega-6 to know your EFA status. Most health experts do agree on an average of a 1:1 to 4:1 ratio of omega-6s to omega-3s.

If you do opt for a fish oil supplement to help balance your ratio or for therapeutic use, be mindful of the source. Look for fish oil that:

- is of nutraceutical-grade or pharmaceutical-grade
- is third-party-certified for purity and quality
- is free from pesticides and heavy metals such as mercury, PCBs and dioxins—small fish tend to be less toxic
- is custom-made in small batch production
- is stored in a dark bottle (to prevent it from interacting with light)

What about fish itself? Try to buy wild fish rather than farmed fish. As mentioned in a previous chapter, farmed fish are grown in captivity and can contain the same growth hormones as farmed chicken and beef, raised solely for the purpose of profit. Choosing natural, wild-caught fish is better for you and also for the environment. If you are concerned about the mercury levels in fish, I recommend you visit www.gotmercury.com. As a basic rule, the smaller the fish, the better it is. Bigger fish have more time to accumulate a higher level of toxicity from the polluted ocean floor.

> *I will now pay much more attention to where the fish I purchase for our family comes from!*

The following diagram shows examples of health habits with corresponding hack levels. To download the *Hack Your Health Habits Worksheet*, visit

www.hackyourhealthhabits.com/worksheets

READY #HEALTHHACKER?
EXAMPLES OF LEVEL 1, 2 AND 3 HACKS FOR THIS CHAPTER

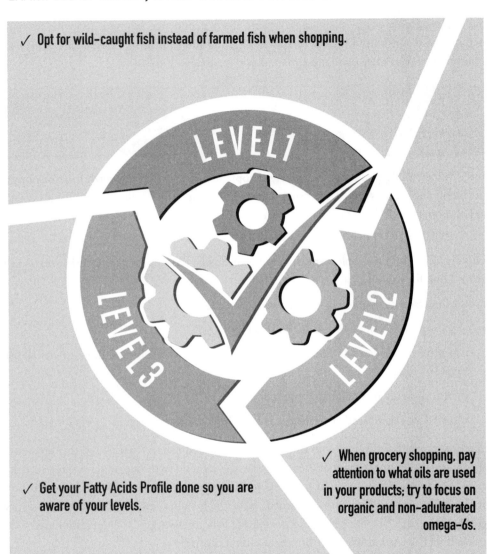

✓ Opt for wild-caught fish instead of farmed fish when shopping.

LEVEL1

LEVEL2

LEVEL3

✓ Get your Fatty Acids Profile done so you are aware of your levels.

✓ When grocery shopping, pay attention to what oils are used in your products; try to focus on organic and non-adulterated omega-6s.

HACK YOUR HEALTH PROGRESS

||||||||||||||||||||||||||||||||||||||||||||||||||||||||||||

CHAPTER 26

27

PROBIOTICS
Keep Your Bugs Happy!

"We now know that probiotics can affect gene expression."

— S. D. Annamalay

THINK IT OVER

- How do probiotics work to maintain gut health?

- Is yogurt a comprehensive source of probiotics?

- What effects do antibiotics have on the gut?

You have probably seen the commercials on TV for brands promoting the merits of healthy bacteria in yogurt for digestive health—even going as far as calling their products "probiotic yogurt." However, many people are still unaware of the role probiotics play and probably don't fully understand the extent of their benefits. Is yogurt a good enough source of probiotics? Should one take a probiotic supplement? What do the different strains mean, and what dosage should be taken? There is a lot of confusion and many myths about these good bugs, so let's dig in!

WHY DO WE NEED PROBIOTICS?

Probiotics play an important role in maintaining our gut flora. The human intestinal tract is home to approximately 100 trillion microorganisms, from more than 1,000 diverse bacterial species.[1]

Collectively, they are tremendously important for overall health. You have probably heard about "good bugs" and "bad bugs." The good bugs are the good bacteria that do a variety of positive things for us. For instance, they help us digest food, synthesize certain vitamins and play an important role in immune defense.

Good bugs need good foods to help them grow. Stress, changes in the diet, contaminated food, chlorinated water, use of certain medications and numerous other factors can alter the bacterial flora in the intestinal tract. The bottom line is that these good bugs are our friends, and we need them to stay happy by taking good care of them. A diet high in processed foods and sugar will feed the bad bugs and create dysbiosis, an imbalance in normal gut flora. This can really affect one's overall health, considering approximately 70 percent of our immune defense comes from the gut![2] More on this in **Chapter 39: Immune System—Is Yours Strong Enough?**

THE MANY BENEFITS OF PROBIOTICS

The health benefits of probiotics seem to be endless. By adding more probiotic foods into your diet, you could see all of the following benefits:

- stronger immune system
- improved digestion
- increased energy from production of vitamin B12
- better breath because probiotics destroy Candida
- healthier skin, since probiotics naturally treat eczema and psoriasis
- reduced colds and flu
- healing from leaky gut syndrome and inflammatory bowel disease
- weight loss

HOW PROBIOTICS WORK

As you will learn in Section 8, our intestinal tract is comprised of various parts, and these various parts contain different concentrations of bacteria. The majority of these bacteria reside in the large intestine. The large intestine is said to have between ten and one hundred billion bacteria, whereas the small intestine has only about ten thousand. Due to this, a common misconception is that supplementing with probiotics has very little effect on our gut microbiota, as a measly 25-50-billion colony-forming unit (CFU) can be seen quite small when compared to the hundreds of billions of bacteria found in the large intestine.

Although the majority of our bugs are found in the large intestine, the aim of probiotics is to populate the *small* intestine, where nutrients from food are absorbed into the bloodstream and where antibiotics tend to have the biggest effect, leaving us susceptible to health complications. The small intestine's membrane is only one cell layer deep, meaning that it is easier for bacteria to latch on and colonize it, By comparison, the large intestine can be up to 200 cells deep, making it more difficult for bacteria to latch on. Supplementing with a high-quality probiotic of a 25-100 billion CFU, therefore, has a great impact on repopulating the small intestine with the necessary bacteria to function optimally.

Here's how probiotics work: They help good bacteria create a barrier, or film-like coating, over the inner lining of the intestinal wall. This film keeps toxins and bad bacteria from gaining access to the wall—and through it, to your bloodstream.

One of the ways in which probiotics may help is by promoting healing and repair of the digestive tract. When the digestive tract is inflamed—due to the conditions mentioned above or infection and irritation by alcohol, painkillers, or antibiotics—it can become abnormally permeable, which is a major cause of the development of food sensitivities and autoimmune issues. This sequence of events can also cause other inflammatory diseases such as arthritis or cardiovascular diseases, conditions which have also been shown to improve with the help of probiotics.

The most proven benefit of probiotics is in cases of diarrhea—especially those brought on by bacterial infections. If you suffer from food sensitivities, chances are probiotics will help you, too. Many food reactions are not solely due to a sensitivity to the food, but also to the feeding of unfriendly bacteria, which then produce substances that activate the immune system in the gut.

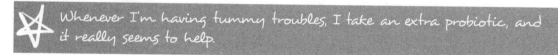

Whenever I'm having tummy troubles, I take an extra probiotic, and it really seems to help.

In addition, a 2014 meta-analysis of 20 trials done on adults and children concluded that probiotics reduce the duration of cough and cold symptoms by 30 percent, whereas 200 mg of vitamin C showed only an 18 percent reduction in children and only 14 percent in adults.[3] This clearly demonstrates the effectiveness of probiotics on the immune system.

More probiotics benefits include the fact that they:

- regulate local and systemic (i.e. full body) immune function
- break down nutrients for metabolite pathways, as well as for glycemic control, cholesterol and the amino acids that enhance gut health
- support the mucosal barrier
- enhance nutrient utilization and absorption
- prevent neoplastic changes
- regulate motility (i.e. gut muscle action)
- regulate appetite (i.e. leptin and ghrelin)
- prevent infection—systemic and gastrointestinal

FERMENTED FOODS AND YOGURT

Contrary to popular belief, yogurt may not be an ideal source of probiotics. Due to the process of pasteurization, the number of bacteria found in yogurt is greatly reduced. For this reason, companies that claim their yogurt has active cultures actually add live bacteria to the yogurt after the pasteurization process is complete. Depending on the brand, the type of strains of bacteria and the CFU will vary, making it difficult to keep track of the probiotic count one is ingesting and whether they provide enough variety. Another issue is that conventional yogurts are loaded with sugars and artificial sweeteners, and sometimes fillers such as cornstarch, which, in turn, are shown to cause gastrointestinal issues and feed the bad bacteria in our gut. For these reasons, it is best to try to make your own yogurt from home using grass-fed, organic dairy and bacteria cultures that can be purchased from any health food store.

Fermented foods are a helpful option to support gut health. Indian and Chinese cultures have been feeding their bodies with these fermented foods for centuries. Fermentation is done to preserve food, as well as enhance taste and flavors. These foods create good bacteria and are rich in enzymes that strengthen the immune system, help with the absorption of vitamins and minerals, and keep our brains sharper. New research shows that fermented foods such as sauerkraut, kimchi, kombucha—fermented for a long time so sugar content is lower—and pickled veggies, apple cider vinegar and tempeh help colonize the gut with healthy bacteria.[4]

> ✦ Mmm, I love kimchi in wraps or salads!

To get the maximum benefit of fermented foods, it is important to read product labels and choose only those that contain active, live cultures—preferably raw—and unpasteurized, perishable ingredients. Fermented vegetables and dairy products like kefir are the most popular options. When it comes to dairy, look for fermented, grass-fed options. Fermented foods can also be made at home, though the probiotic content will vary by batch. Home fermentation is a safe way to ensure that you are ingesting beneficial bacteria. You can use starter cultures such as SCOBY (Symbiotic Culture of Bacteria and Yeast) to easily ferment vegetables or brew kombucha from home.

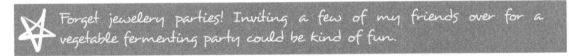

> ✦ Forget jewelery parties! Inviting a few of my friends over for a vegetable fermenting party could be kind of fun.

WHAT ARE PREBIOTICS?

Prebiotics are fiber-rich foods that on which good bacteria feed and grow. In order to be considered "prebiotic," food must be non-digestible by host enzymes, leading to fermentation in the gastrointestinal tract by bacteria. This means that prebiotic foods pass through the upper part of the gastrointestinal tract and remain undigested, as the human body can't fully break them down. Once they pass through the small intestine, they reach the colon, where they're fermented by the gut microflora. There they become "fuel" for the beneficial bacteria that live within your gut, making them happy and enabling them to do their job.

Some of the associated benefits of adding prebiotic foods to your diet include:

- lowered risk for cardiovascular disease

- improved digestion

- lowered stress response

- improved hormonal balance

- improved immune function

- lowered risk for obesity and weight gain

- lowered inflammation and autoimmune reactions

The following are prebiotic-rich foods:

- asparagus
- dandelion greens
- garlic
- kefir
- legumes
- acacia gum (or gum arabic)
- Jerusalem artichoke
- raw jicama

- banana
- eggplant
- honey
- leeks
- onion
- chicory root
- peas

Prebiotics and probiotics together play a fundamental role in preserving health by maintaining the balance and diversity of intestinal bacteria—especially increasing the amount of good bugs. Although, it is always best to get your prebiotics through food, there are supplements available when a person needs a high intake of prebiotics. Fructooligosaccharides (FOS), inulin, high-soluble fibers like Larch arabinogalactans and modified citrus pectin are all beneficial.

WHAT TO LOOK FOR IN A GOOD PROBIOTIC

In order to maintain colonization in the digestive tract, probiotics should be taken regularly. General maintenance recommendations call for ingesting a minimum of 12.5 to 25 billion CFU per serving per day, but, this can vary, based on an individual's specific health condition. For instance, a person who has immune or gut issues may need a higher CFU count in order to help repopulate and rebalance their gut.

To leverage your natural gut flora, lactic-acid-producing strains like lactobacillus and acidophilus are needed in the small and large intestine, respectively. By leveraging the hierarchy present in the gut, a good formulation will ensure that there is a critical balance to help replenish and maintain beneficial strains.

When you start using probiotic supplements, pay attention to how you feel. Are you noticing a reduction in gas and bloating? Are you becoming more regular? Typically, when taking probiotics, signs of digestive discomfort are supposed to decrease. However, if you feel that bloating or flatulence are increasing, it may be a sign that you have an underlying condition that requires gut-healing before you can introduce new strains of bacteria. One such condition is SIBO (Small Intestinal Bacterial Overgrowth), which we will cover in **Chapter 38: Your Gut—Understanding How It Works and What Could Go Wrong.** Also, people diagnosed with SIBO cannot easily handle probiotics that contain arabinogalactan.

Keep in mind that quality does matter—make sure that you use a probiotic brand that has many different strains to give you the variety of bugs that you need. It's also a good idea to cycle your probiotic strains to make sure you get as much variety as possible. Finally, remember to incorporate fermented foods into your diet!

PROBIOTICS, PREGNANT WOMEN AND KIDS

The importance of supplementing with a good probiotic becomes emphasized in certain periods of one's life. This is true for women during pregnancy and children during the first few years of their life, as the child's gut microbiota is forming. It has now been shown that, during the third trimester of pregnancy, a small number of flora from the small intestine of the mother is collected by dendritic cells and macrophages, and then transferred to the breast tissue via the lymphatic system, so that the newborn has exposure to some good flora during nursing. This is one of the reasons why breastfeeding is highly recommended. This is why it is strongly suggested women supplement with probiotics especially during pregnancy, to ensure adequate levels of healthy bugs in the child's small intestine.

Prior to birth, a newborn's gut is almost sterile. However, from the moment the infant enters the world, his or her microbiome begins to develop. The baby's first flora is acquired from the environment which the baby is born into. This highlights the importance of a vaginal birth, as much of the mother's healthy microflora—predominantly lactobacilli, streptococci and enterobacteria—is passed onto the newborn during this process.

In the instance of a C-section birth, the newborn's first encounter with bacteria is through the hospital environment—these bacteria play an important role for infants' intestinal colonization. Some authors have suggested that this lack of exposure of the mother's flora may be a predetermining factor for a number of complications later on in life. These can include allergies, autoimmunity and inflammatory bowel disease, but also vascular disease, some cancers, depression and anxiety.

For women who are delivering via a Caesarean (C-section)—either by choice or by lack thereof—taking a vaginal swab about an hour prior to giving birth, diluting it in water and squeezing the solution into the baby's mouth upon birth may be the best way to ensure the newborn is still being exposed to some of the mother's flora. Intestinal microbiota acquires adult characteristics and is fully formed by two years of age.

WHAT ABOUT TESTING?

Out of the 100 trillion bacteria in the gut, we probably understand only 1,000 of these bacteria, meaning, we are still in the infant stages of understanding our microbiome. Still, testing is available to discover imbalances anywhere in the Gastrointestinal (GI) tract process. This helps us discover issues like indigestion, malabsorption, Irritable Bowel Syndrome (IBS), altered GI and immune function, bacterial or fungal overgrowth, or chronic dysbiosis.

Bacterial cultures of fecal material (collected by a stool sample) are able to give us information on organisms that constitute part of the normal aerobic or commensal flora—meaning the ones that are not recognized as major pathogens. It will also monitor for "opportunistic" pathogens, which may overgrow during periods of stress; their presence may be an indicator of gut dysbiosis. Results should always be interpreted in the context of a person's symptoms and overall health status.

ANTIBIOTICS—THE ULTIMATE BUG-KILLER

One of the many factors to consider when taking an antibiotic are their potential side effects. According to the Centers for Disease Control (CDC), antibiotics are prescribed unnecessarily almost 50 percent of the time.[5] While effective in killing pathogenic bacteria, antibiotics are essentially non-selective and will kill off beneficial gut bacteria, as well. Because there is no distinction between the good and bad bugs, taking antibiotics repeatedly may wreak havoc on the body's digestive and immune system.

There is also the risk that one may develop bacteria that are resistant to common antibiotics over time, which could be dangerous when trying to treat more serious bacterial infections down the road. In addition, recent studies show that good bacteria in our gut have the capability of influencing our gene expression. If good bugs are removed, gene expression may be affected in the long run, resulting in "bad" genes being turned on and leaving us more susceptible to certain illnesses.

Even if you haven't been prescribed antibiotics yourself, you can experience their harmful side effects. How is this possible? Conventionally raised meats are full of antibiotics. In fact, a whopping 60 percent of all antibiotics used in the United States' are used on livestock.[6] Due to their deplorable living conditions, livestock need antibiotics to prevent illness. When we consume these meats, we unintentionally consume antibiotics that have a negative effect on our bodies. Consequences include gut dysbiosis and the disruption of many other systems that are modulated by the gut. This will be further looked at in Section 8.

It is highly recommended that you avoid the use of antibiotics unless absolutely necessary. If you have to take them, make sure you take high dosages of high-quality probiotics to aid in repopulating the good bacteria in your gut that will have been destroyed by the antibiotics. Now I know what you may be thinking: Wouldn't taking an antibiotic with a probiotic defeat the purpose? Yes and no; you do not want to take them together. Rather, make sure you take your probiotic two hours before or two hours after taking an antibiotic to ensure that they do not interfere. Many companies have a specific formula for antibiotic therapy support as it is so crucial to replenish those bugs to prevent further complications in the gut down the line.

SKINNY BUGS VERSUS FAT BUGS?

Yes, you read right! Thin people have different intestinal bugs than obese people. Researchers at the Genome Sequencing Centre at Washington University have demonstrated that there are notable differences in the bacteria of a lean person versus the bacteria of an obese person.[7] Lean individuals in the study had a higher ratio of a kind of bacteria called Bacteroidetes in comparison to another kind called Firmicutes. While obese subjects were found to have much higher levels of Firmicutes when compared to levels of Bacteroidetes. The ratio of Firmicutes-to-Bacteroidetes has been shown to be critical for determining health and risk of diseases. And, if that was not enough for us to pay attention to this ratio, recent studies show that higher levels of Firmicutes actually have the potential to turn on genes that increase risks of obesity, diabetes and even cardiovascular disease.[8]

IN CONCLUSION

Probiotics and fermented foods have been a part of the human diet for thousands of years. It is important to ensure that we are getting an adequate supply of them to keep our good bacteria happy. As mentioned in this chapter, insufficient gut bacteria come with a slew of health effects, including digestive disorders, skin issues, Candida, autoimmune diseases, weight gain and even compromised gene expression. Modern-day science is linking more and more widespread chronic conditions to gut health, so a happy gut is truly a happy you!

The following diagram shows examples of health habits with corresponding hack levels. To download the *Hack Your Health Habits Worksheet*, visit

www.hackyourhealthhabits.com/worksheets

READY #HEALTHHACKER?
EXAMPLES OF LEVEL 1, 2 AND 3 HACKS FOR THIS CHAPTER

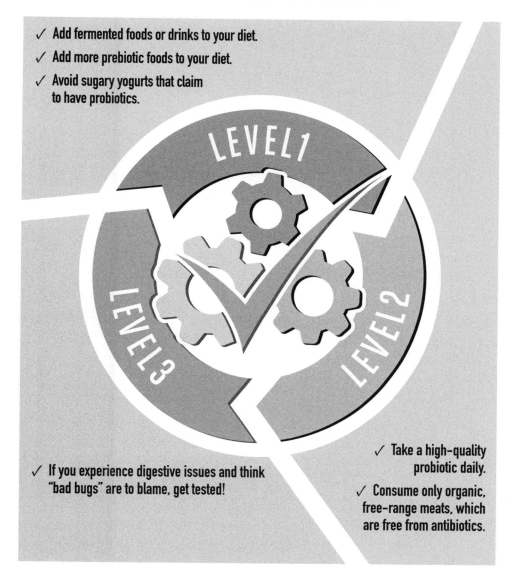

✓ Add fermented foods or drinks to your diet.

✓ Add more prebiotic foods to your diet.

✓ Avoid sugary yogurts that claim to have probiotics.

LEVEL 1

LEVEL 2

LEVEL 3

✓ If you experience digestive issues and think "bad bugs" are to blame, get tested!

✓ Take a high-quality probiotic daily.

✓ Consume only organic, free-range meats, which are free from antibiotics.

HACK YOUR HEALTH PROGRESS

||||||||||||||||||||||||||||||||

CHAPTER 27

SECTION 6

Get Fit and Strong in Less Time

Feel like you never have the time to workout? Fear no more! While exercise might be a foundation for good health, you don't need spend countless hours in a gym each day to stay fit. In Section 6, you learn why shorter, more functional workouts are actually better for you and how you can turn exercise into a habit that you actually enjoy.

THE GOAL OF FITNESS
Use It or Lose It

THINK IT OVER

- **What does being fit mean to you?**

- **Do you truly understand the benefits of exercise on your overall health?**

- **Is fitness integrated into your weekly calendar, or is it just an afterthought?**

When you think of a fit individual, what do you envision? It's likely you imagine a good-looking person with a toned, sculpted and lean body. This isn't surprising as fitness is most often associated with physical appearance. For women, that means a flat tummy, long, sculpted legs, a rounded bum and toned arms. For men, that means a hefty chest, pumped-up arms and washboard abs. There is nothing wrong with these images; in fact, these bodies are likely healthy and fit. However, there *is* an issue with society's current perception of fitness.

In today's world, we tend to view fitness as looking a certain way. Corporations are making billions of dollars off of selling a vision of fitness based purely on appearances. They prey upon our insecurities, urging us to try weight loss pills, shakes, waist-cinchers, fat burners, metabolism boosters and super detox teas. They use gorgeous models with flawless bodies, and promise that we can "Drop 2 sizes in 2 weeks!" or "Get beach-body ready in no time!"

But, that's not what fitness is about. Fitness is about so much more than weight management or a quick fix. We need to remember that, just because someone looks fit, doesn't mean that they are healthy. Those pumped-up arms could be the result of steroid use, that flat tummy might be the result of starvation, and that gorgeous body could be the result of winning the genetic lottery. In order to understand fitness, we need to realize that it extends far beyond appearances.

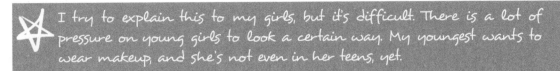

I try to explain this to my girls, but it's difficult. There is a lot of pressure on young girls to look a certain way. My youngest wants to wear makeup, and she's not even in her teens, yet.

To get a better picture of what true fitness is, let's first define health. The World Health Organization came up with a comprehensive definition in 1948, defining health as: "a state of complete physical, mental and social well-being and not merely the absence of disease or infirmity."[1] This definition is good but is still somewhat vague. What exactly does "complete well-being" mean? Does it mean being symptom-free? Based on this, how could we explain it when a person who goes in for a routine check-up feeling great, but then leaves with a cancer diagnosis? Or, what about a very athletic person who eats great, regularly trains and ends up dropping dead of a heart attack?

The challenge, when it comes to health, is how exactly do we measure it? Is health being able to run a marathon, lift weights, or perform yoga poses? Is it an "all clear" on routine blood tests? Is it eating right and taking your vitamins? Yes, technology has come a long way, and it is now much easier to get a diagnosis, but our society has often placed the focus on treating the symptoms and not so much on finding and resolving the cause of disease. Moreover, our testing focuses on measuring "sickness" parameters, rather than "wellness" parameters. The parameters are things such as inflammatory markers and liver enzymes rather than examining nutrient levels and cofactors for optimal body function. We tend to take a reactive approach to health when we should really be focusing on a preventative approach.

With the above in mind, exercise becomes more about optimal health, better functioning, and longer life expectancy than merely physical appearance. It becomes a science that we need to truly comprehend and apply if we want to be healthy. From an evolutionary standpoint, our bodies are made for movement. They are not meant to be sedentary for long periods of time. Exercise does more than just burn fat or build muscle; it impacts our bodies on a cellular level. It benefits the brain and endocrine system in more ways than any other stimulus out there. No shake, diet pill, or waist-cincher can achieve the same result. The benefits of exercise are vast! Here are just some of the ways physical activity can benefit us.

MENTAL HEALTH

Regular exercise

- improves cognitive function and memory
- effectively treats anxiety and depression

- releases endorphins and improves mood
- improves sleep quality
- helps foster new and healthy relationships
- makes you a positive role model for family and friends
- increases self-esteem and self-confidence
- makes you more productive and efficient at work
- improves energy levels
- increases blood supply to the brain
- makes you happier

HEART HEALTH

Regular exercise

- reduces your resting heart rate
- reduces the workload on the heart
- improves muscular and cardiovascular endurance
- reduces your risk of cardiovascular disease
- reduces your blood pressure
- improves cholesterol levels
- decreases blood triglycerides

JOINT, BONE & MUSCLE HEALTH

Regular exercise

- increases blood supply to muscles
- improves flexibility through increased mobility
- stimulates bone growth and improves bone strength and density
- gives you stronger ligaments, tendons and joints
- helps relieve arthritis pain
- improves balance
- increases lean body mass
- improves your day-to-day functional strength
- improves posture

- makes you stronger
- protects against injury
- improves recovery time when rehabilitating injuries

LUNG HEALTH

Regular exercise

- improves V02 max, your body's upper limit for consuming and distributing oxygen for the purpose of energy production
- increases lung capacity
- increases EPOC, your excess post-exercise consumption

HORMONE HEALTH

Regular exercise

- improves glucose metabolism
- improves insulin sensitivity
- effectively manages type 2 diabetes
- boosts metabolism and enables more calorie burning when at rest
- increases mitochondrial (the powerhouse of a cell) function for more efficient fat burning
- lowers body fat levels
- helps you become a better fat burner
- improves leptin sensitivity (leptin is our satiety hormone)
- helps prevent obesity
- helps prevent muscle loss when losing weight
- increases thyroid hormone
- increases growth hormone levels
- boosts testosterone production and increases sex drive
- enhances immune function

DETOXIFICATION

Regular exercise

- gets the bowels moving for more effective elimination

- prevents lymph from becoming stagnant

- helps eliminate toxic substances through sweating

AGING

Regular exercise

- increases longevity

- makes you look younger

- reduces your risk of breast and colon cancer

- can help you quit smoking

Yes, this is a long list! You may have read it and said to yourself, "Yeah, I know all this!" Yet, there are some people who prefer to gamble with their health rather than make a concerted effort to *prevent* potential health problems by exercising regularly. There's a huge difference between knowing and doing. In fact, after more than two decades of seeing patients who do not exercise, it still baffles me that while we all know about the benefits of exercise, people are still not making time for it.

There are many reasons why exercise should become part of your daily routine that goes beyond the typical goal of wanting to lose weight. A fitness regimen, powered by the goal of attaining a certain physique, is not going to last long. *Fitness should be viewed as a crucial aspect of physical and emotional well-being.*

 This is so motivating. I've always viewed exercise as a way to maintain my weight. I never realized just how integral it is to every single aspect of my health.

HOW TO BECOME FIT

To start, find a fitness atmosphere that best suits your needs and lifestyle. Once you've found an atmosphere, develop a workout plan that will vary in intensity so the body does not adapt to it. Some may prefer staying fit through regular team sports and drills, while others may prefer a gym membership and sessions with a personal trainer, or to attend fitness classes. It's important to find a workout environment that feels comfortable for you and that motivates you. If the gym stresses you out, don't force yourself to go. There are plenty of things you can do outdoors or inside your home.

The same goes for types of exercises; some may prefer body-weight-oriented exercises like yoga, while others may prefer higher intensity level workouts like boot camps or CrossFit. Identifying what works for you is an important part of developing a fitness regime. If you don't enjoy the exercise you are doing, there is a lesser chance you will stick with it. There are so many different ways to stay fit—find something you will love doing that will keep you active!

Next, change your mindset about exercise. Stop viewing exercise as a chore, or a punishment for eating junk food. How many times have you heard someone say: "I've got to hit the gym later—someone brought donuts to work this morning?" Fitness should not be a punishment for what you've eaten, but rather a reward for everything your body is capable of doing.

Think back to the many benefits of exercise listed earlier on in this chapter. A workout isn't punishing our body, it's rewarding it! After a workout, you should feel better, think clearer and sleep better. When we shift our perspective of exercise from a punishment to what it really is—a reward—we become much more inclined to participate in physical activity rather than dread it. Celebrate what your body can do.

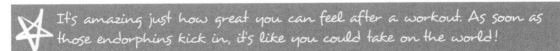

It's amazing just how great you can feel after a workout. As soon as those endorphins kick in, it's like you could take on the world!

Fitness isn't just a look. It's also a mindset. How fit are you?

The following diagram shows examples of health habits with corresponding hack levels. To download the *Hack Your Health Habits Worksheet*, visit

www.hackyourhealthhabits.com/worksheets

READY #HEALTHHACKER?
EXAMPLES OF LEVEL 1, 2 AND 3 HACKS FOR THIS CHAPTER

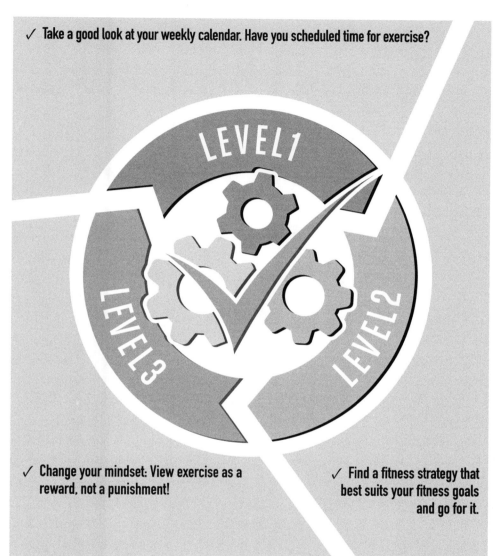

✓ Take a good look at your weekly calendar. Have you scheduled time for exercise?

LEVEL 1

LEVEL 2

LEVEL 3

✓ Change your mindset: View exercise as a reward, not a punishment!

✓ Find a fitness strategy that best suits your fitness goals and go for it.

HACK YOUR HEALTH PROGRESS

||||||||||||||||||||||||||||||||||||

CHAPTER 28

BEYOND BEING FIT
Be Functional

"Nothing will work unless you do."

— Maya Angelou

THINK IT OVER

- What is functional fitness?

- Are you practicing "safe form?"

- Do you know what tools or programs are available to measure your body functionality?

Have you heard the expression "fundamentals first?" Top-level coaches and professionals use this expression to advocate starting with the basics. What does this mean? While we may *think* that we are ready to sign up for an advanced Pilates or CrossFit class, failing to master the basics beforehand puts us at risk of injury. "Fundamentals first" requires you to perform the movement with correct form before moving onto a high-performance class or even adding weight to a complex movement that you have not yet mastered.

Here is something I see all the time as a chiropractor: Patients who try to get back into shape yet keep injuring their back at the gym. When asked what their routine consists of, they name countless machines they use. However, when I get them to perform a simple bodyweight squat for me, it is evident that their form is off. Due to their improper biomechanics, loading up the weights is doing them more harm than good. No wonder they keep injuring themselves! We can't move into complex heavy movements without getting the basics right.

> ✦ *Argh, I made the same mistake! Recently, I pushed myself too hard strength training and pulled a hamstring. I was limping for days.*

The primary goal of *all* exercise programs should be to *prevent* injury or any abnormal repetitive movements that could lead to injury or wear and tear on the body (e.g. osteoarthritis, disc-degeneration disease, tendinitis, bursitis, etc.). This should be considered even more important than weight loss, muscle building, and performance-enhancement goals, because what good are goals like these if an injury leaves you unable to perform, or creates imbalances in your body?

> ✦ *Very true. My hamstring incident resulted in an inability to exercise for a few weeks. On top of that, I put more weight on my uninjured leg to compensate, which led to lower back and hip problems.*

Exercise is meant to improve daily movement and strengthen muscles to protect joints, bones and ligaments. The types of exercise you do should mimic the functional movements you perform every day. These include movements like bending over to pick up something relatively heavy, reaching overhead, squatting to sit, or twisting. These types of exercises are known as functional fitness exercises. Functional fitness exercises require you to use muscles in multiple areas of the body simultaneously to engage the core. They also train your muscles to work together, simulating common movements you do at home, work, or while playing sports.[1]

One of my older female patients, who has the funniest and most sarcastic sense of humor I know, came in for her appointment one day and told me, "We have a problem. My back goes out more than I do!" Have you ever bent down to pick up something off the floor only to have your back "go out" on you? It's these kinds of occurrences that make functional exercise so important—especially nowadays when most people are seated at a computer from 9 a.m. to 5 p.m. In case you didn't already know, our bodies were not built to be hunched over and staring at a computer all day. These positions leave our bodies with abnormal physical strains and imbalances, which will be discussed more in the next chapter.

WHAT ARE THE BENEFITS OF FUNCTIONAL FITNESS TRAINING?

Functional exercises tend to use multiple parts of the body at once. Instead of only moving the knees, for example, a functional exercise might involve the shoulders, spine, hips and ankles. As mentioned, this type of training, when done properly, can make everyday activities easier, reduce your risk of injury and improve your quality of life. Functional training may be especially beneficial for older adults to improve balance, agility and muscle strength, as well as reduce the risk of falls. Multifaceted physical movements, found in activities such as Tai Chi and yoga, involve varying combinations of flexibility training and resistance that can help build functional fitness.

It's a good idea to start with exercises that use only your own bodyweight as resistance when beginning an exercise program. As you become fitter and ready for more difficult movements, you can add more resistance in the form of weights, resistance bands, or performing movements in the water. As your workouts become more functional, you should see improvements in your ability to perform your everyday activities. That's quite a return on your exercise investment!

THE IMPORTANCE OF NATURAL MOVEMENT PATTERNS

As I mentioned earlier, most of our bodies are no longer moving the way they are meant to. From driving commutes to long hours at a desk to leisure time dominated by screen time, many of us live increasingly sedentary lives. We no longer scavenge or grow our food, build shelter, or otherwise work physically to ensure our survival—in other words, we no longer perform the primal movement patterns for which our bodies were designed. If we neglect our natural roots, our bodies are going to pay dearly for it. And, that is why issues such as poor posture, lower back pain, neck pain and poor circulation—just to name a few—have recently become so prevalent.

Functional exercises—like squatting, lunging, lifting overhead, picking up a weight, pushing or pulling our own body weight or an object—mimic our natural movement patterns and, therefore, keep our muscles and joints functional. This decreases our risk of injury or pain while improving flexibility, strength and functionality.

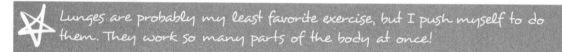

Lunges are probably my least favorite exercise, but I push myself to do them. They work so many parts of the body at once!

SCREENING TOOLS

There are various screening tools available to assess your body's functionality, such as the Functional Movement Screen (FMS). This screening process looks at "fundamental movements, motor control within movements, and our ability to perform basic movement patterns."[2] Its goal is to "determine movement deficiency and uncover asymmetry." Another tool is the Selective Functional Movement Assessment (SFMA), which is a diagnostic system, designed to clinically assess seven fundamental movement patterns in those with known musculoskeletal pain.

The assessment provides an efficient method to systematically find the cause of symptoms by logically breaking down dysfunctional patterns and diagnosing their root cause as either a mobility problem or a stability/motor control problem. Based on an individual's results, the trainer or clinician can recommend corrective exercises to improve mobility and motor control for better functionality.

When it comes to fitness, don't be afraid to ask for professional help. Finding someone who is trained to detect these abnormal movement patterns can help correct or prevent pain and discomfort. These screens can be done with any qualified FMS and SFMA practitioners.

REMEMBER, FUNDAMENTALS FIRST

Like I mentioned at the start of this chapter, in my 20+ years of chiropractic practice, I have seen so many people—with the best intentions—injure themselves while exercising and become incredibly discouraged because of it. Our body needs to be prepared for exercise. We have to go at it slowly, wisely and consistently if we want to function optimally and with minimal pain. As the great author and motivational speaker, Jim Rohn said, "Take good care of your body. It's the only place you have to live."

Remember, the goal is to become functional before we get into more complex exercises. We want to ensure that the body is moving in its natural range of motion before putting heavier loads onto it. Let's get back to basics to be fit, functional and injury free!

The following diagram shows examples of health habits with corresponding hack levels. To download the *Hack Your Health Habits Worksheet*, visit

www.hackyourhealthhabits.com/worksheets

READY #HEALTHHACKER?
EXAMPLES OF LEVEL 1, 2 AND 3 HACKS FOR THIS CHAPTER

✓ Get up and move during the day. Set a timer on your computer to remind you to get up regularly.

✓ Incorporate functional fitness moves into your workouts.

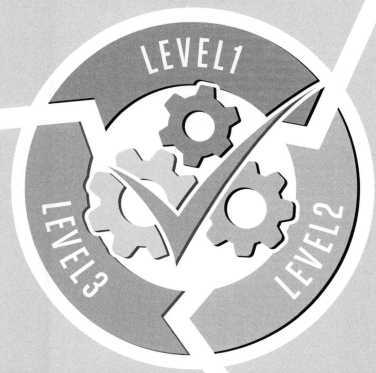

✓ Undergo a Functional Movement Screen and seek professional help to ensure you know the basics.

✓ Sign up for a weekly yoga or tai chi class to help maintain functionality.

HACK YOUR HEALTH PROGRESS

|||||||||||||||||||||||||||||||||||

CHAPTER 29

HIGH-INTENSITY INTERVAL TRAINING (HIIT)
Keep It Short and Efficient

"HIIT me baby one
more time."

— Unknown

THINK IT OVER

- How efficient are your workouts?

- Are exercises like jogging and biking best for fat loss?

- What methods are known to give the best results in less time?

Tired of spending hours at the gym or not having enough time to fit workouts into your day? Well, I have some good news for you: New science is showing that we do not need to spend prolonged periods of time exercising to see benefits. Rather, short bursts of intense exercise—typically lasting from just a few minutes to under a half-hour—are shown to be as effective for fat loss, boosting energy and feeling great.

HIIT stands for High-Intensity Interval Training—sometimes simply referred to as interval training. It consists of bursts of intense movement, followed by a rest or less intense exercise. This type of exercise employs high intensity to improve cardiovascular and muscular fitness, but it doesn't stop there. HIIT rewards the body in many ways, including boosting physical performance, weight loss and many other benefits that go beyond those of steady-state endurance training.

Here's the thing, though—while a HIIT workout can be quick, it does require maximal effort. Sessions can last from 4 to 45 minutes and can include various workout styles such as bodyweight, plyometric (explosive exercises) and resistance exercises. The most popular form of HIIT is known as Tabata. It was researched in 1996 by Professor Izumi Tabata. Research involved Olympic athletes who were asked to perform 20 seconds of ultra-high-intensity cycling, followed by 10 seconds of rest, on a stationary bike. Research concluded that HIIT was more effective at improving aerobic and anaerobic capacities.[1]

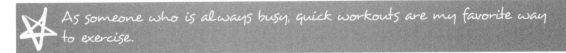

As someone who is always busy, quick workouts are my favorite way to exercise.

WHY HIIT?

Research continues to show that interval training increases the body's calories expended and overall level of fitness more than steady-state exercise. Endurance exercise, such as power walking, jogging, biking and so on, is simply a form of cardio paced at a continuous, steady rate. The oxygen supply meets oxygen demand, and the heart beats at a constant pace, even if it is higher than the normal resting rate. During HIIT exercise, however, your energy output varies, and you become nearly breathless for short periods of time.

This level of intensity expands your body's upper limit for consuming and distributing oxygen (called your VO2 Max) for the purpose of energy production.[2] In addition, the cardiovascular system adapts to aerobic stressors and responds by becoming stronger, more resilient, and better able to handle the stress of greater activity at more intense levels.

This means a stronger heart muscle, improved lung capacity and better overall cardiorespiratory performance. Other physical benefits include increased contractions of skeletal muscles, which boosts blood flow, greater ATP (i.e. energy) production[3], increased reliance on fat as an energy source rather than sugars[4], greater endurance of slow-twitch muscle fibers and increased mitochondrial function (mitochondria are the powerhouse of a cell). The more the body is forced into an anaerobic state—which can be induced by explosive movement—rather than an aerobic state, the more it becomes efficient at creating energy for your muscles at that level of performance.[5]

In the past, it was believed that aerobic activity was the more reliable method for burning fat as an energy source. But, research conducted in 2008 found that fat burning was significantly higher after six weeks of HIIT training.[6] This has an important implication for women trying to control their weight through steady-state exercise. Our bodies are designed to recognize patterns and repetitive activities such as jogging. When steady-state activities are performed, the body will adapt to that steady stimulus and will work to conserve energy rather than expend it. An alternative to running is to perform sprints, bursts of maximal effort runs followed by a few moments of rest and repeat. This will improve performance and burn more energy in the long run.

Already sold? There's more! Another amazing benefit of HIIT training is its ability to burn calories even hours after the workout is completed. Wait, what? After the high-intensity exercise or heavy workout, the body continues to require and use oxygen at an elevated rate—more so than before the exercise session. This sustained energy requirement is known as excess post-exercise oxygen consumption, or EPOC for short. During EPOC, the body works hard to restore itself to its pre-workout status by consuming oxygen at a higher rate, as disruption to the normal state of the body at rest translates to increased energy usage. The body also continues to expend energy to re-oxygenate the blood after your workout is complete.

UP FOR THE CHALLENGE?

There are lots of different styles of HIIT. Here are a few to choose from.

THE TABATA METHOD

This advanced training method, calls for 20 seconds of high-intensity work, followed by 10 seconds of rest for 8 cycles. Total workout time is about 4 minutes, though you could do multiple Tabatas within one workout. Your Tabata could be cardio-based like sprinting, rowing, skipping rope, or cycling; or it could involve bodyweight exercises like squats, push-ups, or pull-ups. You could even combine both within the same workout. The key is to work at maximum effort and at a recommended frequency of 2-4x per week.

Workout Format
3-Minute Warm Up
20-Second High-Intensity Effort
10-Second Rest
Repeat for 8 Cycles
5-Min. Cool-Down

 There are plenty of great Tabata apps on the market. Almost all have an interval timer and audio cues to make your workout easier.

THE GIBALA REGIMEN

Sometimes referred to as "The Little Method," this HIIT protocol is based on a 2009 study conducted by Professors Martin Gibala and Jonathan Little at McMaster University. It calls for 8-12 cycles of 60 seconds of intense exercise, followed by 75 seconds of low-intensity effort for a total of about 27 minutes. It has a recommended frequency of three times per week.

Workout Format
3-Minute Warm Up
60-Second High-Intensity Effort
75-Second Low-Intensity Effort

Repeat 10 to 12 Cycles
5 Min. Cool-Down

TURBULENCE TRAINING

Developed by former athlete and exercise physiology researcher, Craig Ballantyne, Turbulence training combines weight training with cardio-style exercises. This intermediate-level workout alternates 8 repetitions of various weight-training exercises with 1 to 2 minutes of cardio-based exercise for a maximum of 45 minutes. It has a recommended frequency of 3x per week.

Workout Format
5-Minute Warm Up
8-Rep Set of Full-Body Weight-Lifting Exercise
1 to 2 Minutes of Mountain Climbers
Repeat Through Full Body Routine

READY TO HIIT THE GYM?

HIIT is an incredibly effective style of training for improving your fitness in a short period of time, but it is also extremely challenging. Always be sure to check with your health-care professional before starting any new exercise program. Remember, when it comes to any type of exercise, form is vital, if you want to avoid injuries!

The following diagram shows examples of health habits with corresponding hack levels. To download the *Hack Your Health Habits Worksheet*, visit

www.hackyourhealthhabits.com/worksheets

READY #HEALTHHACKER?
EXAMPLES OF LEVEL 1, 2 AND 3 HACKS FOR THIS CHAPTER

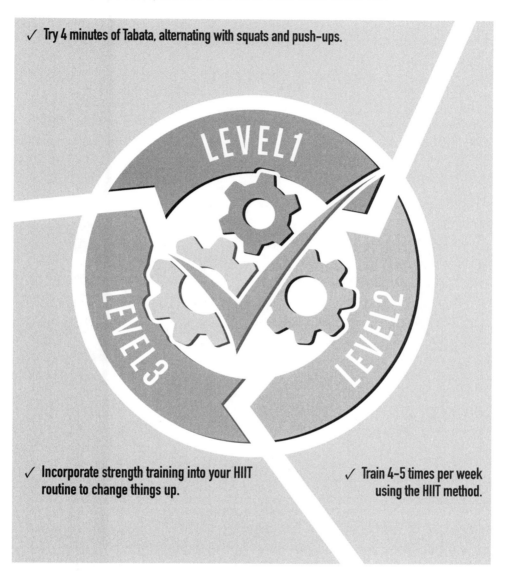

✓ Try 4 minutes of Tabata, alternating with squats and push-ups.

✓ Incorporate strength training into your HIIT routine to change things up.

✓ Train 4–5 times per week using the HIIT method.

HACK YOUR HEALTH PROGRESS

CHAPTER 30

STRENGTH TRAINING
Strong Is the New Sexy

"The only bad workout is the one you didn't do."

— Unknown

THINK IT OVER

- Do you feel intimidated by lifting weights?

- Do you regularly incorporate strength training into your fitness routine?

- What strength training techniques can help improve your overall health?

Whether you're looking to lose weight, keep your energy levels high, gain strength, or keep your muscles healthy and strong, strength training is one of the best exercises you can do.

 For the longest time, I believed cardio was the only way I was going to lose weight, but it wasn't until I started strength training that I really noticed a change in my body.

THE MANY BENEFITS OF STRENGTH TRAINING

Strength training (or resistance training) involves muscular contractions and extensions against gravity using weights, bands, or even your own bodyweight to develop or maintain lean muscle tissue. Lifting weights has been shown to halt and even reverse sarcopenia, which is the reduction of skeletal muscles that occurs as we age. It has also been shown to improve overall mood and increase cognitive function. In addition, strength training is known to produce a greater level of excess post-exercise oxygen consumption (EPOC) than aerobic exercise.

As we learned before, EPOC is what occurs after a workout. Your body works hard to replenish oxygen in order to bring itself back to its normal state—the way it was before you worked out. This takes a lot of energy, and some studies show that it can boost your metabolism for up to 48 hours after your workout is done.[1]

Another great benefit of strength training is its ability to improve posture, which we will discuss in great details in **Chapter 33: Straighten-Up! Is Your Posture Wearing You Out?** Stronger muscles help you sit and stand straighter and more comfortably. This improves muscle stability and makes you less likely to slouch.

What's more, developing strength can enhance the performance of your everyday tasks like taking out the garbage, walking the dog, or picking up after your kids. Working muscles through a full range of motion increases flexibility and reduces the risk of injuries or pain. Strong muscles, tendons and ligaments are less likely to give way under stress. These aren't the only benefits of strength training, though. There are several more, including the fact that it:

- reduces the risk of diabetes
- lowers risk of cardiovascular disease
- lowers high blood pressure
- lowers risk of breast cancer
- decreases or minimizes the risk of osteoporosis by building bone mass
- reduces inflammation
- reduces symptoms of PMS (Premenstrual Syndrome)
- reduces stress and anxiety
- decreases colds and illness
- boosts energy
- increases mental alertness

HOW DOES STRENGTH TRAINING WORK?

Before we actually start lifting anything, the first thing we need to do is have a basic understanding of how our muscles work and why lifting weights can benefit them. We have hundreds of muscles in our body, and they all work cohesively to help our bodies perform daily tasks. For example, when you bend your arm, your bicep contracts and your triceps elongates in order to let your elbow bend. When you extend your arm, the exact opposite happens.

These muscles are made up of many smaller muscle cells, more commonly known as muscle fibers, which are long and cylindrical, and about the size of a single strand of hair.

These fibers can be divided into two categories:

- **Slow twitch (or type I fibers)** – These are used for aerobic exercises where we need to convert oxygen into fuel over long periods of time. They are very resistant to fatigue, but do not move very quickly. These are meant for endurance exercises like running long distances.

- **Fast twitch (or type II fibers)** – These fire very quickly, but also fatigue quickly, so they don't last long. It gets a bit more complicated because there are actually two types of fast-twitch fibers. Type II fibers have some endurance qualities. They are used for things such as longer sprints. Meanwhile, type II fibers are our "super-fast" fibers, used only when a super-short burst is needed—like during HIIT training, in a sprint, or a really heavy lift.

Oftentimes, people believe that we can increase the amount of muscle fibers we have by weight training. In reality, we're born with a set amount of muscle fibers. We can't actually increase the number of muscle fibers, but we can increase their *size*. This is called hypertrophy, and two factors contribute to it:

1. Repeated use of the muscle causes the muscle tissue to break down, and it is then rebuilt by the body. The rebuilt muscle becomes stronger and, through repeated exposure, lifting a certain amount of weight becomes easier.

 So, that's why my muscles will hurt after some workouts!

2. An increase in repetitions (or "reps") leads to an increase in the glycogen storage in your muscle, which gives muscles the "pumped up" appearance.[2]

STRENGTH TRAINING AND WEIGHT LOSS

One misconception about lifting weights, especially for women, is that pumping iron will make you big and bulky. The truth is, women don't have the genetic makeup to get "bulky" from just a few strength training sessions a week. This would happen only if a woman takes anabolic steroids, which I definitely do not recommend—as you could end up looking like a female version of the famous bodybuilder Arnold Schwarzenegger, among many other serious issues.

 I used to think that strength training would make me bulkier. I'm actually leaner now.

When it comes to weight loss, regular strength training decreases adipose tissue—your fat stores. This is key to fat loss and the main reason why strength training has been shown to be more effective than cardio. Cardio is great for maintaining a healthy heart, but not so much for creating fat loss. This is because aerobic activity burns off water weight and even some muscle mass, but does not have a huge impact on body fat. Those relying on aerobic exercises to lose weight will often be what is called "skinny fat"—where a person looks thin but has a high body-fat percentage and a low muscle mass.

Compound weight-lifting exercises—that use multiple muscle groups like deadlifts or squat-to-presses—tap into fat stores for energy and help in the development of muscle.[3] This results in a more toned and sculpted figure. Due to an increase in muscle tissue and a decrease in fat, the number on the scale may not drop as quickly as someone who sticks to only cardio. This is because the body is burning fat tissue and building muscle, and muscle weighs more than fat. While your weight may not fluctuate as much, you will see inches coming off your frame and your overall body composition improving.

 I went from a size 10 to 6, without budging much on the scale!

STRENGTH AND MUSCLE IMBALANCE

Another reason proper strength training should be included in your workout regime is its ability to improve muscle imbalances. There are two scenarios that can potentially be the cause of muscle imbalance. The first is a *biomechanical* cause due to repeated movements using isolated muscle groups or sustained postures over a long duration of time—such as sitting and typing for eight hours a day. The second cause is a *sensorimotor* imbalance due to an interference in the transmission of signals between the brain and that specific muscle.[4]

Muscle imbalances are even more common now with our more sedentary lifestyles. When a person sits all day at work, for example, the hip flexors will become shorter. When such a muscle is shorter than its optimal length, it not only affects the opposing muscle, but can have repercussions on the entire musculoskeletal system. Common muscles that cause lower back pain and postural problems are tight hamstrings, hip flexors and upper-middle back muscles. Slouching and carrying your head forward are also side effects of sitting for prolonged periods of time, which can cause loss of neck curvature, leading to headaches and many more health issues.[5]

CORRECTING MUSCLE IMBALANCES

In order to correct muscle imbalances, it is important to strengthen the major muscle groups and their antagonistic (or opposite) muscles. An example of this would be the quadriceps and hamstrings.

It is also important to strengthen the two musculoskeletal groups that play a key role in good posture:

- **Core** – The "core" consists of the abdominal muscles (i.e. rectus abdominis, transverse abdominis, internal and external obliques) and your lower back muscles (i.e. paraspinals, quadratus lumborum). Most people neglect their back muscles while performing core exercises by mistakenly assuming the core only consists of the rectus abdominis, or the "six pack." By performing proper core-strengthening exercises, you will teach your body to maintain proper postural alignment for the duration of all your exercises. You will also improve your static posture for sitting or standing in place.

- **Glutes** – The glutes comprise of three main muscles: the gluteus maximus, minimus and medius—a.k.a. your 'butt' muscles. To improve the length and tension relationship between your hip flexors and your glutes, you should focus on proper glute exercises such as squats and lunges. These muscles are typically weak and can cause tightness in your hip flexor muscles, which can lead to injury.

MY 20 TIPS FOR OPTIMAL STRENGTH TRAINING

1. **Hire a trainer** – It's worth the money, especially if you're not comfortable or familiar with strength training. This can help you learn what kind of routine works best for your goals and may even help reduce the risk of injury.

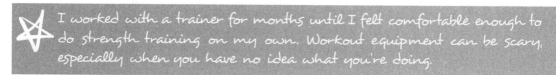

I worked with a trainer for months until I felt comfortable enough to do strength training on my own. Workout equipment can be scary, especially when you have no idea what you're doing.

2. **Always warm up** – Strength training is a high-effort physical activity. It is crucial that you warm up by increasing your body temperature and blood flow, by doing some activity that allows you to get your body moving in preparation for weight training. This might include light jumping jacks, air squats and light push-ups.

3. **Stretch** – In addition to warming up, it is also important to perform short dynamic stretches—stretching as you are moving—to help the muscle groups you will be working on move more easily. However, stretching too much before strength training is not recommended, as it can impede muscle contraction and the proper breakdown of muscle fibers. A good way to warm up is by performing the specific exercise you plan to do with very light weights.

4. **Use good technique** – Above all, remember that good technique is crucial to your progress and to the prevention of injuries. Aim for the right form using the proper weight.

5. **Switch up your angles** – One important strategy with weight training is to be able to work your muscles at different angles to stimulate muscle growth and balance the development of the muscle. For example, the pectoral muscle (or chest muscle) can be worked on at three different angles using the same weight machine: a bench press. You can work the top part of the muscle with an incline bench (i.e. with the bench set at a 45-degree incline); you can work the more central part of the muscle with a flat bench, and you can work the lower part of the pectoral muscle with a declined bench. These three different exercises will fully challenge the different muscle fibers.

6. **Use tempo** – Tempo is another way to challenge your muscles. For example, a "5-2-5" tempo for bench press means you push for the count of five seconds, hold for two seconds, and

lower for the count of five again. You will be amazed at how much harder it makes lifting the weight! It's a great way to challenge your muscles.

7. **Add resistance** – Remember that strength training is also called "resistance training"—for a good reason. If you can complete a set of 25 repetitions, you're not using enough weight. More weight is needed to create enough resistance for your muscles. For strength training to be beneficial, you actually need to create micro-tears in your muscles, which will trigger them to self-repair, and in turn, makes them grow stronger.

8. **Count repetitions and sets** – Repetitions are the number of times you do a movement with a weight, while sets are how many times you do those repetitions. For example, you can do squats for 12 repetitions and three sets, equaling 36 total squats. Sets of 12 repetitions are the most common, but you can do drop-sets by decreasing the number of repetitions with each set while increasing the weight. For example, you could do 12 bicep curls with a 10-pound dumbbell on the first set, 10 bicep curls with a 12-pound dumbbell on the second, and eight bicep curls with a 15-pound dumbbell on the third. By doing drop-sets, you will fully challenge your muscles, and leave them close to exhaustion. Also, for optimal results, it's important to alter the sets and repetitions because muscles have memory, and they will quickly adapt to your routine, which will slow your progress. In other words, you want to avoid plateaus.

9. **Integrate supersets or giant sets** – If you're in a hurry or want to try something quick and different, do supersets or giant-sets. A super-set consists of two exercises alternated twice without rest. For example, when working your chest, you could do a set of bench presses, followed by a set of push-ups, then repeat. For your giant-set, which consists of three exercises done three times without rest, you could add sets of dumbbell flies to push-ups and bench presses.

10. **Know your concentric exercises versus eccentric exercises** – Concentric exercises shorten your muscles while eccentric exercises elongate your muscles. Both are important. The preacher curl is a good example of an eccentric exercise because it stretches the biceps to its full length in the down position. A good example of a concentric exercise is the concentrated bicep curl, where the muscle remains contracted for most of the exercise. It's important to have a mix of the two types of exercises in your workouts to effectively maximize the challenge to your muscles. I strongly suggest that you start with the eccentric exercises in order to engage the muscle through its entire range and then move on to concentric ones.

11. **Use cable exercises** – These are good to incorporate into your workout. You can use cables in lieu of dumbbells or barbells since these offer consistent tension throughout the movement and also increase the use of surrounding stabilizing muscles.

12. **Integrate unilateral and bilateral exercises** – In a unilateral exercise, you use one side of your body at a time, while in a bilateral exercise you use both sides. Since most people have a dominant side, it's important to integrate both types in order to balance your musculature and to effectively use your core muscles.

13. **Vary your exercises** – It's crucial to alter your workout regularly. Some people do the same things at the gym for years and wonder why they don't see the results they want. As I mentioned earlier, muscles adapt quickly, so you need to keep finding new ways of challenging them—even just to maintain your current muscle tone. I know, it may sound complicated, but it also keeps you from getting bored or staying at a plateau.

 I've found tons of different exercises on social media sites like Pinterest and YouTube. There are plenty of workout videos you can do in your own home, too.

14. **Don't forget to breathe** – Don't forget to breathe! Exhale during more demanding concentric muscle movements. By doing so, you will prevent excessive internal pressure that restricts blood flow back to the heart, which could make you feel lightheaded or dizzy.

15. **Keep it short** – Your strength-training workout shouldn't exceed one hour. If you strength train for longer than that, you have a greater chance of getting injured, and your muscles will be too tired or depleted to be productive.

16. **Don't forget to cool down** – This is very important as it helps your muscular system and cardiovascular system return to a resting state. Five to ten minutes on a stationary bike, for example, is a good way to cool down. You should do most of your stretching in the cool-down phase and focus particularly on the body parts you have worked that day.

17. **Recuperation is key** – You need to give your muscles time to recuperate and regenerate. As mentioned earlier, when you train with weights, you actually create micro-tears in your muscles. When given time to heal, your muscles will repair and grow stronger. If you don't give your body the time to regenerate, these muscles lose some of the benefits of strength training. Too many people do too much and then get discouraged when they get injured. Sometimes less is more.

18. **Keep a fitness journal** – I know… groan! But a log book helps you keep your commitment to fitness and measures your improvement. Keeping track of the weight you use allows you to always be ready. This saves you time and pushes you to the next level. Lots of apps exist that can track all this information for you, which can make tracking convenient and efficient.

19. **Use your own bodyweight** – No weights? No problem. Never underestimate the capacity of using your own bodyweight as resistance. Whether you are doing 10 push-ups, 30 squats, or a one-minute plank, your body may be more challenging than you think!

20. **Have fun!** Hundreds of great and varied workout examples are out there! The key is to change it up and have fun with them. Add variation to your routine, otherwise, your body will adapt, which will slow your progress and diminish your results.

AFTER YOUR WORKOUT

DOMS is an acronym for Delayed Onset Muscle Soreness. It's the soreness that you feel in your muscles that doesn't show up until a day or two after you work out. It's a normal part of the process of repairing your muscles from the damage to the fibers you created while exercising. Expect to be sore a few days after doing an exercise for the first time, or after not doing it for a while.

As your muscles get used to that movement and adapt to being put under stress, they will get less and less sore every time. One way to make the soreness go away, at least temporarily, is to continue exercising. This increases blood flow to the muscles and helps them heal. However, remember they still need some rest to heal. So, if you're sore from heavy squats, don't turn around and do heavy squats again. Try doing squats with no weight or stretching to help bring the soreness down.

The following diagram shows examples of health habits with corresponding hack levels. To download the *Hack Your Health Habits Worksheet*, visit

www.hackyourhealthhabits.com/worksheets

READY #HEALTHHACKER?
EXAMPLES OF LEVEL 1, 2 AND 3 HACKS FOR THIS CHAPTER

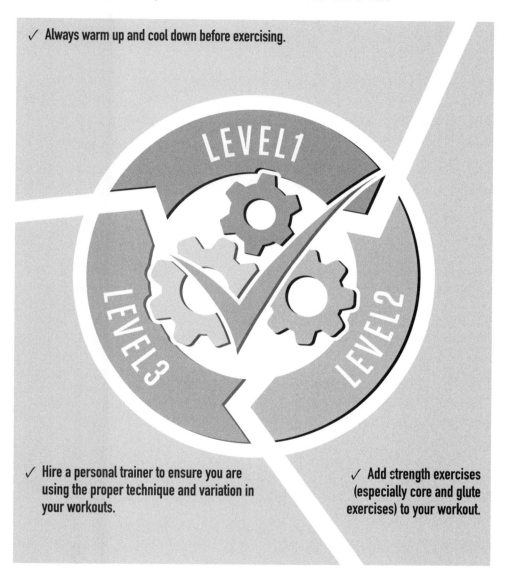

✓ Always warm up and cool down before exercising.

✓ Hire a personal trainer to ensure you are using the proper technique and variation in your workouts.

✓ Add strength exercises (especially core and glute exercises) to your workout.

HACK YOUR HEALTH PROGRESS

||||||||||||||||||||||||||||||||||||||||||||||||||||||||||||||||||||||||||||||

CHAPTER 31

YOGA

32

You Don't Have to Be a Pretzel

"Log out. Shut down.
Do Yoga."

— Unknown

THINK IT OVER

- Do you know the benefits of yoga for the various functions of the body?

- What are the different types of yoga and what are they meant for?

- What type of yoga best suits your lifestyle?

Originating in India, yoga has been practiced for centuries as a method of physical, spiritual and emotional expression. While the people of India have long known about the healing power of yoga, the practice and its benefits are fairly new to the West. Most of us know it as a method of relaxation; however, studies show that the benefits of yoga stretch far beyond stress relief.

The practice has been shown to reduce blood pressure, relieve anxiety, heighten concentration, improve flexibility, increase strength, decrease muscle and joint pain and improve bodily systems.[1] Yoga consists of a variety of different postures and breathing techniques that promote calmness of the nervous system, muscles and joints. Whether you're a beginner or have been practicing for many years, everyone can reap the many benefits of yoga.

My place of work offers a weekly yoga class during lunchtime. It's a great way to de-stress midday and rejuvenate for the afternoon.

YOGA BENEFITS FOR PAIN AND PHYSICAL WELL-BEING

As mentioned, yoga provides many physical benefits. Here is a long list of everything yoga can help you with:

- **Yoga improves flexibility and prevents cartilage degeneration** – Tightness and the inflexibility of muscles and connective tissue may cause issues such as pain, increased risk of injury and poor posture. Regular yoga stretches and poses will improve muscle flexibility and decrease the risk of injury or strain.

- **Yoga builds muscle strength** – Although yoga does not require lifting heavy weights and is known as a calmer exercise, supporting your bodyweight in certain positions will definitely fire up your muscles. Building lean muscle tissue also has the added benefit of granting a boosted metabolism, more energy, and a decreased chance for conditions such as arthritis or chronic lower back pain.

- **Yoga improves posture and protects the spine** – Bad posture can cause back, neck, and other muscle and joint issues. As you slouch, your body may compensate by flattening the normal curves in your neck and lower back, which can cause pain and degenerative arthritis of the spine. Yoga can help in maintaining the natural curvature of the spine and can help promote good joint mobility and flexibility in the vertebral joints.

- **Yoga promotes better blood circulation** – The relaxation exercises you learn in yoga can help your circulation, especially in your limbs. Practicing yoga also helps improve oxygenation of your cells by encouraging blood in the legs and pelvis to flow back to the heart, where it can be pumped to the lungs to be freshly oxygenated. Twisting or inverted poses can help with this as well.

- **Yoga stimulates the lymphatic system** – By stretching, twisting, breathing deeply, and moving the body in certain positions, you increase drainage of lymph. This helps the lymphatic system fight infection and dispose of the toxic-waste products of cellular functioning.

- **Yoga gets the digestive system moving** – Yoga, like any physical exercise, can ease conditions such as constipation, since moving the body facilitates more rapid transport of food and waste products through the bowels. Yoga also relieves stress, which has been shown to be a huge contributing factor in chronic constipation and Irritable Bowel Syndrome (IBS).

- **Yoga eases pain** – Any physical activity has been shown to strengthen weak muscles, improve ligament function, decrease inflammation, and therefore reduce pain. Yoga benefits the body by relaxing tense muscles, allowing proper blood flow, and easing pain caused by conditions such as fibromyalgia, arthritis, carpal tunnel, and many other chronic conditions.

YOGA BENEFITS FOR MENTAL AND EMOTIONAL WELL-BEING

Along with its physical benefits, yoga also rejuvenates the mind and our emotional connectedness. With our constant on-the-go lifestyles, it is easy to get stuck in a chronic state of fight or flight. Yoga helps relax tension and bring our stress response back to neutral. Other ways yoga benefits our mental well-being include:

- **Better concentration** – Yoga requires you to focus on deep breathing and clear your mind of any thoughts or stresses that occur during the day. This focus on relaxation has a spillover effect into other areas that require concentration as well. Regular yoga practice can "improve coordination, reaction time, memory and even IQ scores," as the less distracted you are by thoughts, the more mindful you can be.

- **Helps balance the nervous system** – Yoga shifts the balance from your sympathetic nervous system (or the fight-or-flight response) to the parasympathetic nervous system (or the rest-and-digest response). The latter is calming and restorative; it lowers breathing and heart rate, decreases blood pressure, and increases blood flow to the intestines and reproductive organs. Additionally, removing spinal tension takes stress off the spine and allows the body to relax more easily.

- **Better sleep** – Studies suggest that regular yoga practice results in better sleep—which means you will be less tired and stressed and more likely to function more efficiently.

- **Increased self-esteem** – Yoga is a way of giving yourself important self-care and time. The more you get into the practice and its teachings, the more you will value your well-being and integrate its philosophy into your own.

- **Reduced adrenal exertion and reduced stress** – A regular yoga practice has been shown to reduce the secretion of cortisol and adrenaline, which are the hormones responsible for our fight-or-flight response in acute or chronic stressful situations. Excessive cortisol has been linked to major depression, cognitive decline, osteoporosis, high blood pressure, insulin resistance and metabolic syndrome. One study found that a consistent yoga practice improved depression and led to a significant increase in serotonin, the happy hormone that regulates mood. It also decreases levels of monoamine oxidase, an enzyme that breaks down neurotransmitters. This helps alleviate stress and provides peace of mind.

Surprised? A regular yoga practice can lead to improved physicality, emotional control and mental function.

Confused about all the different types of yoga out there? Not sure where you should start? Here are a few of the different styles of yoga to help you decide. You may have to try a few different classes to figure out which one(s) is (are) right for you!

HATHA YOGA

Hatha (*ha* meaning "sun" and *tha* meaning "moon") is a very general term that can include many types of yoga combined. If a class is described as hatha style, it is probably going to be slow-paced and gentle and can provide a good introduction to basic yoga poses.

KUNDALINI YOGA

The emphasis in *Kundalini* yoga is on breathing in conjunction with physical movement. The intention of this kind of yoga is to free the energy in your lower body and allow it to move upward toward your upper glands and chakras (or energy centers). Kundalini may include rapid, repetitive movements rather than static poses. There are thousands of kriyas (yoga sets of poses) in kundalini yoga, and meditation is always an integral component of it. Some *kriyas* and meditations may also involve the use of sounds or mantras.

VINYASA YOGA

Like Hatha, *Vinyasa* is a general term used to describe many different types of yoga combined. As vinyasa means "breath-synchronized movement," it tends to be a more vigorous style of yoga based on a series of poses called "sun salutations," where your movements are matched to your breath. Toward the end of a Vinyasa class, there is also intense stretching.

ASHTANGA AND POWER YOGA

Ashtanga, which means "eight limbs" in Sanskrit, is a fast-paced, intense style of yoga. With this yoga, a regular series of poses is generally performed in the same order and ideally in a heated room to simulate the warm temperature in India where yoga originated. Ashtanga yoga is physically demanding, due to the constant flow from one pose to the next. This type of yoga has also been the inspiration for Power Yoga, based on a flowing style, but without the strict set of regular poses. Be prepared to sweat in these classes!

 This type of yoga will definitely get your muscles working!

HOT YOGA

Hot yoga is practiced in a 95-to-100-degree-Fahrenheit room. The principle is that the heat helps loosen tight muscles and cleanse the body through profuse sweating. It can take time to become acclimatized to the heat of the room. However, you not only get the benefits of doing yoga but also get the benefits of sweating and allowing your body to detoxify. Make sure to drink lots of water to stay well-hydrated!

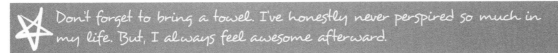 *Don't forget to bring a towel. I've honestly never perspired so much in my life. But, I always feel awesome afterward.*

ANUSARA YOGA

Founded in 1997 by John Friend, *Anusara* yoga focuses on physical alignment and a philosophy derived from tantra, emphasizing the intrinsic goodness of all beings. Anusara classes are usually light-hearted and accessible to those of varying abilities. Poses are taught in a way that opens the heart physically and emotionally. Props are often used.

JIVAMUKTI YOGA

This style of yoga emerged from teachers at a well-known New York yoga studio. Inspired by Ashtanga yoga, but wanting something a little different, *Jivamukti* yoga founders David Life and Sharon Gannon created a yoga that emphasized chanting, meditation and spiritual teachings alongside movements from Ashtanga yoga.

IYENGAR YOGA

Based on the teachings of Yogi B. K. S Iyengar, this style of yoga is all about body alignment. In yoga, the word "alignment" is used to describe the precise way your body should be positioned in each pose in order to avoid injury and obtain maximum benefits. Iyengar yoga usually emphasizes holding poses over long periods of time versus moving quickly from one pose to another. This type of yoga also incorporates the use of props such as yoga blankets, blocks and straps to bring the body into alignment.

Whatever type of yoga you choose, notice how it works your body, mind and soul. When you do start a yoga practice, go at your own pace; yoga is not a competitive sport.

The following diagram shows examples of health habits with corresponding hack levels. To download the *Hack Your Health Habits Worksheet*, visit

www.hackyourhealthhabits.com/worksheets

READY #HEALTHHACKER?
EXAMPLES OF LEVEL 1, 2 AND 3 HACKS FOR THIS CHAPTER

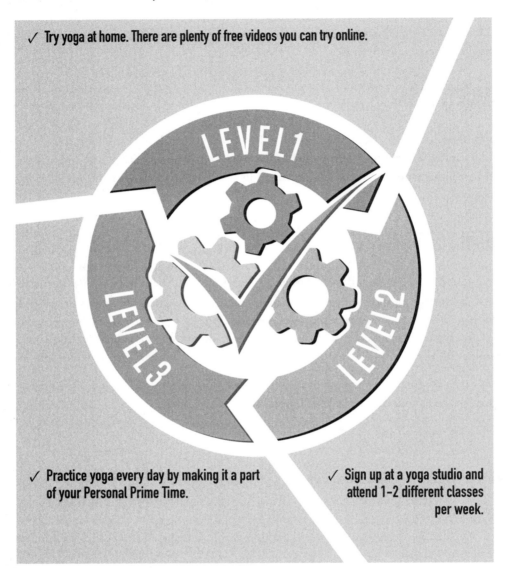

✓ Try yoga at home. There are plenty of free videos you can try online.

LEVEL 1

LEVEL 2

LEVEL 3

✓ Practice yoga every day by making it a part of your Personal Prime Time.

✓ Sign up at a yoga studio and attend 1–2 different classes per week.

HACK YOUR HEALTH PROGRESS

CHAPTER 32

STRAIGHTEN-UP!
Is Your Posture Wearing You Out?

"Posture is the window to
the spine."

— C. J. Mertz

Sit up straight! Parents tend to nag their kids all the time about bad posture but funny enough, they are just as bad. I can't tell you the amount of times I have come out of an adjustment room to find my patients hunched over their phones or slouched in a waiting room chair. Meanwhile, many wonder why they experience pain and discomfort.

Although often overlooked, good posture is at the top of the list when it comes to maintaining good health. It is right up there with eating well, exercising often and getting adequate sleep. Surprised? You're not alone. Many fitness advisers and seekers fail to recognize the importance of good posture in their workout regimes.

In my opinion, maintaining good posture is one of the best-kept secrets in the field of health. I so often hear people say "I know I have bad posture... oh well!" Bad posture is not just about looks; it's about an abnormally functioning spine and, therefore, an abnormally functioning nervous system. Remember your anatomy? Your spine protects your nervous system, and your nervous system controls every cell, tissue and organ in your body—kind of important, right?

WHAT IS POSTURE?

Posture refers to the body's alignment and positioning. Whether we are standing, sitting, or lying down, the force of gravity exerts a force on our joints, ligaments and muscles.[1] Good posture entails distributing the force of gravity throughout our body, so no one structure in the body is overstressed. It ensures that our bones are properly aligned, so our muscles, joints and ligaments work efficiently. It also ensures that our vital organs are in the right position so that they can function properly.

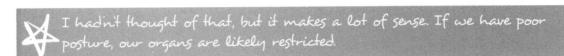
I hadn't thought of that, but it makes a lot of sense. If we have poor posture, our organs are likely restricted.

ANTERIOR HEAD SYNDROME AND OTHER NEGATIVE EFFECTS OF POOR POSTURE

As mentioned earlier, the spine covers and protects our nervous system, so it is crucial that we maintain good posture to prevent spinal decay, and to make sure that there is proper communication between the brain and body. The spinal column has three normal curvatures: the neck lordosis, the thoracic kyphosis and the lumbar lordosis. These curves are there to help evenly distribute the weight of the human body, without losing balance and without placing extra pressure on the spine.

The cervical spine supports the weight of the head. Have you ever heard of Anterior Head Syndrome, a.k.a. "text neck?" Maybe you haven't, but I can guarantee that you've seen it. It is developed from the position most people assume when texting or on their computers.

Why is "text neck" a big deal? Imagine holding a bowling ball with your arm out. No matter how strong you are, your bicep will tire and eventually drop the ball. Same goes for your neck and shoulders. Your head is about the same weight as a bowling ball. When your head is constantly held in a forward position, neck and shoulder muscles become tight, and the normal curve of your neck starts to diminish. In some cases, your back can even start to round. In essence, your spine is "dropping the ball."

In addition to this, Anterior Head Syndrome can result in the following:

- flattening of the spinal curve
- spinal degeneration
- disc herniation
- soft tissue damage
- loss of lung volume capacity
- gastrointestinal problems

- onset of early arthritis

- nerve damage[2]

To make things worse, Anterior Head Syndrome is being seen in younger and younger generations, due to the popularity of smartphones and other mobile devices. Why is this an issue? Youth are in the midst of development. Stressors on their skeletal structure can cause postural alterations as they age, which can impact their health in the short and long term.

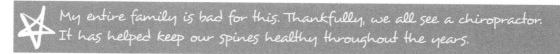

My entire family is bad for this. Thankfully, we all see a chiropractor. It has helped keep our spines healthy throughout the years.

The spine covers and protects the nervous system, which innervates every cell, tissues and organ in the body. This means that the long-term effects of poor posture can affect all the systems in your body. A person who has poor posture may often be tired or unable to concentrate efficiently.

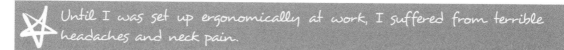

Until I was set up ergonomically at work, I suffered from terrible headaches and neck pain.

THE BENEFITS OF GOOD POSTURE

We've talked a bit about the negative impacts of poor posture, but what about the positive impacts of *good* posture? Studies show numerous benefits associated with standing up straight. These include:

- **Portraying a better, more confident image** – Good posture will boost self-confidence. Try this: In front of a mirror, take a deep breath and stand straight. Then, slump over with poor posture. Repeat a few times. See the difference? Think of the people around you that you see as confident. Many of the people I think of do stand tall and have very good posture.

- **Improved circulation and digestion** – When it comes to the digestive system, proper posture allows the internal organs in the abdomen to assume their natural position without undue compression. Compression can interfere with the normal flow and function of the gastrointestinal system. An improper, slouched posture has been postulated as a contributing factor to several digestive problems from acid reflux to constipation and even hernias.

- **Making you look slimmer and younger** – Good posture can make you look slimmer and younger, and even make your clothes fit better.

- **Helping your muscles and joints** – Good posture helps us keep bones and joints in correct alignment so that our muscles are used correctly. This decreases the abnormal wearing of joint surfaces that could result in degenerative arthritis and joint pain. It also reduces the stress on the ligaments holding the spinal joints together, minimizing the likelihood of injury. Good posture allows muscles to work more efficiently, allowing the body to use less energy and preventing muscle fatigue. It also helps prevent muscle strain, overuse disorders, and even back and muscular pain.

- **Changing your frame of mind** – Posture also affects your frame of mind, and your frame of mind can affect your posture! So, when you are well, feeling happy, and on top of things, your posture tends to be upright and open. In contrast, people who are depressed and in chronic pain often sit or stand slumped. Next time you feel depressed or you're anxious about something, try changing your posture—stand up straight and breathe deeply. Good posture in sitting and standing makes it easier to breathe fully and naturally, helping both relaxation and concentration. Many Eastern practices such as yoga and tai chi work on posture.

- **Keeping your spine and nervous system healthy** – Maintaining correct posture is a simple but very important way to keep the many intricate structures in the back and spine healthy. Not maintaining good posture and adequate back support can add strain to muscles and put stress on the spine. Over time, the stress of poor posture can change the anatomical characteristics of the spine, leading to the possibility of impeded nervous system function. Sitting and standing with proper postural alignment will allow you to work more efficiently with less fatigue and strain on your body's ligaments and muscles. Being aware of good posture is the first step in breaking poor postural habits and reducing stress and strain on your spine.

LIFESTYLE TIPS FOR LIFELONG GOOD POSTURE

So, how can you improve your posture? There are plenty of things you can do. Consider the following:

- **Maintain a good weight** – Excess weight, especially around the midriff, pulls on the back, weakening stomach muscles. This can lead to an increased lower back lordosis.

- **Develop a regular program of exercise** – Regular exercise keeps you flexible and helps tone your muscles to support proper posture.

- **Buy good bedding** – A good medium-firm mattress will support the spine and help maintain the same shape as a person with good upright posture. However, a mattress that is too firm may place unwanted pressure on your hips and shoulders when sleeping on your side. It is important to remember that we spend seven to nine hours in bed, so it is worth investing in a good mattress. To put things in perspective, many people invest a great amount in a car, which we may spend minimal amounts of time in. And, we spend seven to nine hours of each day in bed, yet are reluctant to invest a few thousand dollars in a mattress.

- **Pay attention to injuries from bumps, falls and accidents** – Injuries in youth or young adulthood may cause growth abnormalities or postural adaptations to the injury or pain that can show up later in life.

- **Be conscious of your workstation** – Is your chair high enough to fit your desk? Do you need a footrest to keep pressure off your legs? It is important to be seated or standing in a neutral body position in which your joints are naturally aligned and there is the least amount of stress and strain on your muscles, tendons and joints.

LET'S GET ERGONOMICALLY CORRECT

You may have heard the phrase "sitting is the new smoking." As a chiropractor, I must admit that there is truth behind the sentiment. Surprisingly, inactivity accounts for 5 percent of global mortality and poses a greater risk than being overweight or obese.[3]

This is striking! You would think obesity is already a big risk factor for disease, but in reality, inactivity is even bigger!

This shouldn't really come as a shock, considering many people spend their day sitting at a desk. The fact of the matter is that daily movements we used to have back in the days have been replaced with a sedentary lifestyle that is costing us our health. In addition, being sedentary greatly impacts our posture. In fact, sitting for the majority of the day may be a contributing factor to headaches, neck pain, back pain, loss of spine curvature and sore hips. Therefore, proper desk ergonomics is crucial for reducing the impact of sitting for long hours and the negative health effects that come with it.

Here are some more guidelines to help you maintain a neutral body position when sitting at your workstation:

- Ensure that your hands, wrists and forearms are straight, in line and roughly parallel to the floor. The keyboard and mouse should be at the same level to avoid repetitive reaching.

- Ensure your head is leveled, forward facing and in line with your torso.

- Your shoulders should be relaxed and upper arms should hang normally at the side of the body.

- Ensure your elbows stay close to the body and are bent between 90 and 120 degrees. Rest them softly on a padded elbow support, if you have one on your chair.

- Your lower back should be in a comfortable, neutral position with an adequate lumbar support.

- Your thighs and hips should be parallel to the floor and supported by a well-padded seat that does not press hard on the back of your knees, as it can irritate your sciatic nerve.

- Keep your feet fully supported on the floor with your knees close to a 90-degree angle. Use a footrest if you have to.

Always remember: Regardless of how good your posture is, working in the same posture or sitting still for prolonged periods is not healthy. Make sure to stretch your fingers, hands, and arms, and rotate your torso periodically. And, don't forget to take breaks! Stand up every now and then to stretch or walk around for a few minutes.

There is another benefit to moving around throughout your day: A well-described phenomenon called non-exercise activity thermogenesis (NEAT) suggests that moving around more is a powerful way to stimulate your metabolism and circulation. So, go ahead and fidget, walk around and stretch. It's good for you!

If you experience pain or discomfort while working, an ergonomic assessment may be a good idea. A professional will be able to assess whether your station is ergonomic and if modifications are needed to reduce the negative impact on the spine. Many workplaces are now switching to ergonomic standing desks and chairs to mimic active sitting.

Active sitting occurs when seating allows or encourages the seated occupant to move. Also referred to as dynamic sitting, the concept is that fostering flexibility and movement while sitting can be beneficial to the human body, making some seated tasks easier to perform. This benefits our posture by allowing our bodies to have a natural range of motion.

If you work from home, the same rules apply; you may want to rethink working in bed with your laptop.

ONE LAST WORD ON GOOD POSTURE

It is important to mention that, although you may not work at a desk per se, your hobbies and daily rituals should include some sort of movement as well. Television watching has been associated with an increase in obesity, diabetes and even early mortality. For example, four hours of TV watching per day increases the risk of early death by a whopping 46 percent, and two to four hours of TV watching per day increases the risk for early death by 13 percent! So, make sure that your hobbies and activities involve a bit of action!

> I've really got to get the girls to cut down on TV time. There are so many other activities they can be doing that are better for their bodies and minds...

Good posture looks and feels good. It plays a critical role in the overall functioning of the nervous system, impacting every cell, organ and tissue in the body, not to mention our energy levels and how we feel. So, straighten up and get checked by your chiropractor on a regular basis to make sure your spine and nervous system are working optimally. There will be more on the impact of your nervous system on your overall health in **Chapter 45: The Nervous System—Is Yours Turned On?**

The following diagram shows examples of health habits with corresponding hack levels. To download the *Hack Your Health Habits Worksheet*, visit

www.hackyourhealthhabits.com/worksheets

READY #HEALTHHACKER?
EXAMPLES OF LEVEL 1, 2 AND 3 HACKS FOR THIS CHAPTER

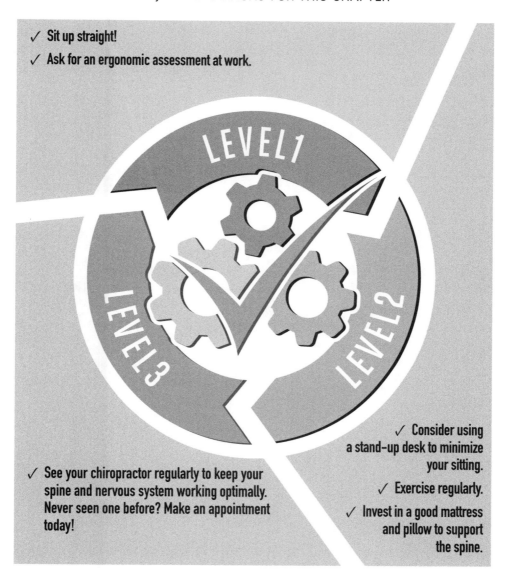

✓ Sit up straight!

✓ Ask for an ergonomic assessment at work.

✓ Consider using a stand-up desk to minimize your sitting.

✓ Exercise regularly.

✓ Invest in a good mattress and pillow to support the spine.

✓ See your chiropractor regularly to keep your spine and nervous system working optimally. Never seen one before? Make an appointment today!

HACK YOUR HEALTH PROGRESS

||||||||||||||||||||||||||||||||||||||||||||||||||||||||||||||||||||||||||||||||

CHAPTER 33

SECTION 7

Get to Know Your Hormones and Feel Better

Are your hormones out of whack? Chronic stress and hormonal imbalances affect not only the body but also the mind, impacting your health in many ways. In Section 7, you will learn all about your hormones: what roles they play, signs and symptoms of imbalances and simple lifestyle changes you can implement to keep them happy!

YOUR ADRENALS
Stress is Not Overrated!

"Dear stress, let's break up."

— Love, Me

THINK IT OVER

- What is the role of well-functioning adrenals on your overall health?

- Do you know the different stages of stress and are you currently in one?

- Are you aware of what supplements and botanicals can help support healthy adrenal function?

Stress. Everyone has felt it at some point. That feeling of being so overwhelmed and overworked that you can barely eat or sleep. Stress has become ingrained in our culture. We associate it with hard work and success, assuming that we can't have one without the other. Though some stress is necessary, we often bite off more than we can chew. We fail to realize that the more stressed we are, the less efficient we are.

✴ *My mind goes blank when I'm stressed. I can't focus on anything.*

We also choose to ignore the negative effects that stress has on our bodies. But, how successful are you, if you are so stressed out that you can't enjoy your life? Excessive stress can lead to a multitude of symptoms, including adrenal fatigue, exhaustion, anxiety, sleep disturbance and hormone imbalances.

This chapter will focus on one of the biggest impacts stress has on the body—adrenal fatigue. Adrenal fatigue is a common effect of stress. In fact, here is a typical scenario I often see in my office: A busy mom with a demanding career comes in complaining of waking up at 2 a.m. ready to go and unable to get back to sleep. She is fatigued during the day, has lost her sex drive, is feeling down and is gaining weight around the tummy area. For the last several years, she has been going hard with work deadlines, playing taxi for the kids' sports activities, helping them with their homework every day and doing the lion's share of the cooking and cleaning. Basically, she goes from morning to night with little rest and downtime. Her adrenals are tapped out, and so is she. Does this sound like you? Could your adrenals be fatigued?

WHAT ARE ADRENAL GLANDS AND WHAT DO THEY DO?

The adrenal glands (also known as suprarenal glands) are the triangle-shaped endocrine glands that sit on top of your kidneys. Similar to ovaries, testicles and the thyroid, the adrenal glands are hormone-producing glands. They're responsible for regulating our stress response and even play an important role in the maintenance of a healthy immune system. They are also key contributors to proper thyroid function, the balance of hormones, maintaining an ideal weight, stabilizing emotions and controlling cravings.

Most people do not realize just how important the adrenal glands are to their overall health and well-being. Multiple studies have proven that the health of the adrenal glands will dictate a person's overall health and ability to recover from many types of chronic illnesses. Since chronic stress is the main cause of overactive adrenals, it is important that one finds a way to control and minimize stress. Moreover, proper nutrition, adequate rest and exercise are also very important.

TYPES OF STRESS

There are two main types of stress: acute and chronic stress. Each affects us differently.

1. **Acute Stress** – An example of acute stress would be narrowly missing a car accident or watching the final four minutes of your kid's overtime hockey game. During acute stress, the brain sends a message through the spinal cord to the adrenal glands. The adrenal glands begin secreting hormones such as epinephrine and norepinephrine (also called adrenaline), triggering a quick, acute and immediate response. This response will generally consist of an increase in heart rate, blood pressure and perspiration, dilation of the bronchioles, decreased digestive system activity and an increased metabolic rate. The adrenaline also causes the liver to convert stored glycogen into glucose (sugar) for rapid energy. Think of it this way: if you are getting chased by a bear, it's not the time to pee and poo; you need all your systems focused on getting you out of there!

2. **Chronic Stress** – You might be chronically stressed if you are dissatisfied with your job or regularly take care of a sick family member. Similar to acute stress, chronic stress starts in the brain. The brain sends messages to the anterior pituitary gland and adrenal cortex, which

stimulates the secretion of mineralocorticoids. Mineralocorticoids are responsible for the retention of sodium and water by the kidneys, as well as regulation of blood volume and blood pressure. Also, during long-term stress, proteins and fats are converted to glucose or broken down for energy, leading to an increase in blood glucose. This may explain why people under constant stress find it difficult to lose weight. Stress also has a big impact on the immune system. Those under chronic stress are often more susceptible to colds and infection.

If you remember our Productivity and Energy Management Chapter, we talked about eustress and distress, which were terms coined fifty years ago by the "father of stress," Dr. Hans Selye. Selye also came up with the concept of General Adaptation Syndrome (GAS), which is the process our bodies go through when adapting to stressors.[1] According to Selye, the body undergoes three universal stages of coping:

1. **Alarm** – In this first stage, the body considers a stressor to be dangerous and stimulates an increase in cortisol production. But levels of DHEA (a natural steroid also produced by the adrenals) stay normal. This thrusts your body into fight-or-flight mode.

2. **Resistance** – In this second stage, the body remains on guard in the continued presence of a stressor, but is weakened. Cortisol is chronically elevated, but DHEA levels decline, which may lead to mood swings, anxiety attacks or even depression. This can be taken as a warning sign that some relaxation and downtime is required before a burnout. The adrenals will adapt to this stage by going through a stage called the 'pregnenolone steal' phase or also called the 'adrenal steal' phase. Pregnenolone is derived from cholesterol and is the precursor for cortisol and sex hormones. However, the body only has so much pregnenolone to go around, and during times of stress, the body will stunt the available pregnenolone into cortisol instead of DHEA. The body will favor making the cortisol it needs to deal with stress over making sex hormones, such as estrogen and testosterone. This stage is represented in the adrenal profile as increased cortisol/low DHEA.

3. **Exhaustion** – At this point, your body loses its ability to combat stressors. The adrenals do not function properly, cortisol and DHEA levels decrease further, and adrenal fatigue settles in. In extreme exhaustion, DHEA levels can even normalize as the adrenal steal is no longer even happening.

General adaption syndrome doesn't just apply to instances where we are in serious danger. The following stressors can prompt the GAS process:

- refined sugars
- nutrient-poor food
- emotional stress
- negative outlook on life
- toxic environment
- drugs

- excess caffeine
- lack of sleep
- chronic infection
- lack of relaxation
- smoking
- too much or too little exercise

(If adrenals are already under a lot of pressure, high intensity or endurance-type of exercises can do more harm than good.)

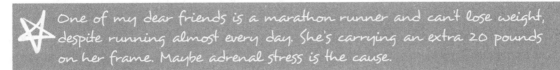

One of my dear friends is a marathon runner and can't lose weight, despite running almost every day. She's carrying an extra 20 pounds on her frame. Maybe adrenal stress is the cause.

SYMPTOMS OF ADRENAL DYSFUNCTION

Symptoms of adrenal dysfunction will depend on whether the adrenal glands are under- or over-activated. Depending on your symptoms, you may be able to discern how your adrenals are functioning.

Hypo-adrenal function:

- unable to stay asleep
- crave salts
- slow to get started in the morning
- afternoon fatigue
- dizziness when standing quickly
- afternoon headaches
- a headache with exertion or stress
- weak nails

Hyper-adrenal function:

- unable to fall asleep
- sweat a lot, even with little activity
- under a high amount of stress
- weight gain
- wake up tired

HOW DO YOU KNOW IF YOUR ADRENALS ARE STRESSED?

Measuring cortisol levels is key to help determine adrenal health. Ideally, cortisol levels should be at their highest in the morning, as throughout the night our cortisol gradually increases, providing us with a source of glucose to keep our blood sugar stable while we are fasting for the hours that we sleep. As the day progresses, cortisol levels gradually decrease. By bedtime, levels should be at their lowest, allowing you to fall asleep and stay asleep. Melatonin (another hormone) works in opposition to cortisol levels, increasing at night and decreasing in the morning, leading to adequate and restful sleep.

We will be exploring the various forms of hormone testing in greater depth in **Chapter 36: Sex Hormones—Happy or Cranky?** In the meantime, when it comes to the adrenals, the best way to test for their function is to do a four-point cortisol test. This measures cortisol level fluctuation at specific times in the day—upon waking up, at lunchtime, at dinner time and before going to bed. Graphing the daily cortisol rhythm can inform us on how well the hypothalamic-pituitary axis (HPA) is functioning. The HPA axis is a set of interactions among three of our endocrine glands: the hypothalamus, the pituitary gland (a pea-shaped structure located below the thalamus) and the adrenals. Hair cortisol levels can also be used to assess overall functioning of the HPA axis over many weeks, and, therefore, can be useful in assessing long-term, or chronic, stress.

General blood chemistry can also help evaluate whether the adrenals are over- or underactive. In the case of underactive adrenals, the results will show potassium and sodium levels outside their normal range and a *decrease* in glucose; while, if the adrenals are in hyperfunction, the results will show potassium and sodium levels outside their normal range and an *increase* in glucose and triglycerides.

Another very simple test that is commonly used to test adrenal fatigue is called postural hypotension, which is a drop in blood pressure, which occurs upon rising from a horizontal position. To perform the test, blood pressure is first taken at rest. This should be around 120/80 to be considered in the healthy range. Then the patient is asked to stand up, where the blood pressure is taken once again. A normal result would show an increase in blood pressure by 10-20 points. If it drops by ten points or more, it is a good indication that the adrenals are fatigued. This test is obviously a generalized measure and is not a precise diagnosis of adrenal fatigue. However, it may be a good starting point or indication that further adrenal testing may be beneficial.

The autonomic nervous system also plays a key role in adrenal health. Keeping the sympathetic and the parasympathetic nervous systems in balance is essential. The sympathetic nervous system is what activates our stress response (fight-or-flight), and the parasympathetic inhibits it (rest-or-digest). In today's world, we are often in a state of arousal, causing our sympathetic nervous system to become overactive. Stuck in fight-or-flight mode, we become what is called sympathetic dominant. Dominance can lead to exhaustion, poor health and accelerated aging. Heart rate variability (HRV) technology are often used by chiropractors and other healthcare professionals to evaluate the body's response and adaptation to stress as it measures and tracks a patient's autonomic nervous system state.

HOW TO MINIMIZE ADRENAL FATIGUE

So, what can you do? There are numerous natural ways to support the adrenals and help balance your autonomic nervous system:

- chiropractic care
- meditation

- yoga and Tai Chi

- proper sleep

- exercise

- avoiding sugar, caffeine and alcohol

- massage therapy

- breathing work

- emotional freedom technique (EFT)

- acupuncture

- laughter

- proper nutrition

- supplementation

Consuming whole, organic foods rich in phytonutrients is great for adrenal support, but supplementation is often needed to support proper adrenal function when the adrenals are taxed. Supplements like B complex, vitamin C, vitamin D, magnesium, zinc and omega-3 fatty acids can be of great benefit. Bovine adrenal glandular concentrate is also available for supporting healthy adrenal function. There are also several botanical adaptogens that can be taken to help support the adrenal glands throughout the stress response process. Adaptogens are medicinal plants that can help the body adapt to stress. Below are suggested adaptogens for the three previously discussed adrenal phases:

- **In the Alarm Phase, consider taking** ashwagandha, 5-HTP, L-theanine, passion flower, valerian root and schisandra.

- **In the Resistance Phase, consider taking** ashwagandha, rhodiola, cordyceps, ginseng, St-John's wort, phosphatidylserine, dark chocolate and melatonin.

- **In the Exhaustion Phase, consider taking** ashwagandha, licorice, Asian ginseng, cordyceps and rehmannia.

Many supplements on the market contain a mix of the above-mentioned herbs, so if you are not sure what phase you are in, I suggest taking a general support formula. If you are taking any medications, check with your natural healthcare practitioner to ensure that there are no interactions, as certain herbs can have drug interactions.

YOUR "NOT-TO-DO LIST"

Everyone needs some downtime—an hour or two when you can get away from the everyday stresses of life. We talked about Personal Prime Time in an earlier chapter, so we know that devoting an hour to yourself each day can drastically reduce stress levels. If you don't have an hour each day, here is a trick I use: I take at least a few minutes to write down a "Not-to-do list," in which I review the things that bring me stress. I go over that list and decide what I can remove, delegate, or ask for help with. Give it a try. You will see it's effective and even therapeutic. On the flip side, you may also want to make a list of things that you enjoy doing most, and make sure to incorporate at least one of these items into your daily routine.

While stress can be an important motivator, to avoid adrenal fatigue we must ensure that we are focusing on the right things and not spending time and energy on unnecessary tasks that do little for us. We can lower our stress levels by making changes to our habits or changing the way we perceive the stressors we encounter. To minimize our stress, we must find balance between our responsibilities, obligations and time for ourselves.

The following diagram shows examples of health habits, with corresponding hack levels. To download the *Hack Your Health Habits Worksheet*, visit

www.hackyourhealthhabits.com/worksheets

READY #HEALTHHACKER?
EXAMPLES OF LEVEL 1, 2 AND 3 HACKS FOR THIS CHAPTER

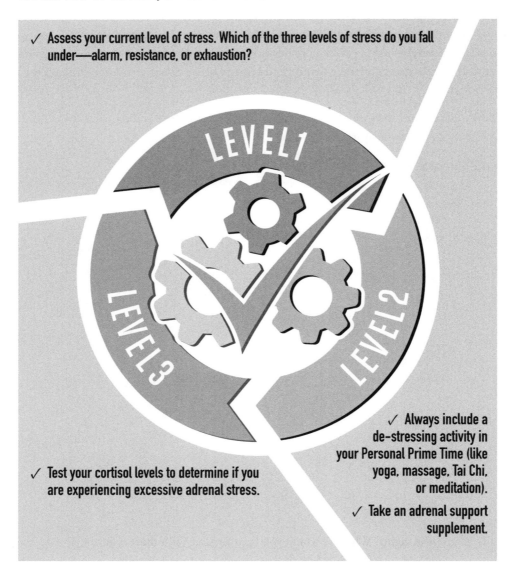

✓ Assess your current level of stress. Which of the three levels of stress do you fall under—alarm, resistance, or exhaustion?

✓ Test your cortisol levels to determine if you are experiencing excessive adrenal stress.

✓ Always include a de-stressing activity in your Personal Prime Time (like yoga, massage, Tai Chi, or meditation).

✓ Take an adrenal support supplement.

HACK YOUR HEALTH PROGRESS

CHAPTER 34

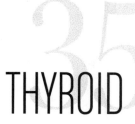

THYROID
Slow and Sluggish = Fatigue and Weight Gain

> "I saw a woman with a T-shirt with 'Guess' on it. I said, thyroid problems?"
>
> — Arnold Schwarzenegger

THINK IT OVER

- Could your thyroid be the reason you are not feeling well?

- Are you experiencing symptoms of thyroid dysfunction, but yet your blood tests keep coming back normal?

- Do you know what vitamins and minerals are key to your thyroid health?

Do you recognize this scenario: You watch what you eat, work out five times a week, but your waistline keeps getting bigger? You're tired no matter how much you sleep. You're cold all the time, your hair is falling out, you're often constipated, plus your brain always seems to be foggy. You go to your doctor and get your thyroid tested but each time your test results come back "normal." You couldn't be more frustrated. You know something is wrong with your thyroid. Well, that's got to be it, right?! Why else would you be struggling with these symptoms?

You're most likely right, and something is probably wrong with your thyroid. It is said that more than 12 percent of the U.S. population will develop a thyroid condition during their lifetime, and, of those, up to 60 percent are unaware of their condition.[1]

WHAT IS THE THYROID?

The thyroid is your master gland of metabolism, which works with a whole team of glands to keep your body running smoothly. In addition to metabolism, the thyroid is also involved in brain development, breathing, heart and nervous system function, body temperature, muscle strength, weight and cholesterol.

In other words, it plays a very important role in your overall health and well-being. In fact, improper thyroid function can lead to many issues like difficulties managing weight, Irritable Bowel Syndrome, infertility, skin disorders, aches and pains, a spectrum of autoimmune diseases and much more. When it comes down to it, if your thyroid isn't functioning well, neither are you.

The thyroid is a butterfly-shaped gland found inside your neck under your larynx, or voice box. It is responsible for producing three very important hormones:

- Triiodothyronine (T3)
- Thyroxine (T4)
- Diiodothyronine (T2)

These hormones play a crucial role in the human body, interacting with all of our other hormones: insulin, cortisol, estrogen, progesterone and testosterone. The fact that all of these hormones are interconnected explains why a dysfunctional thyroid can cause a large amount of seemingly unrelated health problems and diseases.

THE THYROID AND HORMONE PRODUCTION

Currently, the T2 hormone is the least understood of the thyroid hormones and is the subject of several ongoing studies. Previously, the focus has been on the study of T3 and T4 hormones. This isn't surprising when you factor in that 80 percent of the hormones produced by your thyroid are in the form of T4. Additionally, approximately 60 percent of T4 is converted to the T3 hormone, which is 10 times more biologically active than its counterpart.[2]

When the thyroid is working optimally, you will have the correct amounts of T3 and T4. These hormones control the metabolism of every cell in your body. If your T3 is inadequate, either by scarce production or from abnormal conversion rate from T4, your whole system will suffer. Some T3 is also produced in different parts of the body, with the liver playing the major role in the conversion of T4 to T3. So, if the liver is stressed and is overloaded by toxins, the conversion of T4 to T3 will be impeded.

Factors that disrupt T3 production include:

- toxins (e.g., PCBs, BPA, triclosan, dioxins)
- heavy metals
- fluoride (an antagonist to iodine)
- infection or trauma
- certain medications
- radiation
- autoimmune diseases (such as celiac disease)

- elevated cortisol levels

If this was not complex enough, there is also a hormone called reverse T3 (RT3), which decreases thyroid function. A great analogy of this is looking at T3 as the gas pedal of the thyroid and RT3 as the brakes. Elevated levels of RT3 can be a sign of toxicity from heavy metals or a sign of high stress.

The improper functioning of the thyroid can result in two possible outcomes: hypothyroidism or hyperthyroidism.

Symptoms of hypothyroidism include:

- fatigue
- cold intolerance
- menstrual issues
- constipation
- pains

- weight gain
- dry skin and hair
- edema
- muscle and joint aches
- depression

Symptoms of hyperthyroidism include:

- anxiety
- heart palpitations
- sweating
- increase in bowel movements

- irritability
- intolerance to heat
- tremors
- weight loss

MINERALS, CHEMICALS AND THYROID FUNCTION

As with most health conditions, a lack of certain vitamins and minerals can lead to thyroid deficiency. The most important mineral in thyroid function is iodine. The body needs iodine to make thyroid hormones. Iodine also plays a role in fertility and fetal development, protection against breast and prostate cancer, and autoimmune diseases. Unfortunately, most of us are iodine deficient due to the erosion of our soils. Eroded soils lack essential minerals and are depleted of nutrients for basic plant nutrition. Insufficient iodine intake impairs the production of thyroid hormones, leading to hypothyroidism. The best sources of iodine are ocean foods like fish and seaweed.

Other things that affect the absorption of iodine include:

- calcium carbonate
- coffee
- antacids
- grapefruit juice

- soy
- aluminum
- sulphate

Selenium is also an important mineral affecting thyroid function. The thyroid contains more selenium by weight than any other organ. Selenium is a necessary component of the enzymes that convert T4 to T3. Selenium also plays a role in fertility and fetal development, mitochondrial function, calcium homeostasis and antioxidant function. Other minerals that have an effect on thyroid function include zinc, tyrosine, iron, and vitamins C, E, D, B2, B3 and B6. If you are deficient in one or more of these vitamins and minerals, symptoms of thyroid dysfunction are likely to occur.

THYROID NEUROTOXICITY

Bromine exposure is a huge concern when it comes to thyroid neurotoxicity. Bromine is a chemical element found in many baked goods and processed foods today. It's also found in fire retardant and in our mattresses, sofas and carpets—making it very hard to avoid. Individuals overly exposed to bromines are at risk of developing thyroid problems and other health issues. This is because bromines are common endocrine disruptors. They compete for the same cell receptors that are used to capture iodine, which means that, if bromine is present, your body will not hold onto the iodine that it needs. And, as we just learned, iodine is incredibly important in thyroid function.

Another heavy metal to look out for is cadmium. It, too, is known as an endocrine disrupter and tends to concentrate in the kidneys and thyroid. Overexposure can impair conversion of T4 to T3, lead to the formation of reactive oxygen species (ROS) and malondialdehyde, as well as decrease glutathione levels, which damages mitochondria. Those who smoke cigarettes, as well as those who work in the steel, mining, or smelting industries, or those who have been subjected to battery or plastic burning have been exposed to cadmium.

BLOOD TESTS AND THYROID ISSUES

If you suspect that your thyroid gland may be sluggish, ask to get tested, but do realize that most routine blood tests test only for Thyroid Stimulating Hormones (TSH). The issue with only measuring TSH is that you are not getting the full picture of your thyroid function. A complete thyroid blood panel should include free T4, free T3, reverse T3 and thyroid antibodies (TPO and anti-TG) to assess central and peripheral thyroid function as well as thyroid auto-immunity.

The most common cause of hypothyroidism is called Hashimoto's autoimmunity. This is where the body actually mounts an immune reaction against its own thyroid gland tissue, leading to inflammation and destruction of the gland. This is why thyroid antibodies should be measured before it can be concluded that the thyroid is working optimally. Women are typically much more prone to develop a thyroid autoimmune disease. It is also important to test for selenium, iodine, zinc, ferritin, iron magnesium, and vitamin A and D, as all of these vitamins and minerals are important in the functioning of the thyroid, as mentioned earlier.

Although everyone should get their thyroid levels checked, it is especially important for individuals who:

- work in toxic environments or with toxic products like pesticides, metal plating, batteries, plastics, plumbing, or in indoor water treatment facilities

- are on a variety of medications

- have a history of thyroid issues in the family

- are planning on getting pregnant

A urinary iodine plus test should also be done to measure the level of iodine, bromine and cadmium in your body. This will help to determine if your endocrine system is being disrupted or not.

HOW TO NATURALLY BALANCE YOUR THYROID

- Eat organic as often as possible to minimize pesticide exposure.

- Avoid eating from plastic containers; use glass, instead.

- Opt for a water filtration system to decrease fluoride exposure as fluoride counteracts iodine.

- Consume iodine-dense whole foods such as potatoes, strawberries, sea vegetables, beans, cranberries, etc. (But, don't do this if you have been diagnosed with Hashimoto's autoimmune disease, as too much iodine may be contraindicated.) It is best is to get iodine levels tested to know if you have too much or too little.

- Minimize stress to maintain healthy cortisol levels.

- Be cautious about which medications you are using, as some are known to disrupt hormone function.

- Ensure you are getting enough sleep.

- Remain active. Exercise helps improve cellular sensitivity to thyroid hormones.

- Eat vitamin-rich foods and consider taking supplements if you are deficient. For optimal thyroid function, one should take 15-20 mg of iron (You want to have a ferritin level of 50-100 mcg.), 15-30 mg of zinc, 200-400 mcg of selenium, and 2,000 IU of vitamin D (depending on how much sun exposure you get).

- Other supplements like tyrosine, sensoril ashwagandha, guggul extract, pantothenic acid (vitamin B5)—as well as a good multivitamin—can also help balance and support the thyroid.

WHAT ABOUT NATURAL VS. SYNTHETIC THYROID MEDICATION?

The use of synthetic thyroid drugs has become widespread in the treatment of hypothyroid problems. The active ingredient is levothyroxine, which is a synthetic (man-/woman-made) version of the principal thyroid hormone, thyroxine (T4). Also available is a more natural form, which consists of desiccated animal thyroid. It is commonly used by those who are trying a less synthetic approach of treating their thyroid problems when lifestyle modifications and thyroid support supplementation have not been successful to balance thyroid function.

In a study examining the effects of desiccated thyroid versus levothyroxine, 70 patients with hypothyroidism were treated with either the former or latter for 12 weeks, followed by a switch to the other for another 16 weeks. The participants were "blinded" during both phases, meaning they did not know the type of pill they received. After each treatment period, patients were weighed, had blood tests, underwent psychometric testing, and were asked which therapy they preferred. The researchers report that 49 percent of the patients preferred desiccated thyroid extract, 19 percent preferred levothyroxine and 23 percent had no preference. Desiccated thyroid extract use was also associated with more weight loss.[3]

IN CONCLUSION

Many people experience thyroid problems. If you suspect that you are one of them, get tested and start implementing some of the tips suggested above. Also, it is important to remember that we can't treat lab results—we have to treat the whole person.

The following diagram shows examples of health habits, with corresponding hack levels. To download the *Hack Your Health Habits Worksheet*, visit

www.hackyourhealthhabits.com/worksheets

READY #HEALTHHACKER?
EXAMPLES OF LEVEL 1, 2 AND 3 HACKS FOR THIS CHAPTER

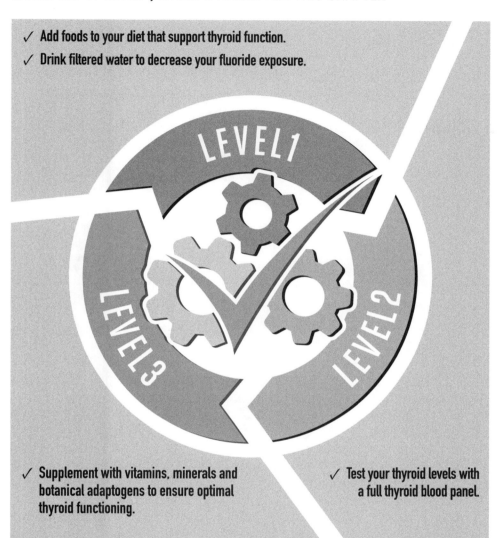

✓ Add foods to your diet that support thyroid function.
✓ Drink filtered water to decrease your fluoride exposure.

✓ Supplement with vitamins, minerals and botanical adaptogens to ensure optimal thyroid functioning.

✓ Test your thyroid levels with a full thyroid blood panel.

HACK YOUR HEALTH PROGRESS

||||||||||||||||||||||||||||||||||||||||||||||||||||||||||||||||||||||||

CHAPTER 35

SEX HORMONES
Happy or Cranky?

"To control your hormones
is to control your life."

— Dr. Barry Sears

THINK IT OVER

- **What are symptoms of sex hormone imbalance?**

- **Do you know what xenoestrogens are and how they are affecting your health?**

- **Are there ways to balance hormones without the use of pharmaceutical management?**

Remember your middle school sex-ed class, where boys were taught about erections and sperm and girls were taught about bras and periods? Amongst the birds and the bees and your classmates' giggles, one key aspect of puberty was left out—the aspect responsible for turning us into functioning, reproductive adults—our sex hormones.

When it comes to sex hormones, many of us are misinformed. We've come to accept heavy, dreadful periods and deathly menopausal symptoms as normal parts of female physiology, and erectile dysfunction as a normal part of men aging. The thing is, they aren't, and this chapter explains why and what you can do about it. Think of it as a sex-ed class for adults.

HOW SEX HORMONES ARE MADE

Hormones are special chemical messengers in the body that control most bodily functions. The hormones that have the biggest impact on us are the steroid hormones. These include estrogen, progesterone, testosterone, DHEA and cortisol. Understanding these major hormones and what they do can help us take better control of our health.

To begin with, it's important to note that *cholesterol*—which is often made out to be the enemy of health—is the precursor to the production of our sex hormones. When cholesterol levels are depleted due to poor liver function or the use of statin drugs, hormone production is disrupted. This puts individuals at a greater risk for not only hormone dysfunction, but also for cognitive impairments, depression and certain types of cancers. In other words, we need to keep our hormones healthy, if we want to function optimally.

Now that we know some of the basics, let's delve a little deeper and expand upon the roles of your sex hormones.

ESTROGEN

Estrogen is not a single hormone as many think; it is a group of hormones that play an important role in the development of men's and women's sexual and reproductive health. What hormones make up estrogen?

1. **Estrone (E1)** is an estrogenic hormone secreted by the ovaries as well as adipose tissue. It is the main form of estrogen in postmenopausal women.

2. **Estradiol (E2)** is produced by the ovaries using cholesterol and is the main estrogen secreted before periods cease at menopause. It is also produced by the adrenal glands. It is responsible for building up the lining of the uterus. It is known as a strong estrogen with a powerful effect on estrogen receptors.

3. **Estriol (E3)** is a relatively weak natural estrogenic hormone and is one of the metabolic products of estradiol. It is the main estrogen produced during pregnancy.

In women, estrogen is produced in the ovaries, adrenal glands and fat cells. Men produce estrogen through a process involving an enzyme called aromatase, which transforms testosterone into estradiol. Estrogen can affect both men and women. However, it is largely responsible for female physical features and reproduction.

Ladies, you will remember going through puberty, seeing your breasts develop, pubic and armpit hair grow, and the start of your menstruation cycle. This was a result of rising estrogen levels. While estrogen is mainly involved in puberty and reproduction, it also affects the urinary tract, cardiovascular health, bones, breasts, skin, hair and even the brain. And that's not all.

Estrogen also plays a role in the:

- formation of female secondary sex characteristics

- acceleration of metabolism

- reduction of muscle mass

- increase of fat stores

- stimulation of endometrial growth

- increase of uterine growth

- increase of vaginal lubrication

- thickening of the vaginal wall

- maintenance of vessel and skin

- increase of bone formation

- promotion of heart health

For many reasons, your body can make too much or too little estrogen. One may even be exposed to too much estrogen via certain foods, medication, etc.—more on this later. When this happens, hormones become imbalanced and symptoms can persist.

Excess estrogen—also called estrogen dominance—can cause:

- acne

- depression

- fatigue

- fluid retention

- loss of libido

- low thyroid function

- low progesterone

- memory loss

- migraine headaches

- heavy and painful menstruations

- PMS

- hot flashes

- weight gain

- insomnia

- estrogen-dominant conditions such as uterine fibroids, fibrocystic breasts, ovarian cysts, endometriosis and cancer

- erectile dysfunction in men

- breast growth in men

Do some of these symptoms sound familiar?

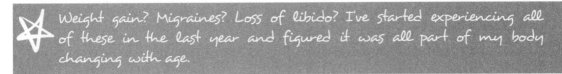

Weight gain? Migraines? Loss of libido? I've started experiencing all of these in the last year and figured it was all part of my body changing with age.

It's surprising that many of these symptoms are considered a normal part of menstruation or menopause, such as the fluid retention, acne, or hot flashes. In reality, they are just signs that our hormones are imbalanced.

On the other end of the spectrum, low estrogen can cause:

- brain fog
- painful intercourse
- recurring urinary tract infections
- vaginal dryness
- thinning of vaginal wall
- hot flashes and night sweats
- infertility
- low libido in men
- excess belly fat in men

Again, brain fog, vaginal dryness and loss of libido are commonly associated with aging, but is that really what aging gracefully consists of? I hope not! Many of these signs are subtle or not-so-subtle indications that our hormones may not be functioning up to par. This shouldn't be taken lightly.

ESTROGEN DOMINANCE: XENOESTROGENS—HOW THEY AFFECT US

A problem today is that we are bombarded by environmental estrogens, also called xenoestrogens or estrogen mimickers. These synthetic chemicals act like estrogen in the body. When you have too much estrogen, you are what is called estrogen-dominant.

Some of the most common female estrogen-dominant conditions are pre-menstrual syndrome (PMS), endometriosis, abnormal PAP tests, ovarian cysts, cystic breasts, uterine fibroids, heavy periods, low thyroid function, cellulite, hormonal acne and severe menopausal symptoms. Also, if you cannot lose weight, there is also a good chance you are estrogen-dominant. On top of that, women who take hormones in the form of the birth control pill or hormone replacement therapy can also become hormone overloaded if they are not being monitored properly, increasing their risks for serious health issues.

Xenoestrogen can be either synthetic or natural chemical compounds and can be found in our food and environment, including in:

- pesticides, herbicides and fungicides

- parabens and phthalates, which are mostly found in cosmetics

- farmed fish, commercially raised meat and dairy

- birth control pills and hormone replacement therapy

- coffee and alcohol

- soy products

Just about every organ and tissue in the body have estrogen receptors. When estrogen circulates in the body, it binds to estrogen receptors and triggers certain effects in that organ or tissue. Xenoestrogen will mimic our natural estrogen and attach to our estrogen receptors, potentially taking the place of a real estrogen molecule, or giving the cell the wrong signals. This disturbs our hormonal system and affects the entire body. Limiting exposure to these chemical estrogen mimickers is key for optimal hormone function and optimal health.

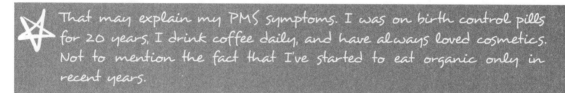

That may explain my PMS symptoms. I was on birth control pills for 20 years, I drink coffee daily, and have always loved cosmetics. Not to mention the fact that I've started to eat organic only in recent years.

PROGESTERONE

Known as the "feel good hormone," progesterone is produced in the ovaries and used in the production of other sex hormones in women. Progesterone receptors can be found all over the body including the brain, skin, thyroid, blood vessels, breasts and bones. An optimal level of progesterone is needed to ensure that these areas function properly. Progesterone is especially high during pregnancy, keeping the uterus from contracting until labor begins. It naturally decreases around menopause when the ovaries stop the production of eggs. However, small amounts are still produced by the adrenal glands. In men, progesterone is converted into testosterone and DHEA.

How will you know if you have too much or too little progesterone?

Symptoms of *excess* progesterone include:

- breast swelling and pain

- depression or low mood

- growing excess facial hair

- fatigue, drowsiness

- overproducing insulin
- low libido
- oily skin
- developing brown spots on the skin

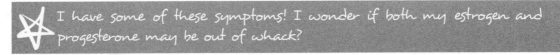

I have some of these symptoms! I wonder if both my estrogen and progesterone may be out of whack?

Symptoms of *low* progesterone include:

- anxiety or difficulty handling stress
- carb craving
- elevated cortisol levels
- estrogen-dominant conditions
- headaches
- heavy periods
- infertility
- osteopenia and osteoporosis
- recurring miscarriages
- water retention
- weight gains around the abdomen
- insomnia

TESTOSTERONE

Testosterone, although known to influence male sex drive and aggression, also plays an important role in female hormone health. It is crucial for women's sex drive, muscle tone, bone health, skin and cardiovascular system. In women, testosterone is produced in the ovaries but most is later converted into estradiol.

Symptoms of *low* testosterone are:

- tiredness
- weakness
- mood swings and depression
- change in sleep habits
- increased body fat and decreased muscle mass

- low sex drive

- erectile dysfunction for men

- weight gain

- anxiety

- hair loss

Normal levels of testosterone will result in:

- well-being (i.e. mild euphoria and a reduction in depression)

- confidence (i.e. reduced social anxiety and greater assertiveness)

- better energy

- greater sex drive and libido

- greater concentration and focus

- body fat reduction and increased muscle mass

Women on high doses of estrogen supplementation, Hormone Replacement Therapy (HRT), may also have an increase in Sex Hormone Binding Globulin (SHBG). SHBG is a blood protein that reduces amounts of free testosterone, as it has a higher affinity to bind to testosterone than estrogen, therefore reducing the amount of testosterone available.

TESTOSTERONE AND AROMATASE

Aromatase is a naturally-occurring enzyme located in multiple tissues in the body. In men, it is located in the brain, muscles and testicles. In women, it is located in the ovaries, placenta and lining of the uterus. It is the enzyme responsible for converting testosterone into estrogen and has been found to increase with the amount of fat an individual has. Poor nutrition and weight gain are a common cause of increased aromatase activity. In addition to this, high-stress levels, lack of exercise, chronic inflammation and insulin dysregulation can also contribute to an increase in aromatase. When one wants to decrease aromatase activity in a situation where aromatase levels need to be decreased, certain foods can help. These foods include flax seeds, resveratrol, green tea extracts, quercetin, iodine, mangosteen extracts and isoflavones.

DEHYDROEPIANDROSTERONE (DHEA)

DHEA is mainly produced by the adrenal glands (just like cortisol) and is used in the production of estrogen and testosterone. It reaches its peak in your twenties and steadily declines after that. This hormone is a very powerful precursor to all of your major sex hormones: estrogen, progesterone and testosterone. When DHEA levels are low, the body does not have enough working material for proper endocrine function, which throws off overall hormone production.

CORTISOL AND THE IMPACT OF STRESS ON SEX HORMONES PRODUCTION

We have already discussed, at great length, the role of cortisol and adrenal function. However, it is also very important to make note of cortisol's impact on sex hormone production. What happens when we are stressed? First, the sympathetic nervous system kicks in by increasing heart and breathing rates, initiating sweating, jacking up blood sugar and inhibiting digestion—or as you may recall, the "fight-or-flight" response. Second, the hypothalamus, which is our hormone command center, gives marching orders to our adrenals to pump adrenaline (a short-term response) and cortisol (a longer-term response). Cortisol has many similar physiological effects to activating the sympathetic nervous system, as it can spike blood sugar, inhibit digestion and even halt immune activities.

So how is the body able to make cortisol? As mentioned in the previous chapter on the adrenals, cortisol is made from the precursor hormone pregnenolone. In times of high stress and higher cortisol production, cortisol will actually steal pregnenolone away from the sex hormone pathways, therefore reducing sex hormone production.

High cortisol levels can also result in high estrogen levels. How is that? When there is an overabundance of stored fat, fat cells produce excess estrogen, which signal to your body to store more fat. One of the main roles of cortisol is to break down fat cells and move triglycerides (fat molecules) into the bloodstream for more energy. This energy is used in "fight-or-flight" responses to stress.

However, since many people are in a constant state of "fight-or-flight" due to high-stress levels, the body often produces an overabundance of triglycerides that go unused. Cortisol causes these unused fats to be redeposited in the adipose tissues surrounding the belly. Talk about a double whammy! Keeping the adrenal glands in check and keeping our body fat low are the best ways for women to avoid hormonal imbalance and keep their hormones happy.

MENOPAUSE

Oh, menopause! I could write an entire book on menopause, but I'm going to keep it short. The secret to a happy menopause is to prepare for it. Make diet and lifestyle changes before you get there. For women who haven't gone through menopause yet, here are five questions you should ask yourself:

1. Am I running on high cortisol and stress that is causing my adrenal glands to tap out?

 Yes

2. Am I exposed to xenoestrogens that could be making me estrogen dominant?

 Yes

3. Is my blood sugar stable?

I'm not sure... I think so!

4. Are my liver and gut healthy enough to process and detoxify my hormones?

 I don't think so. In fact, I've been thinking of doing a liver detox.

5. If I am already having hormonal symptoms and have already made diet and lifestyle modifications, am I using high-quality natural supplements and adaptogens (i.e. herbs) to help balance my hormones?

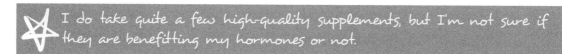 *I do take quite a few high-quality supplements, but I'm not sure if they are benefitting my hormones or not.*

Answering these five questions can bring awareness to potential body signals and lifestyle factors that could contribute to a smoother menopausal experience. This means ensuring that your adrenals are in check, that you minimize your exposure to xenoestrogens and toxins, and that you control your blood sugar.

YOUR HORMONES—GETTING TESTED

There are various methods to test for hormones, the most common being through blood, saliva and urine. Each have their strengths and limitations. For example, blood-serum testing does not effectively test adrenal hormones because free cortisol is logistically hard to test throughout the day—since you would have to get tested four times throughout the day. These methods of testing also lack in measuring the downstream metabolite by-products of hormones, which can lead to a lack in some critical information on how the body is processing and eliminating hormones—especially cortisol and estrogen. So, what is one to do?

The Newer Kid on The Block—the DUTCH Test – The Dried Urine Test for Comprehensive Hormones (DUTCH) measures hormone levels and their metabolites from urine collected at four specific times in a day. Precision Analytical, the maker of the DUTCH test, explains: *"If a hormone group is like a family, then cortisol, estradiol, progesterone and testosterone are like the parents since they are the 'heads' of their respective families."*

The hormone metabolites are like children because they are formed from the parent hormone. Combining data on the parent hormone with information about its metabolites gives a fairly complete picture of hormone function. Or, put a different way: *"The DUTCH test shows how the whole hormone family works together for most of a day, whereas serum and saliva tests only check on the parents once a day. The DUTCH test provides useful information on how your body breaks down parent hormones into metabolites that are excreted in urine."*[1]

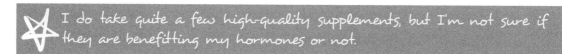 *I'm definitely going to look into this more.*

Unfortunately, not all physicians are aware of this new test, so if you are interested in doing some digging into your own hormone health and finding out how your body is using or breaking down hormones, it's worth finding a natural healthcare professional who uses this method of testing which will help dig deeper in how your body is metabolizing your hormones, giving you greater insight on what lifestyle changes would best fit your current needs.

HORMONE REPLACEMENT THERAPY (HRT)

In 2002, the Journal of the American Medical Association published results of the Women's Health Initiative study that showed the usage of HRT coincided with a 26 percent increase in invasive breast cancer, a 41 percent increase in strokes, and a 29 percent increase in heart attacks—as it doubled rates of blood clots, weight gain, and an increased risk for gallbladder and liver disease.[2]

After these findings were published, the widespread usage of HRT diminished and was followed by Bioidentical Hormone Replacement Therapy (BHRT). The synthetic hormones used in BHRT are called bioidentical hormones because they mimic the hormones naturally produced by the body on a molecular level. Although they are often thought to be a more natural approach to hormone therapy, one has to keep in mind that these too are not completely natural—they are synthesized from a plant chemical extracted from yams and soy.

The jury is still out on whether BHRT is completely safe. More studies definitely need to be done to truly understand the risks and benefits. Keep in mind that the amount of hormones given to women should aim to balance their hormones according to their age and should be adjusted as aging occurs. I personally believe that every woman's situation is different and that everyone should make decisions that are in the best interest of their health. At the same time, I believe that it's important to start with the basics of eating right, exercising, and controlling one's stress when it comes to managing symptoms.

UTERUS AND OVARY REMOVAL—THE HEALTH IMPACT

Many women have gone under the knife to have their uterus and cervix removed in a procedure called a hysterectomy. If the uterus is removed but not the cervix, this is called a subtotal hysterectomy. The ovaries together with the fallopian tubes are also sometimes removed as well; this procedure is called a Bilateral Salpingo-Oophorectomy.

When only the ovaries are removed, the procedure is called an oophorectomy. These are quite common procedures that take place for a number of reasons and are considered "safe" with little or no health effects. However, depending on a woman's age, the removal of her sex organs can very much affect her overall health as the ovaries are the main source of female hormones production. Even after menopause, the ovaries still contribute to a woman's hormonal health, to a lesser extent.

Some of the associated risks of oophorectomy include:

- increased carotid artery thickness

- increased risk of death from coronary artery disease

- decreased bone density, increased risk of osteoporosis and hip fracture

- increased risk of cognitive impairment, Parkinson's, depression and anxiety[3]

- increased risk of all cancers except ovarian cancer[4]

So how about the health effects of hysterectomies when the ovaries are preserved? Does the removal of the uterus affect ovarian function? Unfortunately, research is showing that removing the uterus while sparing the ovaries still does impede ovarian functioning.

A recent study looked at 406 women aged 30 to 47 years who underwent a hysterectomy without the removal of the ovaries, and 465 women with intact uteri. Blood samples and questionnaire data were obtained at baseline and annually for up to five years. The results showed that ovarian failure occurred among 60 of the women with hysterectomy and 46 of the women in the control group. In other words, women undergoing hysterectomy were at nearly a twofold increased risk for ovarian failure as compared with women with intact uteri.

It was further estimated that 14.8 percent of women with hysterectomies experienced ovarian failure after four years of follow-up, compared with 8 percent of the women in the control group.[5] Moreover, what many women aren't told is that the uterus and ovaries share their blood supply, and once the uterus is removed, ovarian function can be negatively affected.

As you can see, removal of female sex organs prior to menopause—and even after it—has a significant impact on hormonal function and overall health. Our sex hormones play a crucial role in the regulation of many systems throughout the body and are necessary for optimal functioning as we age.

HOW TO BALANCE YOUR HORMONES NATURALLY

There are several things you can do to regulate your hormones. Here are my top tips:

- **Prevent "pregnenolone steal"** – Make sure to keep your cortisol levels in check by controlling your stress. It is also crucial to be sleeping at least 7 to 9 hours per night to avoid your adrenals stealing from your sex hormones.

- **Decrease your environmental estrogen exposure** – Avoid products containing environmental estrogens such as cosmetics containing parabens, plastics with BPA, synthetic hormones in dairy and meat.

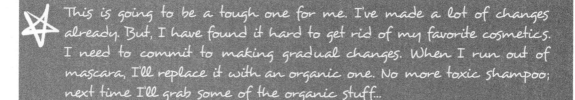

This is going to be a tough one for me. I've made a lot of changes already. But, I have found it hard to get rid of my favorite cosmetics. I need to commit to making gradual changes. When I run out of mascara, I'll replace it with an organic one. No more toxic shampoo; next time I'll grab some of the organic stuff...

- **Detoxify** – The liver acts as a filter, helping us to get rid of toxins, and, when it works overtime with things like alcohol, caffeine and prescription drugs, its ability to cleanse the blood of excess estrogen is compromised. Try your best to avoid or, at least, limit your use of these items. Easy ways to help your body detoxify is to consume organic foods and try to focus on eating cruciferous vegetables like broccoli, Brussel sprouts, cauliflower, cabbage and kale. Also, consider dry brushing, taking Epsom salt baths and using an infrared sauna regularly.

- **Rethink hormone replacement therapy (HRT) and the birth control pill** – Both can really disturb the intricate balance of many of your hormones. Before considering HRT, make sure that you have implemented appropriate lifestyle changes and have balanced your adrenals and your thyroid.

- **Clear your bowels** – Slow colonic transit time (or getting "backed up") could actually lead to an increase in estrogen levels! Vitamin C and magnesium citrate can help speed up colon transit time and get things moving smoothly.

- **Botanical adaptogens** – To protect you from environmental estrogens and hormonal imbalances, you may consider using botanical adaptogens such as indole-3-Carbinol, diindolylmethane (DIM) and sulforaphane.

When it comes to hormones, you've got to take charge! If you are experiencing the symptoms listed in this chapter, your body is telling you something is wrong. Seek help. Consider getting your hormones tested or working with a functional medicine practitioner as they have many tools to help you balance your hormones naturally.

The following diagram shows examples of health habits with corresponding hack levels. To download the *Hack Your Health Habits Worksheet*, visit

www.hackyourhealthhabits.com/worksheets

READY #HEALTHHACKER?
EXAMPLES OF LEVEL 1, 2 AND 3 HACKS FOR THIS CHAPTER

✓ Add broccoli, cabbage, or kale to your lunch or dinner.

✓ Assess your current level of xenoestrogen exposure. What can you do to minimize it?

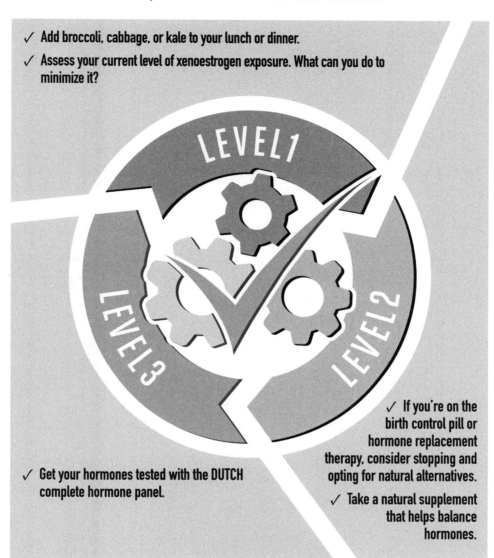

LEVEL 1

LEVEL 2

✓ If you're on the birth control pill or hormone replacement therapy, consider stopping and opting for natural alternatives.

✓ Take a natural supplement that helps balance hormones.

LEVEL 3

✓ Get your hormones tested with the DUTCH complete hormone panel.

HACK YOUR HEALTH PROGRESS

||||||||||||||||||||||||||||||||||||||||||||||||||||||||||||||||||||||||||||||||||||||||

CHAPTER 36

BLOOD SUGAR

How Is It Impacting Your Weight and Your Health?

"Eat less sugar, you're sweet
enough already."

— UNKNOWN

THINK IT OVER

- Have you ever experienced symptoms of hypo- or hyperglycemia?

- Have you had your blood sugar levels measured recently?

- Do you know the negative health effects of artificial sweeteners?

Today, it is said that the average American consumes 32 teaspoons of sugar per day.[1] That's just over half a cup. Stop and think about it.

Sugar is added to coffee and tea, baked into pastries, cakes and cookies, and sprinkled over breakfast cereal for added "flavor." It's even hidden in dressings, sauces, soups, bread, pasta and grain products. A little sugar here and a little sugar there can quickly become 32 teaspoons. This is highly problematic as sugar is said to be eight times more addictive than cocaine and has serious implications for our health.

 The amount of sugar in soda and juice is extraordinary.

Elevated blood sugar levels can cause insulin resistance, metabolic syndrome, cardiovascular diseases, cognitive decline, pancreatic cancer and type 2 diabetes. In order to survive, our bodies try to naturally maintain a balance (or homeostasis) of blood glucose levels. As a result, a person who has stable blood sugar levels should not experience a surge of energy right after consuming a meal, nor a drop in energy as these are respectively indicative of reactive hypoglycemia and insulin resistance issues.

However, when overloaded with more sugar than can be metabolized, homeostasis is difficult to maintain. Those with healthy blood sugar levels can handle spikes and keep ourselves in homeostasis. Those unable to keep blood sugar levels balanced likely suffer from either hypoglycemia (low blood sugar) or hyperglycemia (high blood sugar).

What's the difference? People who suffer from *hypo*glycemia tend to have symptoms such as:

- impaired mental function
- lethargy
- shakes or twitches
- loss of muscle strength
- irritability or aggression
- sweating
- paranoia
- feeling a surge of energy after meals

Meanwhile, those with *hyper*glycemia tend to have:

- trouble concentrating
- heart problems
- obesity
- kidney damage
- worsening vision or even eye damage
- intestinal issues—chronic constipation or diarrhea
- skin and vaginal infections
- nerve damage resulting in loss of hair
- cold or insensitive feet, or erectile dysfunction in men

The symptoms listed above occur when blood sugars levels are consistently high. A drastic spike in blood sugar levels (which lasts a shorter period of time) can sometimes result in different symptoms like:

- loss of consciousness (in extreme situations)
- a loss of appetite

- increased thirst

- blurred vision

- frequent urination

- headaches

It's astonishing the number of bodily systems that are affected by high blood glucose. Robert Lustig, a professor of Clinical Pediatrics in the Division of Endocrinology at the University of California and a pioneer in decoding sugar metabolism, says that your body can safely metabolize approximately six teaspoons of sugar per day.[2] Remember when I said most Americans consume 32 teaspoons per day? Since most Americans consume way more than six teaspoons, the excess sugar is often metabolized into body fat, which has led to debilitating chronic metabolic diseases.

ARE ALL SUGARS DANGEROUS?

There are many different types of sugar, some of which are more dangerous than others:

- Glucose refers to the "simple" sugars found in all foods that contain carbohydrates. Your body breaks down carbohydrates into glucose to use for immediate energy, while the excess is stored in the form of glycogen in the muscles or fat.

- Fructose is another simple sugar. It's commonly referred to as fruit sugar because it's mostly found in fruits. Honey is also considered a fructose.

- Sucrose typically combines glucose and fructose to become a "complex" sugar. Examples of this include white and brown sugars. Processed sugars, or refined sugars, come from sugarcanes or sugar beets that are processed to extract the sugar.

- High-fructose corn syrup is a chemically produced sugar that's cheaper than regular sugar and is found in many processed foods.

Are these sugars healthy? Glucose and fructose, in their natural states, are quite safe—to a certain extent. However, those trying to lose weight or who have blood sugar issues should limit their fruit and simple carbohydrate consumption. Furthermore, we also have to be wary of refined and chemically produced sugars as they can wreak havoc on our health. Consuming too much of them can truly contribute to the health problems discussed earlier in this chapter.

WHAT ABOUT ARTIFICIAL SWEETENERS?

Artificial sweeteners like Splenda, NutraSweet, Sweet 'N' Low, Saccharin, Sorbitol or Sucralose should also be avoided. Though they might not have the same effects as sugar consumption, they come with a whole new set of health problems—health problems, dare I say, that are even worse than what sugar or high fructose corn syrup can do!

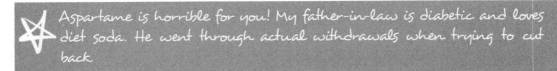

They have been shown to increase the very things that they are said to help prevent: obesity, metabolic syndrome, type 2 diabetes and cardiovascular disease. They are also known as neurotoxins and have been shown to contribute to gut dysbiosis and interfere with metabolic functions.[3]

SUGAR AND INSULIN RESISTANCE

The constant roller coaster of spikes and dips in blood sugar produces what we call AGES—Advanced Glycation End Products. They are one of the causes of cellular oxidation and inflammation and can lead to insulin resistance if not attended to. A good analogy to better illustrate the effects of glycation on the cells is to think of how rust forms on a car. Similarly, AGES "rust" the cell.

The overconsumption of carbohydrates and refined sugars has led to an increase in diabetes, heart conditions, cancers and many other lifestyle-related illnesses. Thus, when striving for health, energy and vitality, it's important to understand blood sugar and its effect on our overall well-being.

The hormone insulin is a key player in the regulation of blood sugar. Insulin's job is to stimulate the uptake of glucose into the cells and promote the production of glycogen.

Glycogen is a source of stored glucose in the cells—mostly liver and muscles. Insulin also promotes the formation of lipids, triglycerides and proteins. When the system is functioning optimally, the body can easily convert glucose into energy. In other words, it is insulin *sensitive*, which is the case in healthy, active people. The opposite of this is insulin *resistance*.

Individuals who are overweight and tend to make poor lifestyle choices can develop a resistance to insulin. Insulin resistance occurs when the amount of insulin secreted is not enough to move glucose into cells. This means the body must produce more insulin to metabolize the amount of sugar it's presented with, resulting in chronically high insulin levels. Insulin resistance puts a strain on the pancreas, which can negatively impact your waistline, energy, mood and overall health. It can also result in the development of type 2 diabetes. Another common issue that comes along with insulin resistance is its ability to inhibit the conversion of the thyroid hormone T4 to T3, so many diabetics or individuals with insulin resistance will often end up with thyroid issues.

What are the symptoms of insulin resistance? Well, to start, constant cravings for sweets or caffeine shows that the body is going through spikes and drops of blood sugar, and is looking for something to regain energy. This can cause fatigue, poor concentration, irritability, and other symptoms such as:

- weakness
- fogginess
- weight gain

- insomnia
- greater appetite
- anxiety

- ADHD
- puffiness in the skin
- depression

- heart palpitations
- water retention

Insulin also plays a key role in the body's ability to burn fat. When insulin and blood sugar levels are too high, the body is unable to burn fat and stores fat into cells. This is why so many people struggle with losing weight. Many start the day with a high-carb breakfast (e.g. toast, bagels, pancakes, cereals), which is problematic as carbohydrates turn into sugar. High-carb breakfasts spike our insulin levels and can cause us to crash by mid-morning.

What do we tend to reach for when crashing? Something sugary like a muffin or a chocolate granola bar, which perpetuates the cycle and keeps us in fat-building mode. The cycle also suppresses the body's ability to turn fat into energy, causing people to feel lethargic and experience more mood swings. The less active people are and the more sugars they consume, the less energy they have to complete their daily activities, and the more they pack on pounds. It's a very vicious cycle in which many people are trapped.

When we eat right and exercise, insulin is our friend. It helps us build muscle, regulate our blood sugar levels and absorb energy. It's the poor choices we make that turn insulin into a bad guy. Too many refined sugars, carbohydrates and processed foods, not enough sleep, and high-stress levels all contribute to poor insulin regulation. The harsh reality is that the body was never designed to handle the carbs and sugar that the average person consumes. If we want insulin to work in our favor, we need to make healthier choices.

SUGAR AND LEPTIN

Excess sugar not only affects insulin, it also affects leptin. Leptin is a very influential hormone produced by fat cells. It is how fat cells communicate with the brain to let it know how much energy is available and what to do with it. If the system is working properly, excess food energy will surge leptin levels, signaling to the brain that fat is no longer needed and to stop eating. It also tells the brain that you are full. Leptin resistance occurs when the brain no longer receives the satiety message, and you continue eating even if you have already fueled up. You become leptin-resistant the same way that you become insulin-resistant—by continuous overexposure to high levels of the hormone. Yes, yet another double whammy!

TYPE-3 DIABETES

For years, the primary cause of Alzheimer's disease was unknown. But a growing body of research suggests there's a powerful connection between your diet and your risk of both Alzheimer's disease and glaucoma—a condition that causes damage to your eye's optic nerve. Alzheimer's disease is now being called "type-3 diabetes" by some experts.

Why this connection? Researchers have learned that the pancreas is not the only organ that produces insulin—the brain does as well. And "this brain insulin is necessary for the survival of your brain cells."[4]

Insulin helps with neuronal glucose uptake and the regulation of neurotransmitters, like acetylcholine, which is crucial for memory and learning. This is why reducing the level of insulin in your brain impairs your cognition. Other research shows that type-2 diabetics lose more brain volume with age than expected, particularly gray matter. This kind of brain atrophy is yet another contributing factor for dementia.

"Brain diabetes" may also be responsible for glaucoma, according to recent research. Fluctuations in insulin production in your brain may contribute to the degeneration of your brain cells, and studies have found that people with lower levels of insulin and insulin receptors in their brain often develop Alzheimer's disease.

SLEEP, STRESS AND SUGAR

Sleep plays a major role in controlling satiety, appetite and even insulin levels. It also affects ghrelin, which is known as the hunger hormone. Studies show that sleeping less than seven hours per night can significantly increase ghrelin levels, causing cravings and an increased appetite. The less you sleep, the higher the secretion of ghrelin and the greater the chance of gaining weight.

Another shocking fact is that the more fat cells you have, the more the body produces ghrelin. Due to this, individuals who are overweight are more likely to feel hungry even when full, and this results in eating more and storing more fat. To get out of this cycle, it's important to get at least seven to eight hours of undisturbed sleep per night. This helps the body rejuvenate and regulate its hormones, so that ghrelin isn't overproduced.

As discussed in prior chapters, stress also affects blood sugar control. In stressful situations, our adrenal glands secrete cortisol, which when partnered with adrenaline creates that "fight-or-flight" response. Cortisol's main function is to raise blood sugar levels by converting glycogen from your muscles back into sugar for immediate energy. This provides you with fuel for sudden and unexpected situations, like running away from a harmful situation. As our blood sugar increases in response to our cortisol levels, our insulin levels also rise. Our body was designed to handle short bursts of stress. Unfortunately, in this day and age, many people are chronically stressed, which is something our body wasn't designed for. Chronic stress keeps our cortisol and insulin levels elevated, which is the perfect recipe for weight gain.

New research has also shown that there is a connection between insulin dysfunction and mood disturbances such as depression. According to the research, blood sugar irregularities can take a toll on the human brain and neurotransmitter function.[5]

METABOLIC RISK FACTORS

As if all this was not enough, the combination of these lifestyle stressors can eventually lead to an overarching condition known as metabolic syndrome. The five conditions described below are metabolic risk factors. You can have any one of these risk factors by itself, but they tend to occur together. In order to be officially diagnosed with metabolic syndrome, you must have at least three of the metabolic risk factors.[6]

- **A large waistline** – This also is called abdominal obesity or "having an apple shape." Excess fat in the abdominal area causes a greater risk factor for heart disease than excess fat in other parts of the body.

- **A high triglyceride level** – Triglycerides are a type of fat found in the blood, and, when they are too high, chances for heart disease and stroke are increased. Triglycerides can be increased due to a diet high in refined carbs, sugars and unhealthy trans fats.

- **A low HDL cholesterol level** – HDL sometimes is called "good" cholesterol. This is because it helps remove cholesterol from your arteries. A low HDL cholesterol level raises your risk for heart disease.

- **High blood pressure** – Blood pressure is the force of blood pushing against the walls of your arteries as your heart pumps blood. If this pressure rises and stays high over time, it can damage your heart and lead to plaque buildup.

- **High fasting blood sugar** – Even mildly high blood sugar may be an early sign of prediabetes. Tests such as the fasted serum glucose test can help identify if blood sugar is abnormally high so that the necessary precautions can be taken to prevent it from becoming higher.

TESTING FOR BLOOD SUGAR?

When testing, blood sugar levels are not the only thing to be measured; you should measure insulin levels and hemoglobin A1c (which is a measure of glycation), as well. Other tests should include measuring High Sensitivity C-Reactive Protein, which is a good marker for inflammation. It can also be important to test levels of cytokines, interleukins and TNF-alpha since they are inflammatory markers as well. Other markers like ferritin levels, fibrinogen activity and homocysteine can also be tested to indicate inflammation or oxidative stress response.

HOW TO KICK THE SUGAR ADDICTION

Reading about the effects of sugar and stress is enough to make someone stressed. But don't be too discouraged. There are solutions. There might not be a magic pill, but eating a proper diet and exercising daily is the only magic you need! Eating right and moving your body is the best treatment for restoring the body's ability to respond to insulin.

When trying to kick your sugar addiction, keep these tips in mind:

- **Address hypoglycemia** – People who are hypoglycemic are often not hungry in the morning and sometimes are even nauseated. It is suggested that they should try their best to eat, even a small amount. They should start with small bites to engage their parasympathetic (rest-and-digest) system and gradually finish their meals. After 2 or 3 days of stabilizing their blood glucose, they will take themselves out of sympathetic (fight-or-flight) overdrive, and will no longer wake up with nausea or loss of appetite.

- **Drink water** – Keeping the body hydrated helps it function optimally. It also allows more waste to be eliminated rather than being stored.

- **Eat healthy fats** – Increase your consumption of healthy fats, such as omega-3, saturated and monounsaturated fats. Your body needs health-promoting fats from animal and vegetable sources for optimal functioning. Some of the best sources include organic butter from raw milk, (unheated) virgin olive oil, coconut oil, raw nuts like walnuts and macadamias, free-range eggs, avocado and wild sockeye salmon.

- **Substitute natural sugars for artificial ones** – Natural sugars do not spike the blood glucose level as much as refined sugars. They also provide some nutrients and minerals the body can use. Reach for things like raw honey or maple syrup. Stay away from artificial sugars.

- **Use herbs and spices** – Cinnamon not only has a sweet taste to it but is actually good for helping to balance your blood sugar levels. You can also use fenugreek, bitter melon, or bilberry as they too have been shown to impact blood sugar levels.

- **Exercise** – Craving something sweet? Exercise. Exercising replaces the "sugar rush" with an endorphin rush and gives your body the energy boost it's looking for.

- **Don't smoke** – Smoking contributes to insulin resistance. Quitting is recommended to keep the sugar levels under control, as well as to improve your overall health.

- **Monitor your sugar levels** – Consider buying a blood glucose monitor to measure your blood sugar levels. Most monitors are around $100. A little pricey, but a worthy investment. Many people are surprised by how high their blood sugars actually are. Measuring your levels can help gauge where you are at and how much sugar needs to be cut out of your diet.

SUPPLEMENT RECOMMENDATIONS TO HELP STABILIZE BLOOD SUGAR

Although diet and lifestyle changes should be your main method of stabilizing blood sugar, there are also supplement options that can help such as:

- chromium
- probiotics
- magnesium
- alpha-lipoic acid
- vanadium
- vitamin C
- selenium
- Chirositol®
- vitamin D
- CoQ10
- EPA/DHA
- biotin
- zinc

Maintaining a normal and stable blood glucose level is key when it comes to weight management and improving your overall health. Ultimately, too much sugar leads to inflammation, and inflammation leads to chronic diseases. The choice is yours.

The following diagram shows examples of health habits with corresponding hack levels. To download the *Hack Your Health Habits Worksheet*, visit

www.hackyourhealthhabits.com/worksheets

READY #HEALTHHACKER?
EXAMPLES OF LEVEL 1, 2 AND 3 HACKS FOR THIS CHAPTER

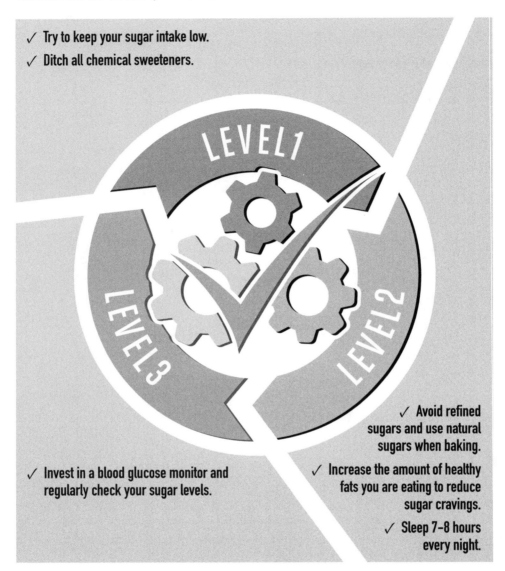

✓ Try to keep your sugar intake low.
✓ Ditch all chemical sweeteners.

✓ Avoid refined sugars and use natural sugars when baking.
✓ Increase the amount of healthy fats you are eating to reduce sugar cravings.
✓ Sleep 7–8 hours every night.

✓ Invest in a blood glucose monitor and regularly check your sugar levels.

HACK YOUR HEALTH PROGRESS

|||||||||||||||||||||||||||||||||||||||||||||||||||||||||||||

CHAPTER 37

SECTION 8

*Get Your Gut and Immune
System Performing Optimally*

Do you know what vital role your gut plays in
moderating your overall wellness? From your mood
to your immunity, your digestive tract is a lot more
than just a food processor! Section 8 discusses the
conditions associated with a troubled digestive
system, and explores why healing the gut is the
foundation for improving many chronic
health conditions.

38

YOUR GUT
Understanding How It Works and What Could Go Wrong

"All diseases begin in
the gut."

— Hippocrates

THINK IT OVER

- What is the role of the gut and digestive tract in modulating overall health?

- What are the most common gut issues, and what can be done to improve them?

- What are the best health strategies for restoring and maintaining gut integrity?

When you think about the gut, you might just think of it as part of your "digestive factory," processing the food you ingest. However, this is only a small fraction of what your gut and digestive system are responsible for doing. The gastrointestinal tract, also called the GI tract for short, is an organ system that takes the food we eat, processes it to extract and absorb nutrients, and then excretes the remaining contents as feces and urine. In addition, it acts as a moderator for various important bodily functions. The gut is quite literally the core of our well-being. From immune cells to neurotransmitters (our chemical messengers), a properly functioning GI tract allows our health to thrive. In the same sense, an improperly functioning gut can cause a variety of illnesses and health conditions.

THE NERVOUS SYSTEM AND THE GUT

Contrary to popular belief, the gut actually possesses its own nervous system comprised of its own neurons and has the ability to produce neurotransmitters. This is called the enteric nervous system, which functions independently of the central nervous system (i.e. the brain and spinal cord).[1] Yes, that's right, your gut quite literally has the means to act as a second brain. The brain and the gut communicate via two pathways: neural communication through the vagus nerve that runs down from your brain to your gut, and systemic communication, which include the hypothalamic–pituitary–adrenal (HPA) axis, neurotransmitters, bacterial metabolites and cytokines.

We have known for a long time that the vagus nerve plays a significant role in communication between the brain and the gut. However, the importance of the systemic communication between the two organs has been recently reinforced as evidence has shown that the brain and gut still continue to communicate even when the vagus nerve is severed. While many believe that the brain is the primary organ in charge of information transmission to the gut, your enteric nervous system actually sends far more information to the brain than it receives from it. This reinforces the importance of gut health even further, as research now shows that problems in your gut can have a direct impact on mental health.

At some point, you have probably heard someone say, "I had a gut feeling." Recent research shows that there might be truth behind this saying. Those butterflies in your stomach actually have a direct correlation with thoughts, emotions and moods.

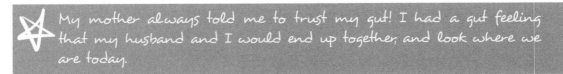

My mother always told me to trust my gut! I had a gut feeling that my husband and I would end up together, and look where we are today.

Although we are not entirely sure how the link between the gut and our mental well-being functions, we know that certain neurotransmitters are largely mediated through the good bacteria found in the gut.

As a matter of fact, the gut produces a large quantity of the body's neurotransmitters. In addition, it also possesses two-thirds of the body's immune tissue, has greater metabolic activity than the liver, and possesses 10 times more microbial cells than human cells. Your gut also possesses its own genome (genetic material) that is 100 times larger than the human genome.[2] Your body is literally filled with bacteria. Before you freak out, rest assured that this is a good thing! These tiny microorganisms that make up your microbiome have an enormous impact on our overall health. Around 100 trillion bacteria live in the gut and provide important benefits:

- They help process the toxins to which we are exposed.
- They balance the nervous system by serving as a source of neurotransmitters.
- They optimize immune function.
- They help absorb vital nutrients.

Most of the time, when we experience problems in some of these areas, we are quick to blame genetics or age, not realizing how our lifestyles play a big role in our gut health. This ultimately determines the functioning of many of the other systems as mentioned above. Studies show that a whopping 70 percent of Americans have digestive-related symptoms and diseases.[3]

The root causes of these gut-related conditions can include excess toxins and allergens including molds, pollens, and chemicals; microbes, ticks, yeast, and parasites; physical and psychological stress; poor diet; and antibiotic overuse. In fact, 40 percent of all adults and 70 percent of all children in the U.S. take one or more courses of antibiotics every year, which wreaks havoc on their gut health and leaves them susceptible to other issues.[4]

THE ANATOMY OF THE GUT

I know what you might be thinking: *"Why in the world do I need to know how my digestion works?"* Well, it's your body. Shouldn't you know what happens to the food you put in your mouth and how it's processed by your body?

The process of digestion starts in the mouth, where large pieces of food are broken down mechanically by the teeth. Saliva is then secreted in order to soften the food, making it easier to ingest. It also helps break down starches into sugar.

Once the swallowed food passes into the esophagus, the food is moved down the digestive tract by muscular movements into the stomach. There, the food mixes with mucus and stomach acids, secreted by the inner lining of the stomach, which are responsible for killing bacteria in the food and breaking down proteins and carbs into simpler substances. This process takes, on average, two hours.

The broken-down substance continues through the digestive tract as it enters the small intestine, a highly coiled structure that stretches about 20 feet long. As it receives food from the stomach, digestive enzymes are secreted—such as the bile produced by the liver—to break down fats. At the same time, pancreatic juices break down proteins and carbohydrates. The inner wall of the small intestine is covered by hair-like organisms (called microvilli) that help absorb the food's nutrients. The average time spent by food in the small intestine is about three hours.

Undigested food then enters the large intestine which is about five feet in length and has three parts: the cecum, the colon and the rectum. The food then mixes with mucus and bacteria that live in the large intestine where it begins the formation of fecal matter. Food generally spends 19 hours in the large intestine—far longer than in the small. The colon absorbs most of the water and remaining vitamins and minerals. The bacteria present in the colon are responsible for the synthesis of the vitamin B and K, and for turning unabsorbed carbohydrates into methane gas, carbon dioxide and hydrogen.

The flora in the large intestine is also responsible for fermenting soluble fibers to produce approximately 20-30 grams per day of the short-chained fatty acids (SCFA). It is estimated that about 5 percent to 10 percent of total body energy comes from SCFAs.

The fecal matter then reaches the rectum and triggers what is called the defecation reflex—the urge to go the bathroom. It then exits by the anus, in what we know as a bowel movement. There we go—the digestive process from top to bottom!

> ⭐ *That's quite the process. No wonder fasting can be so beneficial. If our digestive system is always working, it has no time to rest and heal.*

THE BUGS IN OUR GUT

The amount of energy that we harvest from the food we eat is largely determined by the bugs in our gut. It's important to note that the bugs rely on fiber, and, without fiber, they will starve. In order to keep our microbiome healthy, a diverse range of fiber-rich foods is needed. The wider the variety of foods we eat, the more strains of bacteria we will find in our gut.

Unfortunately, when the gut is not working optimally, a wide array of symptoms can occur. These symptoms include:

- gas, cramping and bloating
- fatigue
- nausea
- food cravings
- frequent infections
- insomnia

- constipation or diarrhea
- inflammation
- headaches
- depression or poor mood
- vitamin deficiencies

Below is an overview of the five most common gut dysfunctions that people face when it comes to digestive problems. These five areas are digestion and absorption, intestinal permeability, gut microbiota and dysbiosis, inflammation and immunity and nervous system balance. Let's get started.

1. DIGESTION AND ABSORPTION

On a mechanical level, the improper breakdown of food through mastication may be a cause of malabsorption and poor nutrient assimilation. As insignificant as this step sounds, chewing food properly actually plays a vital role in easing the rest of the digestive process. Therefore, it is important to avoid eating when in a rush or stressed to ensure relaxed chewing and proper breakdown of food.

Next, adequate levels of bile, enzymes and stomach acid are required for optimal food breakdown. The stomach needs to be acidic—with an optimal pH of 1.5-3.0 in order to do its work and activate pepsin, among other enzymes, to break down protein. If our stomachs aren't sufficiently acidic, we can't digest protein properly, we can't access many of the minerals in our food, and we don't properly trigger vitally important digestive functions further down the process.

The secretion of hydrochloric acid (HCL) is an absolutely essential part of the digestive puzzle. Furthermore, a highly acidic environment is our body's first line of defense against foodborne pathogens. As hard as it is to believe with the heavy promotion of antacids and acid-blockers, most people with heartburn often have low acidity (a.k.a. hypochlorhydria), or too much acidity (a.k.a. hyperchlorhydria). The bottom line is, if you have any kind of digestive dysfunction, the level of HCL needs to be addressed, or you won't get anywhere with your gut healing.

Signs and symptoms of low stomach acid:

- bloating or belching right after a meal
- the sense of excess fullness after eating
- feeling like food sits in the stomach
- itching around the rectum
- weak, peeling, or cracked fingernails
- acne
- undigested food in stool
- dilated blood vessels in the face (i.e., rosacea)
- iron deficiency
- chronic intestinal infections
- food allergies or sensitivities

If some of these symptoms sound familiar, there is a good chance that you are not producing optimal levels of stomach acids. Causes of this can include stress, poor diet, consuming too little calories, usage of Proton Pump Inhibitors (PPIs), *h. Pylori* bacterial infection, H2 blockers (also called H2 antagonists), and other antacids used for acid reflux and ulcers. Antacids have also been shown to inhibit the absorption of many essential nutrients, including zinc, calcium, B12 and iron.

Intrinsic factor, which is a glycoprotein produced by the stomach cells, is necessary for the absorption of vitamin B12. The body can sometimes have antibodies to the intrinsic factor, which can lead to the diagnosis of pernicious anemia.

Consequences of low stomach acid:

- B12 deficiency
- dysbiosis (lack or imbalance of good gut bacteria)
- chronic Candida infections
- mineral deficiencies (like calcium, zinc and manganese)
- Small Intestinal Bacterial Overgrowth (SIBO)
- increased risk of asthma, celiac disease, diabetes, eczema, gallbladder disease, osteoporosis, psoriasis, rheumatoid arthritis and thyroid dysregulation

BETAINE HCL CHALLENGE TEST FOR LOW STOMACH ACIDITY

There is a screening test you can perform at home to test your stomach acidity. It is the betaine HCl challenge test. This test can be performed safely if you follow the directions below. It will cost you around $20 or less to do this test.

Note: *NSAIDs and corticosteroids increase the chances of ulcers in the stomach, and together, with betaine HCl, increase the risk of gastritis. Consult a physician before trying this test or supplementing, if you are on NSAIDs or corticosteroids.*

Each case of low stomach acidity is unique and will require a custom dosage of betaine HCl. But, one way you can find out if you have low stomach acid is by using betaine HCl supplements.

To perform the test, do the following:

1. Buy some betaine HCl with pepsin.
2. Eat a protein-containing meal.
3. In the middle of the meal, take one betaine HCl tablet.
4. Finish your meal as normal, and pay attention to your body and how you feel.

The test will help discover whether you may or may not have low stomach acid. If you *have* low stomach acid, by taking the betaine HCl, your digestion will improve or you won't notice any significant changes. If you *don't have* low stomach acid, you will feel distress characterized as heaviness, burning, or hotness in the stomach.

This test isn't completely foolproof and should be repeated at least one more time on a different day to confirm the first test. One of the biggest causes of false test results is the amount of protein eaten at the meal, so make sure to eat a chunk of meat with the test. If you do get some burning, don't worry—it will pass in about an hour. You can also mix up a half-teaspoon of baking soda with water and drink it to help stop the discomfort.

If you get two positive tests, it may be time to start supplementing with betaine HCl to get your stomach acid levels where they need to be for good digestion. Other supplements that support gastric acid include digestive enzymes, Swedish bitters, gentian root and apple cider vinegar. Relaxation, chiropractic care and acupuncture have also been shown to help.

GASTROESOPHAGEAL REFLUX DISEASE (GERD)

GERD is a digestive disorder that affects the lower esophageal sphincter (LES), the ring of muscle between the esophagus and stomach, creating a reflux of stomach acids into the esophagus and causing a burning sensation. Twenty percent of adults in the U.S. experience symptoms of heartburn weekly, and sixty percent of the population experience it annually. It is quite common during pregnancy, yet in most cases, it's related to dietary choices.[5] Studies also show that obesity plays a role in the onset of its symptoms.

In most cases, GERD can be relieved through diet and lifestyle changes. These changes may entail:

- avoiding wine, chocolate, citrus fruits, tomatoes, peppermint, onion, garlic, high-fat meals and carbonation

- eating smaller portions

- weight loss

- quitting smoking

- elevating the head of the bed

- sleeping on left side, as this can prevent stomach content being pushed into the esophagus

- not eating three hours prior to bed

- following a low-carb diet

- supplementation with gamma-aminobutyric acid (GABA), melatonin, licorice root extract, aloe vera, slippery elm and zinc L-carnosine

PANCREATIC ENZYME DEFICIENCY

The pancreas is most commonly known for its role in blood sugar regulation through its secretion of insulin. But, the pancreas also secretes specific enzymes to break down fats, proteins and carbohydrates.

These enzymes are:

Lipase – Lipase works with bile from the liver to break down fat molecules so they can be absorbed and used by the body.

Protease – Proteases break down proteins. They help keep the intestine free of parasites such as bacteria, yeast and protozoa.

Amylase – Amylase breaks down carbohydrates (or starches) into sugars, which are more easily absorbed by the body. This enzyme is also found in saliva.

Deficiencies in these enzymes can be caused by stress, toxicity, nutritional insufficiency, damaged gut microvilli, free radical oxidation and a pH imbalance. It can result in:

- indigestion or fullness 2-4 hours after a meal

- bloating or flatulence 2-4 hours after a meal

- undigested food in the stool

- fatty stool

- glucose intolerance

- malnutrition and vitamin deficiencies

- slow transit time (no, this does not mean your bus is late; it refers to the time it takes for your food to go from entrance to exit)

- diarrhea

- fatigue
- increased risk for chronic pancreatitis, cystic fibrosis, diabetes, celiac disease, gastric ulcers, autoimmune conditions, Crohn's disease, anemia, bone loss and even neurological problems

Before resorting to medication to restore proper enzyme levels, it is important to know that there are many natural alternatives available that stimulate enzyme functions. Many natural health supplements are now available. Look for ones that have lipase, protease and amylase; there are vegetarian formulas also available. Spices and herbs such as ginger, cumin, fennel, piperine and curcumin can also be effective digestive aids.

BILE FORMATION AND THE GALLBLADDER

Bile is a fluid produced by the liver and concentrated in the gallbladder. It serves to digest lipids in food and increases the absorption of fats and fat-soluble vitamins. Bile acids are produced in the liver and get conjugated by two amino acids—glycine and taurine. They are often referred to as bile salts after they are conjugated. When bile salts are secreted into the lumen of the intestine, fecal bacteria metabolize primary bile acids into secondary bile acids.

Fiber plays an important role in getting rid of harmful toxins, cholesterol and fat, as it forms a tight bond with the bile in the intestine. As soluble fibers cannot be absorbed by the intestinal wall, neither can the bile attached to it. This fiber-bound bile ultimately leaves the body in a bowel movement with its load of toxins, cholesterol and fat in tow.

Many who have had their gallbladder removed face bile-salt insufficiency, and may benefit from taking bile salts supplements to help break down fat more efficiently.

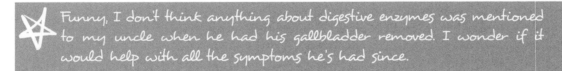
Funny, I don't think anything about digestive enzymes was mentioned to my uncle when he had his gallbladder removed. I wonder if it would help with all the symptoms he's had since.

Signs and symptoms of bile-salt insufficiency can include a sour or bitter metallic taste in the mouth (especially in the morning), incomplete digestion and absorption of fats and chronic diarrhea caused by obstruction (i.e. stones). Causes may include liver toxicity, gallbladder disease, cholecystokinin (CCK) deficiency, bacterial overgrowth and certain medications.

The five F's that represent major risk factors for the development of gallstones are: fair, female, fat, forty and fertile. Foods and supplements that stimulate bile production include radishes, dandelion, bitter greens, artichoke, taurine supplement and limonene.

2. INTESTINAL PERMEABILITY

Intestinal permeability, also called "leaky gut," is a condition that occurs when the tight junctions that make up the wall of the intestines become inflamed and allow undigested food proteins, bacteria and toxins to leak across the lining and into the bloodstream. A protein called zonulin, which is produced by your DNA, is responsible for regulating intestinal permeability by keeping gut cells tightly packed.

Once this protective barrier is compromised, the immune system reacts and triggers body-wide inflammation. When the condition is severe, almost everything that a person consumes becomes an irritant and drives persistent, systemic inflammation, which also increases the risk of developing other chronic diseases. You may remember us discussing this issue when we were talking about Bt toxins and glyphosate and how they quite literally poke holes in our digestive tract.

Other triggers of poor intestinal permeability include poor dietary choices, stress, infections, medication, toxin exposure and low stomach acid. In addition to these, lectins (found largely in nightshade vegetables, grains and legumes) have also been blamed for preventing absorption of nutrients, and compromising the intestinal barrier—causing leaky gut.

But that's not the only concern. If you remember from Chapter 12, we introduced Dr. Gundry's "plant paradox program" which insisted that certain conventional health foods aren't really that healthy at all, due to their high contents of lectins. He claims that lectins impact our health in three ways: by protruding the gut wall, confusing the immune system with molecular mimicry and disrupting cellular communication.

They do this by causing the body to produce the protein zonulin—which opens up the spaces between the cells of intestinal lining—allowing particles to escape and mount an immune reaction. What's more, lectins are nearly indistinguishable from other proteins in the body (what we call molecular mimicry), and can sometimes even bind to cell receptors, acting like a hormone. This, in turn, can disrupt cellular communication and wreak havoc.

Though our guts are designed to have a degree of permeability, when the lining starts to have holes like Swiss cheese, there is a problem.

Leaky gut can manifest as many different ailments, making the diagnosis a challenge for healthcare practitioners. And, unfortunately, many doctors don't seek the root cause of illness, but simply treat the symptoms.

The various conditions linked to leaky gut may include:

- autoimmune disease
- digestive disorders (IBS, Celiac disease and Crohn's) and food sensitivities
- Candida infections
- endocrine disruption
- skin disorders such as acne, psoriasis and eczema
- arthritis
- autism
- depression
- chronic fatigue syndrome

- fibromyalgia
- Parkinson's disease
- kidney disease
- obesity
- diabetes

There are specialized tests to assess intestinal permeability. These tests measure the ability of two types of non-metabolized sugar molecules—lactulose and mannitol—to permeate the intestinal wall. The patient drinks a premeasured amount of the solution, and over the next six hours, a urine sample is collected. The degree of intestinal permeability is reflected in the levels of the two sugars recovered in the sample.

Another test that is a good and a more recent marker of intestinal permeability is a Zonulin Serum test. As previously mentioned, zonulin is responsible for maintaining the tight junctions between gut cells. However, certain situations, such as the presence of gut irritants like gluten and casein, can lead to intestinal permeability, allowing zonulin to enter the bloodstream. Therefore, checking for levels of circulating zonulin is a clinically useful marker for intestinal permeability.

WHAT CAN BE DONE TO PREVENT LEAKY GUT?

- **Remove irritants** – Allergens and irritating foods such as gluten, lectins, dairy, soy, or corn can often cause inflammation and irritate the GI tract. Irritants can also include substances or pollutants we are exposed to in our environment. Find what irritates your digestion and remove them immediately! You will notice a world of difference. Consider doing a Food Sensitivity Test. More on this in **Chapter 41: Food Sensitivities—Is Your Body Angry with What You Are Eating?**

- **Include prebiotic and probiotic foods in your diet** – Remember from our probiotic chapters, prebiotics are the indigestible plant fibers that feed the good bacteria in our gut. Prebiotic foods include bananas, berries, tomatoes, onions, garlic, asparagus, broccoli, etc. Probiotic foods include fermented foods such as kefir, kimchi, sauerkraut and kombucha.

- **Supplement with high-quality supplements** – A high-quality probiotic is essential to restoring healthy gut flora and mending the gut-lining permeability. Additional supplements such as vitamin D, L-glutamine, n-acetyl L-cysteine, magnesium and zinc have also been shown to be effective in restoring and maintaining a healthy gut.

- **Reduce inflammation by eliminating inflammatory foods** – As previously discussed, eliminating the foods that create irritation and, therefore, inflammation is key. Supplementing with natural anti-inflammatory food or supplements like curcumin, resveratrol and green tea extract will help heal the gut.

WHAT ABOUT CANDIDA?

Candida albicans is a common type of yeast overgrowth that occurs on mucous membranes such as the mouth, gut and vagina. (I am sure you have heard of a yeast infection before.) Candida is a fungus that aids with nutrient absorption and digestion when at proper levels in the body. However, when it overproduces, typical Candida symptoms may appear such as chronic fatigue, poor concentration, recurring urinary tract infections (UTIs), hormonal imbalance and IBS-like intestinal distress.

In the digestive tract, if left unchecked, Candida breaks down the walls of the intestinal lining and penetrates into the bloodstream. This releases by-product toxins and other toxins from your system and may be a contributing factor of leaky gut. Candida overgrowth syndrome is the term used when Candida has grown out of control in your body. Make no mistake: This is a chronic health condition. Individuals who have never experienced a serious yeast infection before can develop new sensitivities, allergies, or intolerances to a variety of foods.

What causes Candida infections? There are many possible causes of Candida, including a diet high in the sugar, refined carbohydrates and alcohol that help yeast grow. Other contributing factors include usage of antibiotics, oral contraceptives and corticosteroids, and gut dysbiosis (explained below) may also be contributing factors.

How do you know if you have a Candida infection? Aside from the symptoms listed above, there also exists Candida-specific tests that you can have done. If you have eliminated certain trigger foods like dairy and gluten, and yet still experience symptoms as the ones previously mentioned, there may be a chance that Candida is present. Boosting your immune system through the elimination of refined sugars and carbs and replacing these foods with organic vegetables and healthy oils is a good start to eliminating Candida overgrowth in the body.

3. GUT MICROBIOTA AND DYSBIOSIS

Did you know that there are an estimated 800 different species and 7,000 different strains of bacteria in our GI system, and these bacteria contribute to four pounds of our weight? That is a crazy number of little guys we have in us! Dysbiosis is an imbalance in your gut flora caused by too few beneficial bacteria and an overgrowth of bad bacteria, yeast, or parasites. We need the right bugs, at the right place, and in the right amount for optimal health.

Many bacteria produce enzymes, pigments and toxins. Toxins play an important role in the development of disease. There are two main types of toxins: exotoxins, which are secreted by certain species of bacteria, and endotoxins, which are lipopolysaccharide-protein complexes that form structural components of the cell wall and are liberated when the cell dies.

Bacteria are very complex. In fact, we are still learning about the impact they can have on our health. What we do know, is that both endotoxins and exotoxins can be toxic to the body in different degrees.

Symptoms and Consequences of Gut Dysbiosis

- digestive issues like bloating, belching, constipation, diarrhea, heartburn, bad breath, abdominal pain and indigestion

- lactose intolerance
- immunosuppression
- joint pain
- allergies
- thrush
- fatigue
- sugar cravings (including for alcohol)
- skin problems such as acne or hives
- hyperactivity, learning and behavioral disorders

- inflammation
- chronic fatigue
- fibromyalgia
- yeast infections
- lowered libido
- mental fog
- weight gain
- nail fungi
- depression

WHAT CAUSES DYSBIOSIS?

Imbalances in gut flora are normally a direct consequence of your environment. Common lifestyle stressors that cause these imbalances include the following:

- **Frequent use of antibiotics** – Yes, antibiotics are sometimes needed to kill bacteria that make us sick. But, they are not able to distinguish between the good and bad bacteria in the gut, therefore, you end up losing friendly gut bacteria as well. This can leave you with an unhealthy, imbalanced microbiome. Even if you are not using the medication itself, a large percentage of the animals in conventional livestock are fed antibiotics to prevent illness amongst them. So, if the meat you consume is not certified organic, guess what? You are ingesting those antibiotics, too.

- **Unfiltered water** – If you remember from our toxicity section, chemicals added to our tap water, such as chlorine and fluoride, not only kill waterborne pathogens but also impact your gut bacteria.

- **Antibacterial soaps and cleansers** – A large population of good bacteria lives on your skin. These bacteria ward off invaders before they get into your body. However, with the use of antibacterial and antifungal soaps like triclosan, they die too and are not able to be part of our first line of defense. In addition, these soaps may also cause hormone disruptions.

- **Herbicides and pesticides** – These chemicals designed to kill pests also kill good bacteria in the gut. When you eat non-organic foods that were exposed to pesticides, in particular, glyphosate, they can enter your system and cause an imbalance in your healthy gut bacteria.

- **A nutrient-poor diet** – This is practically the biggest of them all. A poor diet, especially one loaded with processed foods and sugar, is the number one enemy of gut flora. Removing pre-packaged foods, refined sugars, grains and genetically engineered foods, will help maintain healthy gut flora.

- **Mode of birth** – Children delivered through a vaginal birth gain exposure to some vital good bacteria through the mother's canal that children born through C-section do not. These good bugs are needed to develop a strong immune system and gut activity.

WHAT ARE THE BENEFITS OF RESTORING GUT FLORA BALANCE?

In addition to a better functioning digestive system, restoring your gut flora balance can also:

- improved mood and behavioral issues
- boosted immunity
- decreased obesity
- clearer skin
- less risk of cancer

There are also various nutrients found in foods or supplements that can help heal the gut. These are essential fatty acids, glutamine, magnesium, zinc, probiotics and vitamin D.

WHAT IS SMALL INTESTINAL BACTERIAL OVERGROWTH (SIBO)?

Each part of the intestinal tract is colonized by different kinds of bacteria that will serve different purposes. The system works well on its own, but with small intestinal bacterial overgrowth (SIBO), the bacteria in the large intestine travel and populate the small intestine, causing bugs to be where they should not be. SIBO is defined as having more than 100,000 bacterial organisms per millilitre of fluid in the small intestine. SIBO symptoms include gas, bloating, flatulence and loose stools. It has been associated with chronic fatigue, fibromyalgia, restless leg syndrome and rosacea as well.

Consequences of SIBO include:

- carbohydrate and fiber intolerance
- iron, vitamin D and B12 deficiency
- food allergies
- autonomic dysfunction
- restless leg syndrome

- bloating after meals
- fat malabsorption
- systemic inflammation
- chronic fatigue

THE HYDROGEN AND METHANE BREATH TEST

Small Intestinal Bacterial Overgrowth can be diagnosed and assessed through a breath test. The test looks for hydrogen and methane gases in the breath that are by-products of bacterial digestion.

SIBO, as you can see, is a bit complex. Despite being "good," good bacteria should only stay where they belong. In order to control their movement, certain foods must be avoided. Those who have already removed gluten, dairy, and soy from their diets but continue to experience intestinal issues, should try the FODMAP elimination diet.

What is a FODMAP diet? FODMAP stands for Fermentable, Oligosaccharides, Disaccharides, Monosaccharides and Polyols—you can see why the acronym is used. This diet focuses on removing some specific foods like: fructose (in some fruit and fruit juices, honey, processed cereals), lactose (in milk and dairy products), fructans (in wheat, garlic, onion, asparagus, leeks, artichokes, broccoli, cabbage), galactans (in legumes like cabbage and Brussels sprouts) and polyols (like in sorbitol, maltitol, xylitol and erythritol). I know, it can sound overwhelming, but there are great apps out there to help guide you on which foods are good to eat and which foods should be avoided when you are on a FODMAP diet.

The goal of this diet is to address the underlying causes of SIBO, eradicating the bacterial overgrowth and providing nutritional support for optimal digestion. In bad cases, antibiotic therapy may be needed, but first, attempt to treat SIBO with antibacterial natural products like berberine extract, oregano oil, wormwood oil, lemon balm oil and India barberry.

It is important to note, however, that a person with SIBO may not want to take a probiotic as the condition already consists of bacterial overgrowth, and therefore adding more bacteria can worsen the symptoms. It is recommended to heal the gut with foods and gut-healing botanicals such as the ones mentioned above before introducing a probiotic.

4. INFLAMMATION AND IMMUNITY

As mentioned before, gut health plays a crucial role in immune function. In fact, about 70 percent of our immune system is in our gut.[6] In comparison to our skin, which has seven layers to protect us from foreign particles, the gut has only one, making it more easily compromised. Once the barrier of the GI tract is impaired (i.e. through leaky gut syndrome), the body may wrongfully attack food particles, causing inflammation and a weakened immune system. When it comes to staying healthy, protecting our cell barriers and keeping junctions tight is key. Inflammation and immunity will be discussed in greater detail over the next two chapters.

5. NERVOUS SYSTEM REGULATION

The nervous system plays such a huge role in maintaining how our body functions. It is important to keep it balanced by minimizing potential stressors that can cause interferences between the transmission of messages between your brain and the rest of your body—more specifically, the communication between the brain and the gut. As we learned earlier, the gut even has its own nervous system—the enteric nervous system—which is comprised of 100 million neurons that create neurotransmitters and communicate with the brain. This places an even greater emphasis on gut health.

Earlier, we discussed the vagus nerve and its importance in the communication of the gut and brain. The vagus nerve also plays an essential role in the downregulation of stress; also referred to as vagal tone. This controls the parasympathetic nervous system (the rest-and-digest response, as you may remember), which is responsible for calming the body down after a heightened stress state (a.k.a., the sympathetic 'fight-or-flight' response).

When interference of the vagus nerve occurs, the nervous system's ability to restore itself after sympathetic activation is inhibited. In this case, an individual may have trouble getting back into a rested state after being stressed. Getting checked regularly by a chiropractor to remove nerve interferences and balance the autonomic nervous system (i.e. sympathetic and parasympathetic) responses to stress is paramount for proper GI function. More on this in **Chapter 45: The Nervous System—Is Yours Turned On?**

The premise behind chiropractic care is that the body's self-healing and self-regulating, and when working optimally, is in a state of ease. However, interferences caused by various forms of stressors often impede the communication between the brain and body, causing a state of "dis-ease." Balancing the autonomic nervous system will thus help the body move toward ease and away from disease.

It is also helpful to get enough sleep, exercise regularly, meditate and do some deep breathing. Other modalities like massage therapy, acupuncture, yoga and reflexology are great ways to also help balance your nervous system.

INTERMITTENT FASTING AND THE GUT

As you recall, we spoke about the very many benefits of intermittent fasting and how it can be used to improve health. It turns out that fasting also yields benefits for the gut. It gives the gut a much-needed break from digesting food so that it can heal and seal damage in the intestinal lining. Fasting has also been shown to help restore normal gut flora. Fasting can be done on water or bone broth to give the gut a much-needed break, while still providing nutrients to the body.

And, that marks the end of our lesson on the gut. I hope you aren't feeling too overwhelmed. It sure was a challenge to condense so much information. At the time of writing this book, if you searched "gut problems" online, you would have gotten well over 78,100,000 results. There's a lot of information out there!

IN CONCLUSION

As you can see, from the moment you put food into your mouth to the time when it is eliminated from your body, many processes take place, and many potential issues may occur along the way. Rest assured, there exist various tests to measure abnormal GI function in areas such as digestion and absorption, inflammation and immunology, gastrointestinal microbiome and parasitology. Knowing this, if you are experiencing any GI distress, a generalized diagnosis such as IBS is not a comprehensive enough explanation to guide us toward taking the steps necessary to help heal the gut and restore optimal GI health.

Unfortunately, many general practitioners do not have the specific training, tools, or time to help identify potential dysfunctions or deficiencies. In order to address these issues, getting a comprehensive lifestyle evaluation is key to identifying the core problem. From this, you can develop a customized action plan, which includes proper dietary and supplemental changes to help restore and heal the gut for optimal functioning.

TO SIMPLIFY: THE 5 R'S OF GUT HEALTH

- **Remove** – Foods (to which you're sensitive, intolerant, or allergic), pathogenic microflora (i.e. bacteria, fungi, parasites), environmental toxins and pollutants and stress.

- **Replace** – Find out what is lacking—enzymes, HCL bile salts, or fiber?

- **Repopulate** – Use prebiotics and probiotics to restore normal flora balance.

- **Repair** – Repair and heal the gut with adequate supplements and antioxidants. Consider giving your GI tract a break from ongoing digesting with intermittent fasting.

- **Rebalance** – Ensure to reduce levels of stress, get an adequate amount of sleep and eat a balanced diet of whole foods. In addition to that, rebalance the nervous system by removing interferences that block the proper communication between the gut and the brain. These measures will all help in the healing of the gut.

And remember, a healthy gut is a healthy you!

The following diagram shows examples of health habits with corresponding hack levels. To download the *Hack Your Health Habits Worksheet*, visit

www.hackyourhealthhabits.com/worksheets

READY #HEALTHHACKER?
EXAMPLES OF LEVEL 1, 2 AND 3 HACKS FOR THIS CHAPTER

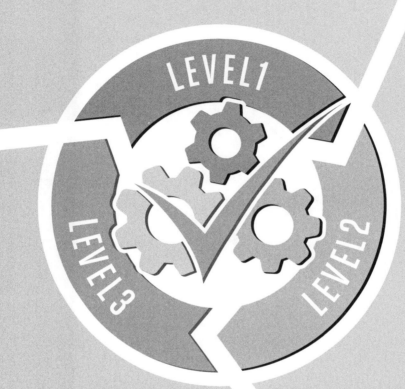

✓ Consume prebiotic foods and a good quality probiotic.

✓ Intermittently fast to give your gut a break from digesting, enabling it to rest and repair.

✓ Do an elimination diet for 28 days to help heal your gut and include vitamins and supplements for support.

✓ Get tested for food sensitivities.

✓ See a chiropractor regularly to remove interferences between the gut-brain connection.

HACK YOUR HEALTH PROGRESS

||||||||||||||||||||||||||||||||||||||||||||||||||||||||||||||||||||

CHAPTER 38

39

THE IMMUNE SYSTEM
Is Yours Strong Enough?

"No doctor has ever healed anyone of anything in the history of the world. The human immune system heals. And that's the only thing that heals."

— Bob Wright

THINK IT OVER

- Do you feel like you are sick more often than others?

- Do you have allergies that have started in recent years and are only getting worse?

- Do you know what supplements you could take to increase the strength of your immune system?

Most know the immune system is the body's primary defense against illness and infection. But, did you know that your daily habits can compromise your immune function? There are more than 200 known autoimmune diseases. Diseases like rheumatoid arthritis, lupus, psoriasis and type 1 diabetes are caused when the immune system views healthy cells as foreign. As a result, it attacks healthy cells, causing a variety of health problems. The stronger your immune system is, the less likely these diseases are to occur. So, how strong is your immune system?

IMMUNE SYSTEM 101

The immune system is comprised of antibodies, white blood cells, and other chemicals and proteins that attack and destroy invaders—such as bacteria and viruses—that they recognize as foreign and different from the body's normal healthy tissues. Other players involved in the immune response are:

- The tonsils and thymus (located in the upper front part of your chest, directly behind your sternum and between your lungs) that produce antibodies.

- The lymphatic system that filters the blood of foreign particles, viruses and bacteria, which are then destroyed by white blood cells.

- Bone marrow, which produces many types of white blood cells that are necessary for a healthy immune system.

- The spleen, which filters the blood by recycling damaged blood cells and storing white blood cells and platelets. It also helps to fight certain types of bacteria and thus aids the immune system.

This complex system is composed of two different parts: the innate and the acquired immune system. The innate immune system consists of physical barriers such as skin, mucous membranes, saliva, urine, tears and stomach acid. These are the body's first line of defense against invaders. They do not target specific bacteria or viruses but trigger a general immune response that stops the invader before it fully enters the body. When a foreign intruder is detected, the body's alarm goes off, and the body sends its own S.W.A.T team: granulocytes (basophil, eosinophil and/or neutrophil), mast cells, dendritic cells, macrophages, natural killer cell (NK) and complement proteins to eliminate the intruders.

If a foreign intruder enters your body and makes it past your innate immune system, your acquired immune system is called into action. Rather than release a general response like your innate system, your acquired immune system will specifically target certain invaders and destroy them by triggering a specific line of defense called lymphocytes. They consist of lymphocytes that will either become B-cell lymphocytes (a humoral immune response) or T-cell lymphocytes (a cell-mediated response).

We could go into far greater depth with both the innate and acquired immune systems, however, for the purposes of this book, let's keep it simple. I am sure you did not pick up this book to get a Ph.D. in immunology. The bottom line is that these two immune responses are there to protect us; think of it as your own personal bodyguards, Mr. Innate and Mr. Acquired.

High stress is very closely related with reduced immunity, as the hormone cortisol (our stress hormone) has been shown to negatively influence natural killer (NK) cells, which are a crucial part of the body's defense. Lack of sleep has shown to have a similar effect; getting enough sleep is needed to maintain the immune system. As your sleep quantity and quality decline, the optimal functioning of B-cells, T-cells and NK-cells decline. Make sure you are prioritizing rest!

THE IMPORTANCE OF ENVIRONMENT AND DIET FOR A STRONG IMMUNE SYSTEM

How does our environment affect our immune system? The environment plays a huge role in your body's ability to ward off illness. From conception on, our immune system is put to work. It is strengthened in a mother's unsterile womb and further strengthened when passing through the vaginal canal. How? During birth, a baby is exposed to its mother's flora, which helps develop his or her own microbiome.

As you've learned, infants who are born through caesarean lack this exposure and may develop a weaker immune system. Breastfeeding also plays a role in strengthening immune function, as breast milk provides a baby with important bacteria from the mother's gastrointestinal tract. Another important factor is an infant's environment as he or she ages. Developing in an environment that is too clean or too antibacterial reduces exposure to important bacteria that assist with immune development.

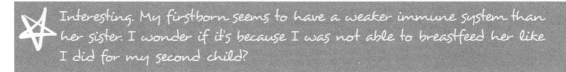

Interesting. My firstborn seems to have a weaker immune system than her sister. I wonder if it's because I was not able to breastfeed her like I did for my second child?

Other factors that affect immune development include poor diet, high stress, dehydration, lack of sleep, lack of exercise, food sensitivities, and use of antibiotics and drugs. Let's take a look at some of these factors a little more closely.

When it comes to immune function, diet is vital. Deficiencies in key nutrients such as zinc, glutamine, amino acids, and vitamins A, C and D limit the body's immune function. What can you do? The sun is one of nature's most potent immune boosters, stimulating the production of more than 200 antimicrobial peptides that kill bad bacteria, viruses and fungi. Vitamin D helps regulate T-cell activity and production. Frequent illnesses may also be associated with a vitamin A deficiency, as vitamin A plays a key role in white blood cell production and the activation of T-cells after an infection has been detected. Vitamin C is also crucial, as it improves the response of neutrophils and lymphocytes. Vitamin C goes hand in hand with zinc, which is responsible for producing T-cells and providing fuel for your thymus gland.

ANTIBIOTIC USE AND THE IMMUNE SYSTEM

Overuse of antibiotics weakens the immune system. How so? As we have discussed in a previous chapter, antibiotics efficiently destroy the bacteria in your body responsible for causing infection. However, while doing so, they also destroy important immune-regulating probiotic gut bacteria. In other words, antibiotics cannot discern between which bacteria are good and which bacteria are opportunistic and making you sick.

If you must take antibiotics, be sure to pair them with a probiotic supplement to modulate the response of intestinal microflora and limit the damage that's done. There's growing evidence that good bacteria never fully recover from the use of antibiotics. In some cases, good bacteria are replaced by resistant organisms. Overuse of antibiotics could be causing the increase in conditions such as obesity, type 1 diabetes, inflammatory bowel disease, allergies and asthma.

FOOD SENSITIVITIES AND THE IMMUNE SYSTEM

Food sensitivities present another serious challenge to the gut, and thus the immune system. A food sensitivity refers to a specific immune reaction to an allergenic food, such as gluten, dairy, corn, soy and lectin. Intestinal inflammation from antigens (e.g. parasites, bacteria, or viruses) may induce breakdown of tight junctions. Food peptides such as casein (from dairy) or gluten (in grain) may induce T-cell induced inflammation. Poor stomach acidity, intestinal dysbiosis and leaky gut all contribute to the increased incidence of food sensitivities.

Essentially, a reaction occurs when undigested food particles make their way into the bloodstream, forcing the immune system to track them down and try to eliminate them. Autoimmune diseases—where the body attacks its own cells and tissues, thinking they are foreign invaders—may also be aggravated by food sensitivities and allergies. This damages cells, tissues and organs in the body. Food sensitivities will be discussed more in **Chapter 41: Food Sensitivities—Is Your Body Angry with What You Are Eating?**

SEASONAL AND ENVIRONMENTAL ALLERGIES—A SIGN OF TOXICITY?

Another huge indicator of improper immune function are seasonal or environmental allergies. Before we delve into this, let's understand what an allergy is and how it is developed. An allergy is your body's natural reaction to particles that it considers foreign or dangerous; these could be airborne particles or even compounds in food. The immune system releases antibodies in response to an allergen, causing an inflammatory response.

This response results in the release of many important chemical mediators, such as leukotrienes and histamines. Histamines can cause airways to constrict and blood vessels to become more permeable, potentially leading to fluid leakage or hives. Leukotrienes cause increased production of mucous, which can cause phlegm or a runny nose. The next time the body is exposed to a specific allergen, mast cells release a multitude of chemical mediators, which trigger allergy symptoms like itchiness, skin flare-ups, breathing issues and so on.

What contributes to priming or triggering allergies?

- toxins
- antimicrobial hygiene products
- C-sections and lowered rates of breastfeeding
- medications, NSAIDS and acid blockers
- pro-inflammatory foods and GMO foods
- stressful lifestyle
- epigenetics and genetics

Most people who suffer from allergies may also experience the following:

- leaky gut
- food sensitivities and or allergies
- bacterial and fungal symbiosis (antibiotics and steroids)
- nutrient deficiencies (vitamin D, magnesium, zinc, B12/B vitamins)
- high stress
- some toxins exposure

SO, WHAT SHOULD ONE DO?

If you are plagued by environmental allergies, consider taking supplements like quercetin, stinging nettle, bromelain, butterbur and vitamin C to reduce your symptoms naturally. Also, consider assessing your antigenic load and making the proper lifestyle changes. Assess things like personal products, cleaning supplies, stress levels, and your consumption of alcohol and sugars. Be wary of taking steroids and NSAIDs regularly, as they affect your gut barrier. Steroids and NSAIDs can be replaced by natural anti-inflammatories like fish oil and immune modulating nutrients like vitamin A, B, C and D.

Stress-reduction techniques and proper exercise will help rebalance the body. Also, be sure to re-inoculate the body by balancing the microbiome with proper prebiotic foods and probiotics. Restore your gut barrier with the help of zinc, carnosine, glutamine, whey, colostrum and magnesium. Consider evaluating your histamine exposure, which we will discuss further in **Chapter 42: Histamine Intolerance—Could It Be Contributing to Your Allergies?**

Keep in mind that when one takes a natural approach to allergies, it can take a few months (up to six) before you see noteworthy results. Unfortunately, there is no quick way to rebalance our systems. Be patient, though. Going the natural route will minimize the drugs you take and ultimately strengthen your immune system.

DID YOU KNOW? THE ROLE OF THE APPENDIX

The appendix is a "safe house" for commensal bacteria. It provides support for bacterial growth and can facilitate the re-inoculation of the colon in the event that contents of the intestinal tract are purged following exposure to a pathogen. The appendix is said to be dysfunctional in "clean" environments. Interestingly, there is a higher rate of appendicitis in industrialized countries, often due to the overuse of antibacterial soaps and disinfectants.

 More reasons to go play in the mud!

IMPACT OF THE GUT ON THE IMMUNE SYSTEM

We have discussed in great detail the importance of gut health in the previous chapter, however, it is important to outline here how dysbiosis can compromise optimal immune function. Dysbiosis is not so much about the microbes as it is about their effect on a susceptible host. In other words, it's about the relationship between host and microbes.

Consequences of dysbiosis:

- **Immunosuppression or activation** – Microbes produce toxins that suppress immune function or have an exaggerated immune response to otherwise normal yeast and bacteria.

- **Inflammation** – Microbes produce metabolites that affect other microbes and damage cells, causing local inflammation.

- **Increased intestinal permeability** – Microbes produce metabolites that damage the intestinal barrier leading to systemic consequences.

Immune-modulating nutrients can be taken to help the immune system and improve gut health. Remember, if you are susceptible to colds, flu, and infections, there is a big chance your gut and immune system are in need of some repair. You can help boost your system with the following immunomodulators (Don't worry, you don't have to take them all.):

- HCl betaine or apple cider vinegar or lemon juice before meal

- digestive enzymes (to help digest protein, carbohydrates and fats)

- omega-3 EPA and DHA (from fish oil)

- alpha-linolenic acid (from flax seeds)

- B complex with biotin

- zinc, vitamin C, vitamin D and vitamin A

- l-glutamine

- prebiotics

- probiotics (lactobacilli, bifidobacteria and saccharomyces boulardii)

- aloe vera

- herbs (astragalus, ashwagandha, echinacea, curcumin, milk thistle and andrographis)

- glutathione enhancers (glutathione, n-acetylcysteine, alpha lipoic acid, whey protein, sulforaphane)

- garlic

- epigallocatechin gallate (EGCG), which is the main polyphenol found in green tea

- cinnamon

- melatonin

- resveratrol

- lactoferrin

- bovine colostrum

- undenatured collagen

Overall, nutraceutical immunomodulators hold great promise as a means to re-inoculate immune systems weakened by lack of appropriate priming from "dirt."

WHAT ABOUT THE FLU SHOT?

When it comes to fighting colds and flu, many argue that the flu shot is the best defense to protect yourself. I don't necessarily agree that it is the best way. I believe that one's best defense against the flu is a strong and optimally functioning immune system. In reality, the effectiveness of the vaccine is dependent on two things: the characteristics (e.g. age, health) of the person being vaccinated, and whether the vaccine is a match with the viruses of that year. Every year, it is a guessing game as to which strain may or may not be floating around during the following flu season. And, even the strains that are covered by the vaccine can, and do, mutate.

Although we are assured that the flu shot cannot cause the flu, it definitely can come with a host of side effects such as fever, vomiting, chest pain and seizures, just to name a few. And, with the presence of some of the additives and adjuvants (a substance that is added to a vaccine to increase the body's immune response to the shot) in the majority of flu shots like formaldehyde, aluminum salts, gelatin, thimerosal, chicken egg proteins and antibiotics. I believe that more long-term research is needed since we currently don't fully understand the long-term effects these ingredients have on the body (toxicity, immune dysregulation, or cancer-promoting).

The bottom line is that the injection of any chemicals directly into the bloodstream should be taken very seriously. The flu shot is a personal decision. Be sure to do your research and look at what the evidence shows in terms of its pros and cons. Unfortunately, you can't always rely on popular media, the government, or the companies that make the flu shot to provide the whole story. There is a lot more to it than meets the eye.

The good news is that there is a lot that you can do to boost your immune system naturally and ensure that you are ready to battle all those nasty viruses out there during the cold and flu season.

- **Wash your hands** – One of the biggest advances in modern medicine is hand-washing. And, it is so simple: soap and water. No need for special antibacterial soap. Just rinse, lather up, scrub for a minimum of 20 seconds, rinse, and dry, and you're ready to go!

- **Get some sleep** – The importance of adequate sleep can't be overstated. Lack of sleep has a huge impact on your immune system and will leave you vulnerable if you come into contact with a virus or harmful bacteria.

- **Eat like your health depends on it** – It is best to stay clear of sugar (especially the white refined stuff) and limit your alcohol intake. Reach for the rainbow. Go for beautiful deep greens (kale, spinach, collards, kiwis) and dark, rich reds (beets, red peppers and berries) and don't forget your oranges (carrots and oranges).

- **Bust a move** – Get moving. Exercise causes changes in antibodies and white blood cells, which, as you've learned, are among the body's immune system cells that help fight disease. These antibodies, or white blood cells, circulate more rapidly with exercise, so they could detect illnesses earlier than they might have before.

- **Reduce your stress** – The science is clear on this one: Stress weakens the immune system, and chronic stress puts your health at risk. So, it goes without saying that reducing your stress will help strengthen your immune system. Ironically, for many, the thought of trying to reduce their stress is, well, stressful.

- **Maintain good gut health** – As learned in the previous chapter, an estimated 70 percent of your immune system is located in the gut, which means that improving your overall digestion is key to better immunity.

- **Get it straight!** – The nervous system controls every cell, tissue and organ in the body. A properly functioning spine and nervous system will ensure proper communication between the brain and the rest of the body, directly impacting immune function.

- **Supplement it!** – There are many natural supplements that you can use that are known for their natural antibiotics properties: oil of oregano, garlic, and immune-boosting vitamins, such as zinc and vitamin A, D and C. Elderberry syrup and echinacea tea can also be beneficial during this time of the year. However, if you have been diagnosed with an autoimmune disease, be wary, as echinacea is not recommended in these cases.

It is important to listen to your body. If you start to feel yourself coming down with a cold or the flu, don't push yourself. Respect your body and take a day off. Drink plenty of fluids (water, herbal teas and coconut water are great!) and rest.

The following diagram shows examples of health habits with corresponding hack levels. To download the *Hack Your Health Habits Worksheet*, visit

www.hackyourhealthhabits.com/worksheets

READY #HEALTHHACKER?
EXAMPLES OF LEVEL 1, 2 AND 3 HACKS FOR THIS CHAPTER

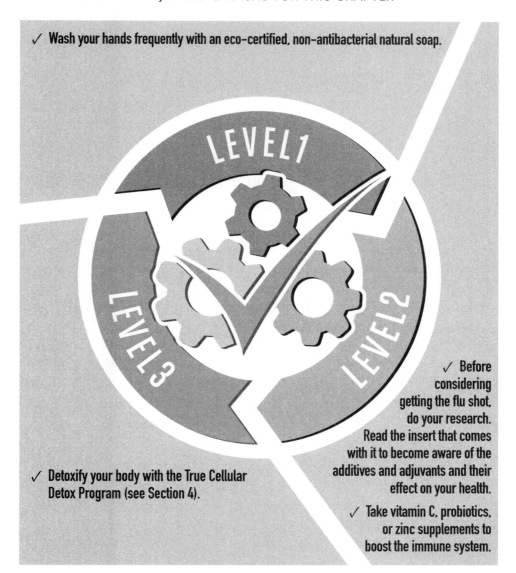

✓ Wash your hands frequently with an eco-certified, non-antibacterial natural soap.

LEVEL1

LEVEL2

LEVEL3

✓ Before considering getting the flu shot, do your research. Read the insert that comes with it to become aware of the additives and adjuvants and their effect on your health.

✓ Take vitamin C, probiotics, or zinc supplements to boost the immune system.

✓ Detoxify your body with the True Cellular Detox Program (see Section 4).

HACK YOUR HEALTH PROGRESS

CHAPTER 39

40
INFLAMMATION
What Does It Mean for Your Health?

"If you don't recognize an ingredient, your body won't either."

— MR. INFLAMMATION

THINK IT OVER

- Do you know if you have inflammation in your body?

- Do you know the effects of inflammation on your health?

- Do you have a history of inflammatory diseases in your family that you should be concerned about?

What is inflammation and how can it affect your health? Inflammation is part of the body's normal physiological attempt to defend itself against foreign invasions and repair itself from injury. When describing what inflammation is to my patients, I always explain that there are two types; the acute and the chronic. Acute inflammation is important, especially if we experience an injury or infection—it's what promotes healing. Heat, pain, redness and swelling best describe the classic inflammatory response. Acute inflammation occurs as a short-term response to a harmful stimulus such as a cut, sprain, or burn. Ever notice that a wounded area swells up and becomes warm? That is the body's way of protecting the area as it begins to heal.

When inflammation persists over time, it becomes chronic. Chronic inflammation is the body's response to ongoing lifestyle stressors like poor diet, lack of sleep and lack of exercise. It occurs when the injury is ongoing or a predisposed immune system fails at counter-regulation. This contributes to the onset of many chronic illnesses. Without getting too technical, chronic inflammation can be explained as an insufficient dampening or excessive up-regulation by intracellular proteins, kind of like a malfunctioning "off switch." Some contributing factors to chronic inflammation include high sugar intake, high intake of trans fats and processed foods, obesity and dysfunction of the mitochondria.

Chronic inflammation can be dangerous. If your body is constantly inflamed, your health will be jeopardized. More and more research is linking chronic inflammation to the development of many illnesses such as cancer, heart disease, diabetes, kidney disease, Alzheimer's, Chronic Obstructive Pulmonary Disease (COPD), fibromyalgia and depression, just to name a few. When dealing with chronic inflammation, one cannot simply focus on the downstream consequences of inflammation. Attention must be paid to the upstream causes of inflammation, by addressing the underlying stressors that initiate or perpetuate inflammation.

Inflamed cells can also cause a multitude of hormonal problems. When the hormone receptors located on the cell membrane become inflamed, communication between the cells and hormones like estrogen, progesterone, insulin, leptin and thyroid hormones can become disrupted. Those with hormone dysregulation are usually prescribed synthetic hormone replacements to remedy the disruption. However, this only contributes to the problem. Unless the inflammation of the cell membrane is addressed and receptors are no longer blocked, prescribing more hormones will often not solve the root cause.

⭐ *So, inflammation could potentially be causing my hormonal issues?*

Ultimately, your health relies on your cells' ability to efficiently get hormones in and get toxins out. Inflammation of the cell can be reduced by avoiding exposure to triggers and by regulating inflammatory mediators with lifestyle and diet. Experts now agree that the less inflammation you have, the more you can dramatically improve cognitive function and fight off degenerative diseases.

Below is a list of symptoms of chronic inflammation:

- low energy
- frequent headaches
- chronic fatigue
- allergies
- food sensitivities
- brain fog

- digestive issues
- high blood pressure
- muscle and joint pains
- weight gain
- mood swings
- autoimmune disorders

Any of these sound familiar? You may want to be checked for inflammation. There are a number of ways this may be monitored through blood tests, but the most common include:

- Complete Blood Count (CBC)
- High Sensitivity C-Reactive Protein (HS-CRP)
- Sedimentation rate

- Homocysteine level

- Blood glucose and insulin

- HbA1c (hemoglobin)

- Nuclear Magnetic Resonance (NMR) spectroscopy, which assesses LDL particles size

Many interesting and well-documented studies found that High Sensitivity C-reactive proteins decreased with the use of a multivitamin, and vitamin C and D.[1]

If you are not finding all the answers to your health challenges with the above-mentioned tests, and you're still experiencing inflammatory symptoms, there are a lot of other tests that can be done. Keep digging!

Here is a laundry list of other things to test for, which could be useful to shed light on your health issues:

- organic acids

- IgG and IgE

- celiac disease

- heavy metals

- zonulin test

- genetic testing of Single Nucleotide Polymorphism (SNPs)

- mycotoxins

There is more on the specifics of these tests in **Chapter 55: Know Your Numbers—Understanding Your Tests Results to Take Control of Your Health**. Another test available, which measures cellular inflammation, is called the Malondialdehyde test (a.k.a. Meta-Oxy test), which determines the amount of cellular damage present in the body. Any certified True Cellular Detox clinic can administer this test.

WEIGHT GAIN AND INFLAMMATION

Fat mass plays an active role in controlling important hormonal production in the body. The more body fat one is carrying, the more inflammation will be present. New research shows that fat tissue acts almost as an endocrine organ, producing powerful hormones that exert a tremendous effect on your metabolism, creating inflammation and increasing the likelihood of chronic disease. As you have learned, fat cells stimulate the production of leptin (the satiety hormone), which happens to also be pro-inflammatory. This causes a vicious circle: Increases in body fat cause higher leptin levels, causing leptin resistance, which inhibits satiety, leading to weight gain and increased inflammation.

Another disadvantage of increased body fat (more specifically, visceral fat, which forms around the organs) is lower production of adiponectin. Adiponectin is a protein that affects how the body utilizes glucose and fat for energy. In obese patients, adiponectin levels have been shown to be reduced, which increases insulin resistance and, thus, increases risk for metabolic conditions. Higher adiponectin levels have been associated with improved sensitivity to insulin and lower blood glucose levels. Adiponectin also has anti-inflammatory properties.

GLUTEN AND INFLAMMATION

Consumption of gluten may be problematic for weight loss, inflammation and overall health. Gluten may interfere with the function of the intestinal protein zonulin and trigger leaky gut syndrome. As discussed in Chapter 38, zonulin is responsible for regulating intestinal permeability by opening up spaces between the cells of the intestinal lining, which occurs in order for nutrients to be absorbed out of the intestine. However, with the presence of gluten, zonulin levels rise, causing the spaces between the cells to open up too much. This opens up the passage for bacteria, toxins and undigested foods to be released into the bloodstream, and can trigger an immune reaction, ultimately causing inflammation. In other words, zonulin is the doorway to leaky gut.

NSAIDS AND INFLAMMATION

NSAIDs, non-steroid anti-inflammatory drugs, are over-the-counter drugs used to treat pain and inflammation. More than 70 million prescriptions for NSAIDs are written each year, and as much as 30 billion doses of NSAIDs (including over-the-counter drugs) are consumed annually in the United States, alone.[2] You know these drugs as aspirin, ibuprofen (Advil or Motrin) or naproxen (Aleve). Researchers have found that those who use NSAIDs on a consistent basis have a higher degree of intestinal tissue damage and increased leaky gut. The reason for this is that NSAIDs work by reducing the production of prostaglandins—hormones created during a chemical reaction at the site of an injury—and by inhibiting Cox 1 and Cox 2 enzymes, which are both needed to produce prostaglandins. Prostaglandins are part of a natural response to stresses, but excessive prostaglandin production can promote inflammation, pain and fever.

You may remember the drug Vioxx, a Cox 2 selective nonsteroidal anti-inflammatory drug. Vioxx worked two ways to cause increased cardiovascular events: It increased plaque formation and blood clotting. Over time, the increase in plaque buildup also increased the risk of myocardial infarction, and it was pulled off the market due to several reported deaths.

While not all NSAIDs are *that* dangerous, they still can cause issues. The most common risk with NSAIDs are GI problems like ulcers or irritable bowel syndrome, but let's also not forget about liver and kidney toxicity issues and allergic reactions. Again, remember that drugs should be used only temporarily as they often don't resolve the root cause of the problem. One has to go upstream with chronic inflammation to find out where the source of inflammation is coming from and why it is there in the first place.

HOW TO DECREASE CHRONIC INFLAMMATION

Looking to prevent or decrease inflammation? Consume more of the following foods:

- fresh whole foods – fruits like berries, vegetables like kale, celery and shiitake mushrooms, gluten-free whole grains like quinoa, nuts and seeds like pumpkin and chia

- omega-3 fats – in wild salmon, flaxseeds and walnuts to help balance your omega-6 to omega-3 ratio

- other good fats – in avocado and coconut oil

- green tea

- garlic

- herbs – basil, chili peppers, curcumin, turmeric, ginger, parsley, rosemary and thyme

To decrease inflammation, reduce or avoid the following:

- processed, packaged and prepared foods

- hydrogenated and trans fats – found in margarine, shortening, lard or products made with them, including commercially baked goods

- omega-6 from adulterated sources such as vegetable oils like canola

- smoking, caffeine and alcohol

- fried foods – French fries, chips, hamburgers, etc.

- sugar and sweets

- synthetic sweeteners – aspartame, Splenda and NutraSweet

- non-organic grain-fed meat

- pasteurized low-fat non-organic dairy products

- wheat products and other grains containing gluten

- nightshade vegetables – potatoes, tomatoes, eggplant and sweet and hot peppers

There are huge benefits to eating an anti-inflammatory diet, and one that is rich in phytonutrients, as they are amazing for calming inflammation in the body (i.e. sore joints, allergies, irritable bowel, etc.). Because of being lighter and of high fiber content, plant-based foods may even help you lose weight, stabilize your blood sugar and reduce acidity in your body. They are also rich in vitamins, minerals and antioxidants, and have been shown to slow down the progression of degenerative diseases.

Sometimes food isn't enough to combat inflammation, and if you are looking to decrease inflammation through the use of natural supplements*, here are a few suggestions of what may help.

*As always, if you are taking medication, please consult with your health-care professional before starting any new supplement. Some supplements can interact with medication and cause adverse effects if not administered properly.

Natural Agents for Modulating Inflammation

- alpha-linolenic acid

- EPA/DHA (ratio of EPA/DHA: 1.5:1)

- GLA (should be taken with EPA to help reduce arachidonic production)

- niacinamide

- alpha-lipoic acid

- n-acetylcysteine

- probiotics

Phytochemical Anti-inflammatories

- salicin (a.k.a. willow bark concentrate)

- quercetin

- boswellia

- curcumin

- licorice root

- grape seed extract

- scute (Chinese skullcap)

- ginger root

- milk thistle

- devil's claw root

- gingko biloba

When it comes to chronic inflammation, we do have some control. We can reduce the inflammation in our body by modifying our lifestyle and minimizing our toxic load. The current North American diet has inflammation written all over it, so food should be our primary approach to decreasing inflammation. Once the triggers and diet are well established, one can use supplements to help modulate inflammation. Once again, I know it may sound cliché, but you really are what you eat.

The following diagram shows examples of health habits with corresponding hack levels. To download the *Hack Your Health Habits Worksheet*, visit

www.hackyourhealthhabits.com/worksheets

READY #HEALTHHACKER?
EXAMPLES OF LEVEL 1, 2 AND 3 HACKS FOR THIS CHAPTER

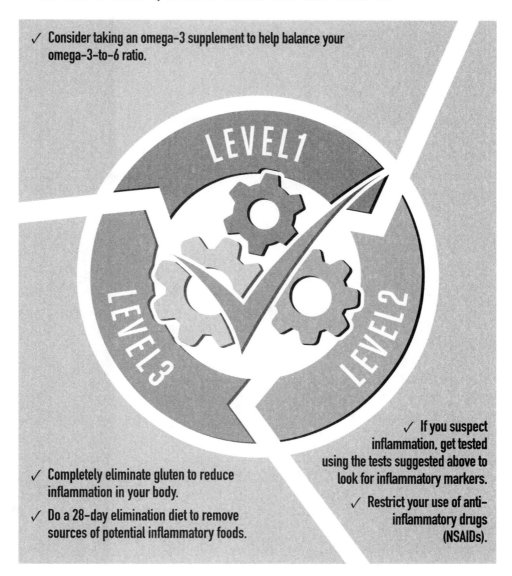

✓ Consider taking an omega-3 supplement to help balance your omega-3-to-6 ratio.

LEVEL 1

LEVEL 2

LEVEL 3

✓ Completely eliminate gluten to reduce inflammation in your body.

✓ Do a 28-day elimination diet to remove sources of potential inflammatory foods.

✓ If you suspect inflammation, get tested using the tests suggested above to look for inflammatory markers.

✓ Restrict your use of anti-inflammatory drugs (NSAIDs).

HACK YOUR HEALTH PROGRESS

||||||||||||||||||||||||||||||||||||||||||||||||||||||||||||||||

CHAPTER 40

41
FOOD SENSITIVITIES
Is Your Body Angry with What You Are Eating?

"Are we allergic to food or
are we increasingly allergic
to what has been done to it?"

— ROBYN O'BRIEN

THINK IT OVER

- Can you identify certain foods that are causing you digestive issues?

- Do you know the difference between food allergies, intolerances and sensitivities?

- Do you understand what the potential health issues are that can arise from the consumption of gluten, dairy and soy?

G as, bloating, discomfort—we've all had one of these symptoms at one time or another. Whether your symptoms happen daily or only after certain meals, they mean something. Indigestion is a telltale sign that you may have a sensitivity or intolerance to what you are consuming. You may be thinking to yourself: *But I'm not allergic to anything that I know of.* Allergies and food intolerances are quite different. Just because you aren't allergic and break out in hives or need an EpiPen to counter the effects some foods have on you, doesn't mean your body won't react to them. People are going gluten- and dairy-free for a reason. If you suffer from frequent gastrointestinal upsets, this chapter may provide you with the answer for which you've been looking.

HOW FOODS REACT WITH THE BODY

Without giving you a long lecture on immunology, let's discuss how the body reacts when a food or allergen is introduced. First of all, there are two types of reactions. You can have an immune-mediated reaction to the food/allergen or you can have a non-immune-mediated reaction. As the name indicates, the first type of reaction involves the immune system, the latter doesn't.

Immune reactions are the following:

- IgE mediated
- Late phase IgE
- IgA mediated
- IgG immune complexes
- T-cell mediated

When it comes to the non-immune mediated reactions, one can experience a toxic reaction or a non-toxic reaction. A toxic reaction occurs in any individual when toxic foods or beverages are consumed. A non-toxic reaction occurs with individual susceptibility and can be either enzymatic (like lactose intolerance), pharmaceutical (like vasoactive amines) or miscellaneous (like an additive intolerance).

According to the Institute of Functional Medicine, here are the definitions of food allergy/sensitivity/intolerance:

- **Food Allergy:** Immunologic IgE-mediated type 1 hypersensitivity, which is an immediate and dangerous allergy (e.g. peanut allergy)
- **Food Sensitivity:** Immunologic reaction to food that is an IgA or IgG-mediated delayed hypersensitivity
- **Food Intolerance:** Non-immunologic reaction to food (i.e. lactose intolerance)

FOOD ALLERGIES AND SENSITIVITIES

Simply put, food allergies and sensitivities are defined as reactions to food or food additives that involve the immune system. Of the two, allergies are more serious. However, both sensitivities and allergies negatively impact the immune system, which will compromise its effectiveness for protecting us from foreign invaders like sickness and disease.

A surveillance team of cells determines whether newly introduced molecules pose a threat to your system or not. New molecules are constantly being introduced into the intestinal tract by the food that we eat. A reaction occurs when your body identifies molecules as potentially harmful or toxic; these molecules are called antigens. The surveillance cells bind to the antigens, activating the immune cells to release histamines and other chemicals, which then signal the scavenger macrophages (one of your body's line of defenses) to come to the site and destroy them. Allergic reactions involving excessive histamine release can cause anaphylactic shock (often causing difficulty breathing), which may lead to a trip to the emergency room or even worse.

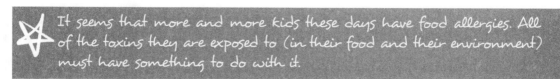

It seems that more and more kids these days have food allergies. All of the toxins they are exposed to (in their food and their environment) must have something to do with it.

People with allergies also often have:

- leaky gut
- bacterial and fungal dysbiosis (which may be caused by antibiotics and steroids)
- nutrient deficiencies (vitamin D, magnesium, zinc, B12/B vitamins)
- high stress
- some toxin exposures

FOOD INTOLERANCES

A food intolerance response is defined as any reproducible, toxic response to food that does not involve the immune system. Food intolerance responses can occur for many different reasons. A food can contain a molecule that your body has difficulty breaking down or digesting, causing an intolerance response as the molecule continues down your intestinal tract. Lactose intolerance is an example of this type of toxic food response. Food intolerances can also be caused by food additives such as sulfites, which are added to processed foods to extend their shelf life.

Below is a list of common components and factors that contribute to certain reactions with food:

- basic contents: proteins, carbs, lectins and histamines
- natural processes: aging, insects, worms, fungi in grapes and tomatoes, fermentation—like in chocolate and tea
- cross-reactivity between pollens and food allergens
- protectants: pesticides, fungicides and antibiotics
- spoilage: bacteria, fungi, toxins, histamines, pathogens and heavy metals
- genetic engineering: soy, coffee, tomato, sugar beets, corn and salmon
- treatments: canning, freezing, heating, salting, smoking, marinating and microwaving
- additives: preservatives (like citric acid, antibiotics and hormones), enzymes (like lactase and bread-amylase) and colorings

That's a long list. However, almost 90 percent of all acute food reactivities are to the following foods or additives: dairy, eggs, peanuts, wheat, soy, gluten, fish and shellfish, tree nuts (e.g. walnuts, cashews, almonds) and corn. I could go on and on about food sensitivities and allergies, but, for the purpose of this book, let's focus on IgG immune-mediated sensitivities and on the most common ones: wheat, gluten, dairy and soy.

WHAT IS WRONG WITH WHEAT?

There are several reasons why wheat is problematic. First, wheat is **modified** – According to the author of the book *Wheat Belly: Lose the Wheat, Lose the Weight, and Find Your Path Back to Health*, Dr. William Davis:

> "Modern wheat has been hybridized (crossing different strains to generate new characteristics; 5 percent of proteins generated in the offspring are not present in either parent), backcrossed (repeated crossing to winnow out a specific trait, e.g., short stature), and hybridized with non-wheat plants (to introduce entirely unique genes)."

Here are some other problems:

Wheat contains **gliadin**, a protein that degrades to exorphins, a compound from wheat protein digestion that affects our mind and stimulates appetite in similar ways to opiates (yes, like the drugs). It can also cause leakiness in the gut and trigger inflammatory and immune responses. Studies are showing that gliadin can also account for an increase in daily calorie consumption—people are eating more.

Wheat contains **gluten**, which gives wheat an elastic property that makes it great for baking—it's what makes bread stick together. Gluten can cause severe digestive issues and can also trigger immune diseases and neurological impairment.

Wheat contains **amylopectin A**, a highly digestible carbohydrate that is no better than table sugar when it comes to raising blood sugar and that contains small LDL particles, which can lead to diabetes and heart disease, among other illnesses.

Wheat contains **wheat germ agglutinin**, a protein that disrupts the intestine and can generate celiac-like destructive changes. In addition to this, wheat germ agglutinin releases foreign substances to the body into the bloodstream, contributing to leaky gut syndrome.

Finally, wheat contains **lectin**. As mentioned previously, lectins are proteins found in plants and animals that bind to sugar. They have an impact on the lining of the gut, which leads to barrier damage. Lectin can also affect appetite by blocking leptin, the satiety hormone.

WHAT IS WRONG WITH GLUTEN?

Gluten is a protein composite found in several types of grains, including wheat but also in spelt, rye and barley. It got its name from its ability to act like a glue and give an elastic property to bread and dough.

Celiac disease is a genetic autoimmune disease, which consists of a severe allergic reaction to gluten, causing the body to attack itself when gluten is consumed. The most common effects is damage to the intestinal walls that can lead to nutrient deficiencies, various digestive issues and anemias. However, in some individuals, celiac-related gut damage is not present and rather can impact the brain, thyroid and even joints. To determine whether one is celiac, a good place to start is to be tested to determine if one has the HLA DQ2 and DQ8 genes. It is important to note that these tests are not fully comprehensive and should not be used exclusively to rule out celiac disease. More extensive testing is available with certain labs.

Some people are sensitive to gluten without being celiac. As previously mentioned, an IgG immune reaction can be mediated by gluten in people who have sensitivities.

Symptoms of IgG Mediated Immune Reaction Food Sensitivity can be:

- systemic – like fever, fatigue, and extreme weakness, sweating or chills

- digestive – like abdominal pain, bloating, nausea, vomiting, or diarrhea

- breathing problems – like asthma or food-induced bronchitis

- pain and inflammation in the joints, muscles and connective tissue – like food-allergic arthritis, pain, stiffness, or swelling

- skin problems – like itching rashes, hives, eczema, or psoriasis

- cognitive – like memory disturbance, brain fog, depression and behavioral problems

Oftentimes, when those sensitive to gluten remove it from their diet, their symptoms will disappear within days. However, for some, it may take months. Those whose symptoms persist may need to follow a stricter diet, known as the FODMAP diet, in order to completely remove their symptoms (which we discussed in Chapter 38).

If you suspect you are sensitive to gluten, avoid the following.

Sources of gluten:

- wheat
- spelt

- barley
- kamut

Hidden sources of gluten:

- food stabilizers
- artificial coloring
- food emulsifiers
- potential gluten cross-reactive foods—whey, casein, oats, yeast sesame and corn

- modified food starch
- dextrins

Replace these ingredients with these non-genetically modified and organic alternatives:

- amaranth

- arrowroot

- buckwheat
- flax
- legumes
- nuts
- quinoa
- sorghum
- tapioca
- wild rice

- cassava
- Indian rice grass
- millet
- potatoes
- sago seeds
- fermented soy
- teff
- yucca

DOES GLUTEN-FREE ALWAYS MEAN HEALTHY?

Nearly every food provider has jumped on board the gluten-free bandwagon, selling everything from gluten-free bread to gluten-free ravioli and cake. People see gluten-free and automatically think they are making a healthy choice. Not quite. Many gluten-free foods are overly processed and include high amounts of sugar, trans fats and refined carbohydrates. Although avoiding gluten can prevent digestive issues, you still need to watch out for the ingredients that contribute to elevated blood glucose and blood pressure.

Many flour-based products are now using gluten-free alternatives such as rice flour, potato flour, corn starch and tapioca starch. Although these alternatives do not contain gluten, they may still have a similar glycemic effect as regular wheat, spiking blood sugar and insulin levels. Insulin blocks mobilization of fat, encouraging fat retention. Sorry, folks, that "guilt-free," gluten-free cookie you ate at lunch isn't that guilt-free, after all!

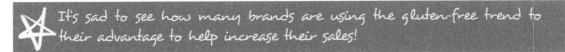
It's sad to see how many brands are using the gluten-free trend to their advantage to help increase their sales!

BENEFITS OF A GLUTEN-FREE LIFESTYLE

When gluten is cut out of the diet, most people no longer suffer from abdominal pain, gas, bloating, constipation, diarrhea, anemia, or skin lesions. In addition, studies show that people with rheumatoid arthritis, multiple sclerosis, Parkinson's disease, seizures, autism, ataxia (i.e. loss of balance), Down's syndrome, lymphoma, osteoporosis and type 2 diabetes may benefit considerably from living a gluten-free lifestyle.

WHAT IS WRONG WITH DAIRY?

When it comes to dairy consumption, there's a lot to be said about whether or not it should be a part of our diets. To sum it up, there are three main issues with modern-day dairy consumption that we will be covering in greater depth. First, we'll go over what is being done to conventional dairy, in terms of its processing. Second, we'll cover the human body's lack of digestive enzymes required to process dairy. And, third, we will touch upon the role of casein in the development of inflammatory and immune conditions.

So, what is being done to dairy? Dairy products are now riddled with allergens and carcinogens. Modern feeding methods have substituted fresh green grass for genetically modified soy or corn-based feeds. In addition, new breeding techniques have created cows with abnormally large pituitary glands, which are capable of producing three times more milk than the old-fashioned scrub cow. Those cows often rely on antibiotics to keep them well. Their milk is then pasteurized and many valuable enzymes are destroyed. Without these enzymes, milk is very difficult to digest. The human pancreas is not always able to produce these enzymes, and this over-stressing of the pancreas can lead to diabetes and other diseases.

Sadly, public health officials and the National Dairy Council enforce rules and regulations that make it very difficult to obtain wholesome, fresh, raw dairy products. This would reduce the concern of pesticides, hormones, antibiotics and the effects of homogenization and pasteurization.

Regulations in the U.S. and Canada are different when it comes to the use of growth hormones. In the U.S., growth hormones are administered to both cows used for beef and dairy. In Canada, growth hormones are approved for use only in beef cows.

THE LOW-FAT CRAZE

Another issue with conventional dairy is our craze with making it 'low-fat', which, by now, we've learned that consuming healthy fat does not equate to gaining weight. So, why, then, are skim milk and fat-free dairy products still so popular?

As we have previously discussed, the notion that fat clogs arteries and causes heart attacks have been instilled in us for decades. It's where the idea that low-fat dairy is a healthier alternative came from. However, recent studies suggest otherwise. Consider this:

- A meta-analysis of 16 studies found that full-fat dairy was either inversely associated with obesity and metabolic disease, or not associated with them at all. In other words, people who ate high-fat dairy foods had the lowest risk of obesity, diabetes and cardiovascular disease.[1]

- Another study showed higher circulating levels of trans-palmitoleic acid (a fatty acid found in full-fat dairy) are associated with healthier levels of cholesterol, inflammatory markers, insulin levels and insulin sensitivity. In one study, people with the highest levels of trans-palmitoleic acid in their blood had a 60 percent lower risk of developing diabetes than those with the lowest levels.[2]

Moreover, studies have found that, when people reduce how much fat they eat, they tend to replace it with sugar or carbohydrates, both of which can have worse effects on insulin and diabetes. Full-fat wins again.

If you are consuming dairy, it is best to opt for whole, organic products instead of conventionally raised ones, which are most likely laden with hormones and antibiotics. Simple daily swaps can help ensure you are getting the benefits of whole dairy. For example, instead of a non-fat latte, choose whole milk.

Better yet, make your coffee at home and put some organic cream in it. Instead of non-fat Greek yogurt, choose whole milk yogurt. Instead of margarine or butter-like spreads made with vegetable oils, choose organic grass-fed butter or ghee. Instead of "light" cheese, choose the real thing.

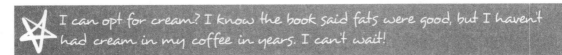

I can opt for cream? I know the book said fats were good, but I haven't had cream in my coffee in years. I can't wait!

STILL NOT PLAYING IN MILK'S FAVOR

The second issue that arises from dairy consumption is our body's inability to process it properly. From an evolutionary point of view, milk is a strange food for humans. Until 10,000 years ago, we didn't domesticate animals and weren't able to drink milk—unless some brave hunter-gatherer milked a wild tiger or buffalo.

If you don't believe that, consider this: The majority of humans stop producing significant amounts of lactase—the enzyme needed to properly metabolize lactose, the sugar in milk—as we age. This occurs sometime between the ages of two and five. In fact, for most mammals, the normal condition is to stop producing the enzymes needed to properly digest and metabolize milk after they have been weaned.

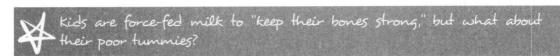

Kids are force-fed milk to "keep their bones strong," but what about their poor tummies?

Our bodies just weren't made to digest milk as adults. Some scientists agree that it's better for us to get calcium, potassium, protein and fats from other food sources, like whole plant foods—vegetables, fruits, beans, whole grains, nuts, seeds and seaweed.

Other Concerns with Milk:

Cow's milk is rich in phosphorous, which can compete with calcium and prevent its absorption. Therefore, milk isn't actually the best source of calcium in terms of absorption. Milk protein also accelerates calcium excretion from the blood through the kidneys.[3]

According to the Food Allergy Initiative, a cow's milk allergy is the most common food allergy in infants and children.[4]

Milk has been well documented as a cause of diarrhea, cramps, bloating, gas, gastrointestinal bleeding, iron-deficiency anemia, skin rashes, atherosclerosis and acne.

New research is showing that our bodies can only effectively process the A-2 casein found in certain forms of dairy. However, it has been found that only Southern European cow's milk contains casein A-2 whereas North American cow's milk contains casein A-1—the type we cannot process. This can explain why many people who cannot properly digest or are intolerant to dairy have no issues with it when they visit Europe![5]

Cow's milk is also an important factor in recurrent ear infections in children and has been linked to insulin-dependent diabetes, rheumatoid arthritis, infertility and leukemia.[6]

MILK ALTERNATIVES ANYONE?

You may be wondering, "Why should there be an alternative to cow's milk? Don't you need its protein?" Several studies suggest that you don't need milk for bone growth, after all. You don't even need a milk substitute. Every nutrient you can get from milk has substitutes—superior substitutes, at that.

Why the addiction to milk? Dairy companies have done a great job at promoting their product. You know the "Got Milk" ad campaigns? And cereals and cookies paired with milk? Even after realizing that traditionally sourced milk is harmful to us, we still crave it.

This addiction to dairy products leads us to our third point—the role of casein, a protein found in dairy products. Dr. T. Colin Campbell, the author of *The China Study*, says that, through his studies, he has found casein to be one of the most relevant cancer promoters ever discovered. Because casein gets digested so slowly, it has the ability to cross the blood-brain barrier and form natural morphine-like substances known as casomorphins that act like opiates in the body as they enter the bloodstream. These attach to opiate receptors in the brain and cause severe addictions to dairy products—hence the reason they keep people coming back for more. Casein can also cause up-regulation of the immune system. This has been shown to aggravate irritable bowel syndrome. Plus, dairy may contribute to even more health problems, like allergies, sinus problems, ear infections, type 1 diabetes, chronic constipation and anemia.

OTHER FACTS ABOUT MILK, CALCIUM AND HEALTH

- Milk doesn't reduce fractures. Contrary to popular belief, eating dairy products has never been shown to reduce fracture risk. In fact, according to the Nurses' Health Study, dairy may increase the risk of fractures by 50 percent. There is no evidence that dairy is good for your bones or prevents osteoporosis. In fact, the animal protein it contains may help cause bone loss. Vitamin D appears to be much more important than calcium in preventing fractures.[7]

- Less dairy means better bones. Countries with the lowest rates of dairy and calcium consumption (like those in Africa and Asia) have the lowest rates of osteoporosis.

- Calcium may raise the risk of cancer. Research shows that higher intakes of both calcium and dairy products may increase a man's risk of prostate cancer by 30 percent to 50 percent. Also, dairy consumption increases the body's level of insulin-like growth factor-1 (IGF-1), which is now known as a cancer promoter.[8]

- Calcium has benefits that dairy doesn't. Calcium supplements—not dairy products—may reduce the risk of colon cancer.[9]

- Not everyone can stomach dairy. About 75 percent of the world's population is genetically unable to properly digest milk and other dairy products—a problem called lactose intolerance.[10]

There's no question that dairy is not for everyone, so it becomes a personal choice. As mentioned earlier, many people are sensitive or intolerant to dairy or compounds found in dairy. For these people, dairy should be avoided. As you may remember in our *Hack Your Health Habits Food Pyramid*, full-fat, organic or fermented dairy was mentioned; however, it was not recommended for those who want to keep inflammation at bay.

FOUR TIPS FOR DEALING WITH DAIRY ISSUES

1. Don't rely on dairy for healthy bones. If you want healthy bones, get plenty of exercise and supplement with vitamin D daily, or get your levels tested to ensure you are not deficient in vitamin D.

2. Get your calcium from food. Include dark green leafy vegetables, sesame tahini, sea vegetables and sardines in your daily diet.

3. Try giving up all dairy if you suffer from sensitivities. That means eliminating milk, cheese, yogurt and ice cream for two weeks and seeing if you feel better. You should notice improvements with your sinuses, post nasal drip, headaches, irritable bowel syndrome, energy and weight. Then, start reintroducing dairy again and see how you feel. If you feel worse, you should try to give it up for good. If you can tolerate dairy, use only raw, organic, grass-fed, dairy products, and try to focus on fermented products like unsweetened yogurt and kefir.

4. If you have to feed your child formula from milk, know that the milk in infant formula is hydrolyzed, or broken down and easier to digest, but it can still cause allergies. Once your child is one year old, switch him or her to real food.

WHAT IS WRONG WITH SOY?

Soy has been called the "wonder food" of the 21st century. From 1992 to 2006, the soy industry went from making $300 million to $4 billion. And from 2000 to 2007, more than 27,000 new soy-based foods were introduced to the market. In a 2008 survey conducted by the United Soybean Board, 85 percent of consumers cited soy products as being healthful.[11]

By doing some research, you can probably find as many good reasons to consume soy products as reasons to avoid them. Two things I will ask you to consider are the sources of the information (Who benefits from it?) and the type of soy involved (e.g. non-fermented and genetically modified). Money talks—the soy industry is a multi-billion-dollar industry, so we have to consider that organizations and administrations do not necessarily have our well-being at the top of their priority list. That being said, their research can, at times, be self-serving.

Soy has been known as a staple in Asian dishes. Contrary to popular belief, Asian diets today include only small amounts of soy, and not the processed kind of soy that North Americans eat. In contrast to the small amount of soy consumed by Asians, if you grab any soy snack and look at the label you will notice it contains about 20 grams of non-fermented, processed soy here in North America. On top of being processed, most soy crops are genetically modified and have been exposed to large amounts of herbicides and pesticides, leading to new compounds entering the body and causing associated concerns.

Today, every part of a soybean is used for profit; as fillers in many foods and products with little regard for its quality. Soy protein isolate, which was initially invented to make cardboard, is now used in many of the food products we eat. And soy lecithin, also a regular ingredient, is actually the leftover waste of the soybean harvesting process.

> ★ There is soy in almost every processed product out there. My niece was sensitive to soy as a baby. My sister-in-law had to completely eliminate it from her diet. Soy can be found in so many foods (even drinks) that you'd never suspect.

Soy is a plant-based protein very commonly used by vegans and vegetarians as a meat substitute. Although it is marketed to us as a "health food," studies on soy consumption beg to differ. An astounding 91 percent of soy grown in North America is genetically modified (GM).[12] Soy is usually genetically modified so that it can resist the toxic herbicide, Roundup. While this is meant to increase farming efficiency and provide you with less expensive soy, the downside is that your soy is loaded with this toxic pesticide. The plants also contain genes from a bacterium that produces a protein that has never before been part of the human food supply. GM soy has also been linked to an increase in allergies.

Here is a summary of non-fermented soy's most glaring problems:

- It contains natural toxins known as **anti-nutrients** – Non-fermented soy foods contain anti-nutritional factors, which interfere with the enzymes you need to digest protein. While a small amount of anti-nutrients would not likely cause a problem, the amount of soy that many Americans are now eating is extremely high.

- It contains **hemagglutinin** – Hemagglutinin is a clot-promoting substance that causes your red blood cells to clump together. These clumped cells are unable to properly absorb and distribute oxygen to your tissues.

- It contains **goitrogens** – Goitrogens are substances that block the synthesis of thyroid hormones and interfere with iodine metabolism, thereby interfering with your thyroid function.

- It contains **phytates** – Phytates bind to metal ions, preventing the absorption of certain minerals, including calcium, magnesium, iron and zinc—all of which are cofactors for optimal biochemistry in your body.

- It is loaded with the **isoflavones** – Isoflavones are a type of phytoestrogen. Phytoestrogens can mimic human estrogen and bind to estrogen receptors in the human body. For this reason, researchers have proposed that soy phytoestrogen be used for natural hormone replacement therapy, as the level of estrogen tends to drop after menopause, causing uncomfortable symptoms like hot flashes. But, soy phytoestrogens are known to disrupt endocrine function and may cause infertility and promote breast cancer in women.

- It often has toxic levels of **aluminum and manganese** – Soybeans are processed by acid washing in aluminum tanks, which can leach high levels of aluminum into the final soy product. Soy formula has up to 80 times higher manganese than is found in human breast milk.

SOY AND FAMILY EXPLAINED

Organic, non-genetically modified, fermented soy has been shown to have some health benefits if consumed in small quantities, but make sure you know the difference between fermented and unfermented soy. Here is a list of frequently consumed soy products:

- **Soybean oil** – Soybeans are super-heated, pressed, mixed with chemicals, and washed in a centrifuge to make this oil. In the U.S., soybean oil accounts for more than 75 percent of the total vegetable fats and oil intake, and it's in all sorts of snack foods and fast foods. Soybean oil is not fermented.

- **Soy milk** – Soy milk is a processed beverage made of ground soybeans mixed with water and boiled, which actually removes some toxins. Soy milk is not fermented. Sugar is also added to improve flavor, and an eight-ounce serving of this drink contains up to 35 milligrams of isoflavones, which may alter your estrogen levels and hinder hormone function.

- **Tofu** – Soy milk is curdled and pressed into cubes of varying firmness to make tofu. Often used as a meat substitute, this product contains anti-nutrients (i.e. enzyme inhibitors). Contrary to popular belief, tofu is not fermented.

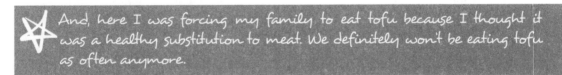

And, here I was forcing my family to eat tofu because I thought it was a healthy substitution to meat. We definitely won't be eating tofu as often anymore.

- **Edamame** – Edamame are whole soybeans, commonly boiled in the pod and eaten as a snack. Most commercial edamame has been preheated to make digestion easier, but it still contains anti-nutrients. Edamame is not fermented.

- **Miso** – Miso is fermented soybean paste used in soups and sauces. This food is rich in good bacteria that helps vitamin absorption. It's high in sodium, but is considered one of the healthiest soy products around.

- **Tempeh** – Tempeh is made when whole soybeans are pressed into loaves and then fermented. Tempeh is rich in B vitamins, minerals and omega-3 fatty acids.

- **Natto** – Natto is made when soybeans are soaked, boiled, or steamed and then fermented. This whole-soybean product is a good source of vitamin K, which helps blood clotting and promotes healthy bones. Some, however, may not like the sticky texture and the rather foul smell!

SOY PROTEIN—QUALITY

Despite popular belief, soy has a low biological value (BV) score, which measures the actual amount of protein deposited per gram of protein absorbed. While whey receives a score of 104 BV, whole eggs 100 BV, and milk 94 BV, soy receives a meager 74 BV. The higher the BV, the better the protein.

Soybeans have been marketed as a complete protein, but they are deficient in the amino acids (which are building blocks of proteins) methionine and cystine. Modern processing of the bean also may denature and break down the amino acid lysine, which will directly impact protein synthesis in our body.

SOY BABY FORMULA

Soy protein isolate is the main ingredient of soy-based infant formulas. Soy formulas are often given to babies with milk allergies, but allergies to soy are almost as common as those to milk. Infants fed soy formulas are exposed to high levels of isoflavones, which are potent anti-thyroid agents that may affect their normal growth and development. Soy formula will also adversely affect hormone levels by exposing infants to up to 2,000 times higher estrogen content than what they should be exposed to. This increases the risk of behavioral problems. Soy formula also exposes infants to potentially high concentrations of aluminum and manganese. Finally, soy formulas also lack cholesterol, which is absolutely essential for the development of the brain and nervous system.

SOY PROTEIN POWDER

Protein isolates from soy used in powder mixes intended for meal-replacement or protein drinks. These isolates are obtained by exposing them to high temperatures that extensively denatures the protein. In its damaged form, the protein is very low in nutritional value.

The soy protein isolates are also high in mineral-blocking phytates, thyroid-depressing phytoestrogen and potent enzyme inhibitors. Also, the high heat used in processing the isolates has been reported to increase the likelihood of forming carcinogenic compounds.

A FINAL NOTE ON SOY

You may still want to use small amounts of organic fermented soy products in your diet; remember that fermented soy products like miso, tempeh and natto can be beneficial for your health. It's all about balancing your diet and ensuring diversity in the foods you eat. Try to pass up non-fermented, processed soy products like milk, burgers, ice cream and cheeses that are disguised as potential health foods. Also, be aware that most of what is labeled as "healthy vegetable oil" is actually soybean oil, so you may have a lot more soy hidden in your current diet than you think!

THREE WAYS TO IDENTIFY FOOD SENSITIVITIES

- **Get tested!** – Blood testing for IgG food allergens can help to identify hidden food sensitivities. While these tests do have their limitations and need to be interpreted in the context of the rest of one's health, they can be useful tools. It's always a good idea to work with a healthcare practitioner trained in dealing with food sensitivities.

- **Go dairy-free and gluten-free for six weeks** – Dairy and gluten are the most common triggers of food sensitivities. Temporarily cutting them out of the diet allows the inflamed gut to heal. This one move may be the single most important thing one can do to lose weight. After six weeks, you may consider re-introducing dairy or gluten one at a time to see how you feel. You may come to the conclusion that you feel better without these foods in your diet. I often have patients who say that they barely have any dairy or gluten products, or that they tried to reduce their consumption of it and did not see much improvement with their symptoms. I like to joke with these patients and tell them that this is like being *a little bit* pregnant; you either are or you aren't. The same goes for eliminating dairy and gluten, as even a little bit can upregulate your immune system. Therefore, it is crucial to ensure we are eliminating it completely to see improvements.

- **Avoid the top food allergens** – If going dairy-free and gluten-free wasn't enough to make you feel better or resolve some of your digestive issues, consider doing a full 28-day elimination diet. Cut out all of the top food allergens like corn, eggs, soy, nuts, nightshades, citrus and yeast (i.e., baker's yeast, Brewer's yeast and fermented products like vinegar). Do this for another six weeks and then re-introduce one food at a time, noticing how you feel. If certain foods trigger problems, consider removing them from your diet.

The following diagram shows examples of health habits with corresponding hack levels. To download the *Hack Your Health Habits Worksheet*, visit

www.hackyourhealthhabits.com/worksheets

READY #HEALTHHACKER?
EXAMPLES OF LEVEL 1, 2 AND 3 HACKS FOR THIS CHAPTER

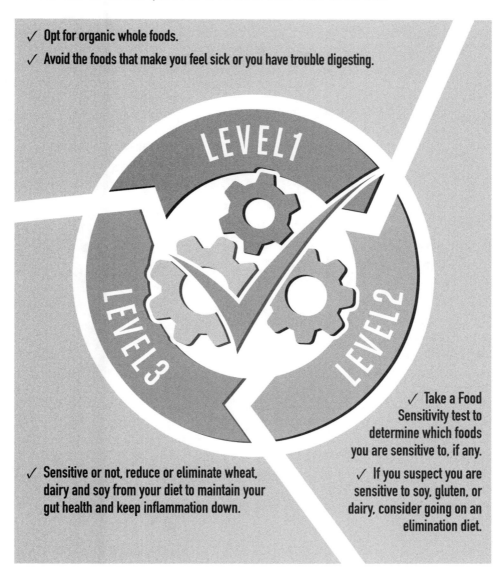

✓ Opt for organic whole foods.

✓ Avoid the foods that make you feel sick or you have trouble digesting.

✓ Take a Food Sensitivity test to determine which foods you are sensitive to, if any.

✓ If you suspect you are sensitive to soy, gluten, or dairy, consider going on an elimination diet.

✓ Sensitive or not, reduce or eliminate wheat, dairy and soy from your diet to maintain your gut health and keep inflammation down.

HACK YOUR HEALTH PROGRESS

||||||||||||||||||||||||||||||||||||||||||||||||||||||||||||||||||||||||

CHAPTER 41

HISTAMINE INTOLERANCE
Could It Be Contributing to Your Allergies?

"Let food be thy medicine and medicine be thy food."

— Hippocrates

THINK IT OVER

- Do you experience a lot of allergy symptoms?

- Do you know what histamines are and how they can be impacting your immune system?

- Can you identify high-histamine foods?

Do you suffer from hives, stomach issues, fatigue, or a chronic runny nose? Does your face flush after drinking red wine? Or, does your mouth itch after eating avocado or eggplant? If so, you may have a histamine intolerance.

Oops, my husband always complains that his mouth gets itchy after eating dates, and I just thought that maybe he was overreacting.

Histamine intolerances are one of the most overlooked health conditions because of their broad and extensive list of symptoms. These symptoms often overlap with other health conditions, making it difficult for health professionals to diagnose.

To put it simply, a histamine intolerance is a resistance to the "normal" levels of histamine in food. This is caused when there is a deficiency of histamine-degrading enzyme called diamine oxidase (DAO).

WHAT ARE HISTAMINES ANYWAY?

Most people have heard about or taken antihistamines before. Antihistamines are medications typically used to overcome allergy symptoms like coughing, sneezing and sniffling.

Don't let the *anti* confuse you though. Histamines aren't all bad. Histamines are important biochemicals used to aid the immune, digestive and central nervous system. As neurotransmitters, histamines communicate signals from the body to the brain. They are kind of like a security system. If they detect a threat, they sound the alarm, swelling and dilating blood vessels and calling white blood cells to attack the threat. This swelling and dilation of blood vessels are known as inflammation.

Inflammation is usually evidence that the body is reacting to a potential threat. Histamines are present when inflammation occurs. Unfortunately, the body can't decipher between an actual threat and an excess of histamines, meaning both can result in inflammation as well as other symptoms. Because histamines travel through the blood, they can affect the skin, lungs and stomach. Even the heart and brain can be affected by histamines.

Symptoms of histamine intolerance include:

- headaches and migraines
- a runny nose
- vertigo
- anxiety
- flushing
- tissue swelling
- digestive disturbances

- sneezing
- congestion
- dizziness
- abdominal cramps
- hives or itchy skin
- fatigue
- hypotension

WHAT CAUSES AN INDIVIDUAL TO BE HISTAMINE INTOLERANT?

The immune system plays an extremely important role in histamine intolerance. As discussed prior, with 70 percent of the immune system located in the gut, the health of our digestive tract is key to sustaining healthy histamine levels. Unfortunately, toxins and chemicals from the environment are very taxing on the gut and consequently on the immune system. This creates sensitivities and allergies to different compounds. There are several causes of high histamine levels, the most common being a diamine oxidase (DAO) deficiency.

The others include:

- leaky gut syndrome
- allergies
- bacterial overgrowth
- alcohol

If you are deficient in DAO, you will likely have symptoms of histamine intolerance. Certain beverages block DAO. These beverages are:

- alcohol
- energy drinks
- mate tea
- black tea
- green tea

Medications such NSAIDs, antidepressants, antihistamines, antibiotics and immune modulators can also lower DOA enzymes that aid in histamine regulation, resulting in higher histamine levels. Certain foods can also contribute to high histamine levels. If you are histamine-intolerant, you should avoid the following foods:

- vinegar-containing foods
- fermented foods like sauerkraut, vinegar and soy sauce
- cured meats like bacon, salami and pepperoni
- nuts like peanuts, walnuts and cashews
- vegetables like avocados, tomatoes, spinach and eggplant
- dried fruit like apricots, prunes and dates
- most citrus fruits
- aged cheese
- smoked fish and certain species of fish
- processed foods of all types as preservatives are high in histamines

DOES EVERYONE HAVE AN INTOLERANCE TO HISTAMINES?

The simple answer is no, not everyone has an intolerance to histamines. When the body is free of most toxins and working properly, it should be able to regulate its histamine levels. That being said, most people carry a heavy toxic load and are likely experiencing some of the symptoms discussed in this chapter.

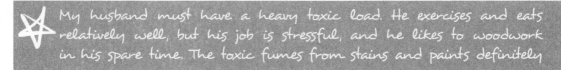

My husband must have a heavy toxic load. He exercises and eats relatively well, but his job is stressful, and he likes to woodwork in his spare time. The toxic fumes from stains and paints definitely *aren't helping. Also, never mind his years as a competitive swimmer soaking in chlorine.*

Eliminating the toxins found in our foods, hygiene products and the environment is key when trying to reduce toxicity levels and overcome histamine intolerances. While eliminating toxins can sound overwhelming, it doesn't have to be. Start by taking a personal inventory of the toxins you are exposed to and attempt to reduce them as much as possible. Next, remove high-histamine foods for one to three months until your DOA levels return to normal and symptoms disappear. Once this occurs, you can gradually reintroduce high-histamine foods into your diet. Try to eat mostly low-histamine foods like:

- freshly cooked meat, poultry
- freshly caught fish
- eggs
- gluten-free grains like rice and quinoa
- fresh fruits: mango, pear, watermelon, apple, kiwi, cantaloupe and grapes
- fresh vegetables (except tomatoes, spinach, avocado and eggplant)
- dairy substitutes such as coconut milk, rice milk, hemp milk, almond milk
- oils like olive oil and coconut oil
- leafy herbs
- herbal teas

TESTING FOR HISTAMINE INTOLERANCE

The two most common ways of testing for histamine intolerance are through an elimination diet or blood tests. As discussed, one method is to completely eliminate certain foods and stimuli, and reintroduce them slowly to see if there is a sensitivity. If symptoms go away and then reappear, a histamine intolerance is likely to blame. Another method is to get a blood test that checks for levels of DAO. A high ratio of histamine to DAO signifies that you are ingesting too much histamine and that you do not produce enough DAO to break it down.

NATURAL SOLUTIONS FOR HISTAMINE INTOLERANCE

As we have learned, histamine intolerances can cause a variety of symptoms. Instead of tackling these symptoms one by one, it is important to take a more functional approach. Getting to the root cause of your problem should not only reduce symptoms, but also ensure that the body is performing optimally. Here are a few tips to help histamine sensitivity:

- **Diet** – Again, use the elimination diet to take allergenic foods out of your system for one to three months. Then slowly reintroduce and monitor how your body reacts.

- **Supplement** – Taking a DAO supplement may get to the source of the issue by aiding in the breakdown of histamine. Quercetin, stinging nettle, bromelain, butterbur and vitamin C have been shown to help decrease histamine levels.

- **Reducing inflammation** – Reducing inflammatory foods, healing the gut and even reducing stress are good places to start when looking to minimize your body's negative response to histamine. Try to eliminate processed foods and replace them with whole, plant-based foods to reduce inflammation.

The following diagram shows examples of health habits with corresponding hack levels. To download the *Hack Your Health Habits Worksheet*, visit

www.hackyourhealthhabits.com/worksheets

READY #HEALTHHACKER?
EXAMPLES OF LEVEL 1, 2 AND 3 HACKS FOR THIS CHAPTER

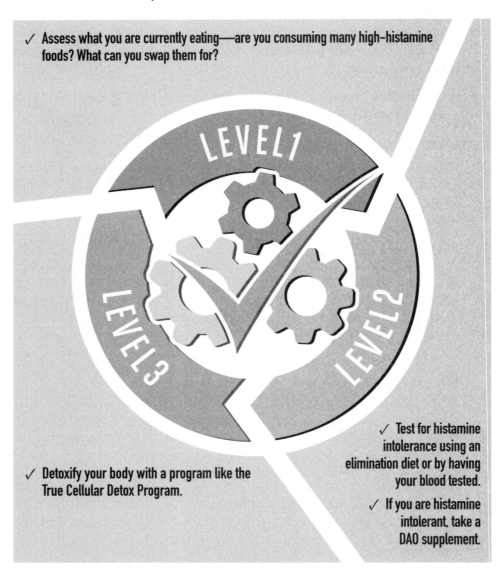

✓ Assess what you are currently eating—are you consuming many high-histamine foods? What can you swap them for?

✓ Test for histamine intolerance using an elimination diet or by having your blood tested.

✓ If you are histamine intolerant, take a DAO supplement.

✓ Detoxify your body with a program like the True Cellular Detox Program.

HACK YOUR HEALTH PROGRESS

CHAPTER 42

SECTION 9

Get Your Brain Turned On to its
Full Power

Feeling foggy, forgetful and unfocused? You're
not alone. Cognitive decline is one of the most
feared conditions associated with aging. Section
9 introduces new habits that can maximize brain
function and enhance communication to the
rest of the body so that you can keep your brain
healthy and sharp. You will also learn more about
the emerging field of epigenetics and what you can
do to lower risk for chronic diseases.

BRAIN 101

How Does Your Brain Work?

THINK IT OVER

- Do you have a good basic understanding of how your brain works?

- Do you know what the three pillars of brain health are?

- Are you aware of which conditions can cause poor oxygen flow to the brain?

> "The chief function of the body is to carry the brain around."
>
> — Thomas Edison

The human brain is often said to be the most complex part of the human body. This three-pound organ is the seat of intelligence, the interpreter of the senses, the initiator of body movement and the controller of behavior. Sitting in its skull shell and surrounded by protective fluid, the brain is the source of all the qualities that define our being. For centuries, scientists and philosophers have been deeply fascinated by the functioning of the brain, viewing it as nearly incomprehensible.

With newer technologies like SPECT scans (single-photon emission computerized tomography), scientists have been able to establish a deeper understanding of the brain. This has shed a light on the brain's relationship to conditions such as dementia, anxiety, depression, or Post Traumatic Stress Disorder (PTSD) and so much more, yet there is still much to be discovered.

Although we consider the brain to be our control system, our daily behaviors and habits have much to do with its efficiency and sharpness. From our nutrition to our physical activity to how much we sleep, we have much more control over our brains than we think. To explore this a little further, let's first have a little lesson on brain anatomy and physiology.

BRAIN BASICS

The brain is comprised of hundreds of billions of nerve cells, called neurons that gather and transmit electrochemical signals called synapses. Neurons are responsible for our thoughts, emotions, actions and sensations through these synapses. There are several different kinds of neurons, with different functions. Sensory neurons send information from sensory receptors located in the skin, eyes, nose, tongue and ears to the central nervous system. Motor neurons send information from the central nervous system to muscles and glands. Interneurons transmit information between sensory and motor neurons.

The largest part of the human brain is the cerebrum, which consists of several parts. The cerebrum is divided into two hemispheres, which are connected by large fiber tracts (called the corpus callosum) that enable the left and right side to efficiently communicate.

The outermost layer of the cerebrum is the cerebral cortex, which consists of four lobes:

- **The frontal lobe** stretches between the temples. Much of our personality comes from this part of the brain. It is responsible for impulse control, emotion, drive, motivation, planning and fine motor coordination. It is involved in ADHD, depression and loss of fine-motor control like handwriting. The prefrontal cortex is said to not be fully developed until the age of 23 for women and 25 for men.[1] Yes, there is a physiological difference! This is a huge indicator of why young teens and adults often partake in risk-taking or impulsive behavior.

- **The temporal lobes** are located to the side, just above the ears, and are responsible for hearing, speech, memory, emotional responses and distinguishing smells. They contain the hippocampus, which is responsible for learning, memory and the sleep-wake cycle. Symptoms of temporal lobe issues include poor memory, difficulty hearing with background noise, tinnitus, disturbed sleep or decreased daytime energy levels and insomnia.

- **The parietal lobes** are directly behind our ears. Their primary function is to perceive sensations like touch and pressure, and to interpret these sensations, judging texture, weight, size, or shape. Another function is to integrate input from the skin, muscles, joints and vision to become aware of the body in its environment. Symptoms of parietal lobe impairment include feeling unstable in darkness or with thick or high-heel shoes on, misjudging where your body is in relation to your environment, being unable to recognize objects through touch, having difficulty perceiving where your limbs are and being prone to falls and sprains.

- **The occipital lobe** is located in the very back of the brain and processes visual information—recognizing shapes, colors and motions. People with impairment to their occipital lobe have difficulty processing visual information and recognizing shape, colors and motions. They may also experience visual hallucinations, visual floaters and visual persistence (i.e. reoccurrence of the image after it has been removed).

Underneath the cerebrum lies the brainstem, which consists of the medulla, pons and midbrain. The brainstem controls the reflexes and autonomic functions (e.g. heart rate, blood pressure), limb movements and visceral functions (e.g. digestion, urination).

Behind that sits the cerebellum. The cerebellum receives input from the sensory systems, the spinal cord and other parts of the brain and then coordinates voluntary movement. Symptoms of cerebellar impairment include episodes of dizziness or vertigo, nausea from visual inputs (e.g. car sickness), poor balance and subtle shakes at the end stage of movement. The cerebellum communicates intimately with the cerebrum. Therefore, it is thought to be the connection between our physical environment (as it relates to movement and position of the body) and our cognition, personality and emotions—providing the mind-body connections so to speak.

Other important parts of the brain include:

- **The basal ganglia** play an important role in planning actions that are required to achieve a particular goal, in executing well-practiced habitual actions and in learning new actions in novel situations.

- **The limbic system** is composed of the amygdala, hippocampus, thalamus, hypothalamus and cingulate gyrus. Each of these parts work together and are involved in processing the senses, emotions, memories, hormone regulation and motivation.

THE THREE PILLARS OF BRAIN HEALTH

There are many things we can do to ensure brain health. However, there are three fundamental facets of neural health and maintenance: oxygen, fuel and stimulation. The healthier your neurons are, the more potential they have to develop a strong communication network with one another. As neuron communication improves, your brain becomes more efficient and functional. This is part of a process called neuroplasticity. In contrast, high blood glucose, poor liver function, overall inflammation, hormone imbalance and lack of neurotransmitters can all *promote* brain degeneration. Let's look into this a little deeper.

OXYGEN

One of the most vital nutrients for the brain is oxygen. It is a vital ingredient in the creation of energy used by the body. All living creatures breathe; thus, we must have plenty of oxygen for the brain, right? Wrong! Just because we breathe to survive does not mean that we are breathing for overall health. We can change how we breathe and, to an extent, change how breathing affects our bodies. Controlled breathing—also known as "paced respiration," "diaphragmatic breathing," and "deep breathing"—have all been shown to decrease stress and anxiety, improve digestion, promote alertness and concentration, cleanses cells, improve quality of sleep and so much more.

How can you tell if you aren't getting enough oxygen? Symptoms of poor circulation and blood flow to the brain include:

- low brain endurance and poor focus and concentration
- the need to exercise or drink coffee to improve brain function
- cold hands and feet
- poor nail health or fungal growth on toes
- having to wear socks at night
- white nail beds instead of bright pink
- cold tip of the nose

Vascular dementia is the second most common form of dementia after Alzheimer's disease and is due to poor blood flow to the brain. There can be many underlying reasons for poor oxygen flow to the brain. However, the most common ones tend to include the following:

- hypothyroidism
- systemic inflammation
- smoking
- low blood pressure
- stress
- anemia
- blood sugar fluctuations

Keeping your blood pressure in check with proper diet and exercise, avoiding smoking or other toxic substances, keeping stress to a minimum, and engaging in deep breathing for at least 10 minutes a day will help ensure that the brain receives the appropriate amount of oxygen it needs for its neurons to function optimally.

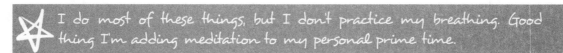

I do most of these things, but I don't practice my breathing. Good thing I'm adding meditation to my personal prime time.

PROPER FUEL

Traditionally, glucose from starchy foods was known as the main source of fuel to the brain. Maintaining a good supply of glucose to the brain without too many dips (i.e. hypoglycemia) and surges (i.e. hyperglycemia) was recommended. However, as you may remember when we discussed ketosis and intermittent fasting, we said that the body's preferred source of fuel is actually ketones (assuming one is already fat adapted). Ketones were compared to burning natural gas, whereas glucose was compared to wood in a chimney—one burns clean and the other leaves a mess! This "mess" creates an inflammation in our bodies.

As the brain is comprised of 70 percent fat, nourishing it with healthy fats not only accelerates ketone production in the brain, but helps with cognitive function as well. By consuming more healthy fats than you consume glucose, you are providing the brain with the proper nutrition it needs to function optimally. However, until the body becomes keto-adapted, the brain will still use glucose as its main source of energy. Therefore, it is important to note that, if a person is not in a state of ketosis from following a ketogenic diet and is not in a state of ketosis, a small amount of glucose is indeed required to ensure the brain has the fuel it requires to function. An absolute physiological minimum has been said to be about 30 grams per day.

It is always better to control blood sugar and glucose levels by means of the diet, but there are some supplements that can support blood glucose regulation:

- banana leaf extracts
- bitter lemon
- vanadium
- vitamin E
- magnesium
- zinc
- niacin
- chirositol

- maitake mushroom
- chromium
- alpha-lipoic acid
- true cinnamon
- biotin
- inositol
- l-carnitine

STIMULATION

The saying "use it or you lose it" truly applies when it comes to neuroplasticity and neural generation. Just like muscles need resistance training to stay strong, the brain's neural connections do, too. The more stimulation and challenge the brain gets, the faster synapses become, the better it acquires information, and the less chance there is of memory loss and brain degeneration. This topic will be further discussed in **Chapter 46: Sharpening Your Brain—How to Mitigate Cognitive Decline**, when we discuss exercises to keep the brain young and sharp.

THE GUT-BRAIN CONNECTION

More and more research lately is showing the reciprocal connection between our gut and our brains. By now, you've learned that the gut has its own nervous system called the enteric nervous system—the largest network of nerves in the human body, which is linked to the brain through the vagus nerve. The vagus nerve is key in balancing our autonomic nervous system, as its downregulating effect allows for a tempered response to stress, acting as a buffer for the fight-or-flight response during stressful situations. Due to the strong connection between the brain and gut, factors such as a poor diet, stress and the use of antibiotics have a negative effect on overall brain chemistry. Remember, a happy gut means a happy brain!

The following diagram shows examples of health habits with corresponding hack levels. To download the *Hack Your Health Habits Worksheet*, visit

www.hackyourhealthhabits.com/worksheets

READY #HEALTHHACKER?
EXAMPLES OF LEVEL 1, 2 AND 3 HACKS FOR THIS CHAPTER

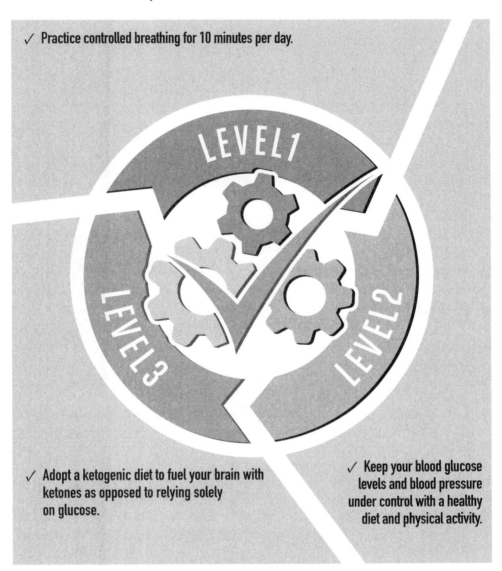

✓ Practice controlled breathing for 10 minutes per day.

✓ Adopt a ketogenic diet to fuel your brain with ketones as opposed to relying solely on glucose.

✓ Keep your blood glucose levels and blood pressure under control with a healthy diet and physical activity.

HACK YOUR HEALTH PROGRESS

CHAPTER 43

44
NEUROTRANSMITTERS
Nutritional Support for Optimal Brain-Body Communication

"Your brain is the organ of
your personality, character
and intelligence
and is heavily involved in
making you how you are."

— Dr. Daniel Amen

THINK IT OVER

- Do you know what neurotransmitters are and their effects on your overall health?

- Do you know the symptoms of imbalance associated with the brain's main neurotransmitters?

- Are you aware of the lifestyle modifications that may help support your neurotransmitters?

The brain and body function optimally when each neuron is properly producing, sending and receiving biochemical messages. Your brain chemistry influences the five major areas of brain function: memory, attention, temperament, personality and physical well-being. The biochemical messages that enable the communication between the brain and the body are called neurotransmitters.

Neurotransmitters are chemicals released by nerve fibers and are responsible for many processes in the body. Different neurotransmitters have different roles and carry various messages between the brain and body, from controlling alertness to assisting in digestion. Having our neurotransmitters functioning well and in proper balance is key to brain health and ensuring that your brain and body are communicating properly.

The brain is a very complex organ, and having it evaluated for dysfunction is not as clear-cut as one would like. For instance, when you have heart issues, an ECG (electrocardiogram) is done. When you have digestion issues, an endoscopy or colonoscopy are done. If you have hormone issues, a hormone-test panel is done. However, when it comes to the brain, there is not a single test that indicates fully what is going on with an individual, for example, in terms of anxiety, depression, obsessive-compulsive behaviors, or personality disorders.

No doubt, brain research has come a long way. There are different brain scans that can be administered to view changes in brain activity or lesions pertaining to neurodegenerative diseases such as dementia. However, we still have a long way to go before we fully understand brain function and disease. This lack of understanding contributes to a feeling of hopelessness experienced by people struggling with neurological disorders.

The goal of this chapter is for you to learn about the most influential neurotransmitters and what they are responsible for in your body, as well as how to know if yours may be out of balance. A better understanding of these neurotransmitters can help you make lifestyle modifications (specialized meal plans, supplements, meditation, etc.) to help restore proper balance.

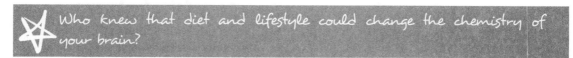

Who knew that diet and lifestyle could change the chemistry of your brain?

Now, for some biology. There are two types of neurotransmitters:

- **Excitatory neurotransmitters:** These types of neurotransmitters have excitatory effects on the neurons; they increase the likelihood that the neuron will fire. Some excitatory neurotransmitters include epinephrine and norepinephrine.

- **Inhibitory neurotransmitters:** These types of neurotransmitters have inhibitory effects on the neurons; they decrease the likelihood that the neuron will fire an action potential. Gamma-Amino Butyric Acid (GABA) is an example of an inhibitory neurotransmitter.

The number of neurotransmitters in the body is well over 100, but for the purposes of this chapter, let's focus on five key neurotransmitters: acetylcholine, norepinephrine, dopamine, GABA and serotonin.

I know, this sounds a bit complex but bear with me. Trying to understand your brain is a worthwhile effort and a good brain exercise in itself.

Important Note: Please be cautious when taking natural supplements in conjunction with prescribed medication. Consult your healthcare professional to discuss whether or not it is safe, as the combination of supplements and drugs can have troubling effects. For example, those on prescription antidepressants are advised to avoid 5-HTP and St. John's Wort. Be aware.

ACETYLCHOLINE

Acetylcholine is one of the most important neurotransmitters in the process of converting short-term memory to long-term, which happens in the hippocampus. Poor acetylcholine activity impacts memory function and may even give symptoms of dementia and Alzheimer's. In addition, this neurotransmitter is responsible for the speed at which electrical signals are processed throughout the body.

Acetylcholine is also responsible for our intuitive, innovative and creative nature. It creates feelings of sociability, adventurousness and enables communication. When levels of this neurotransmitter are low, one may experience the following symptoms:

- loss of visual and photographic memory
- loss of verbal memory
- memory lapse
- impaired creativity
- decreased comprehension
- difficulties with numbers
- difficulty recognizing objects and faces
- slowness of mental response
- poor attention span
- mood swings
- difficulty with directions and spatial orientation

Certain nutritional compounds such as L-huperzine A, L-acetyl carnitine and vitamin B5 can help support acetylcholine pathways functions. Foods high in choline, an acetylcholine precursor, like organ meats, egg yolks, nuts and high-fat dairy products can help balance acetylcholine levels. It is also important to avoid blood sugar fluctuations as they can cause acetylcholine imbalances. Lifestyle practices such as visual meditation, reading, regular exercise, deep breathing and taking time to yourself will help replenish this neurotransmitter.

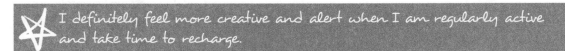

I definitely feel more creative and alert when I am regularly active and take time to recharge.

NOREPINEPHRINE

Norepinephrine, also referred to as noradrenaline, along with epinephrine, is what most of us think of when it comes to a "fight-or-flight" response. As neurotransmitters, it plays a significant role in our attention, mental health and overall happiness. Norepinephrine is released from noradrenergic neurons in the central nervous and sympathetic nervous systems, as well as from the adrenal glands into the blood as a hormone.

Norepinephrine, serotonin and dopamine are neurotransmitters that belong to a group of compounds known as the monoamines, which play a major role in mood regulation. Some of the main symptoms of low norepinephrine-based depression are feelings of fatigue, brain fog and loss of "oomph" for life. As you can see, these symptoms are well associated with depression, which is normally diagnosed as a serotonin deficiency. This explains why most antidepressants work by increasing serotonin levels by preventing its reuptake. Only a few antidepressants work on dopamine or norepinephrine.

ADHD AND NEUROTRANSMITTERS

Another common disorder linked to norepinephrine is Attention Deficit Hyperactivity Disorder (ADHD). While the conventional treatment for ADHD is a prescription stimulant, most of these are based on the theory that those with attention disorders are deficient in dopamine or norepinephrine. These drugs stimulate the release of dopamine and norepinephrine and slow their rate of reabsorption, allowing more to properly bind to receptors. This allows the person to make better use of available norepinephrine and dopamine. However, this comes with a whole slew of side effects such as lightheadedness, nervousness, anxiety, irritability and much more.

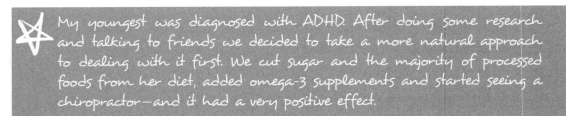

My youngest was diagnosed with ADHD. After doing some research and talking to friends we decided to take a more natural approach to dealing with it first. We cut sugar and the majority of processed foods from her diet, added omega-3 supplements and started seeing a chiropractor—and it had a very positive effect.

The good news is you don't have to rely on drugs to increase norepinephrine to manage ADHD. Dr. John Ratey, clinical professor of psychiatry at Harvard Medical School and best-selling author of *Spark: The Revolutionary New Science of Exercise and the Brain,* has spent decades studying the effects of physical exercise on the brain. He has found that exercise tempers ADHD symptoms by raising both norepinephrine and dopamine, which work to regulate the attention system.

Diet can also have a significant effect on managing ADHD symptoms. While most medical professionals do not see diet as an important factor when it comes to dealing with ADHD, a new body of evidence is starting to show otherwise.

If you want to eat to nourish your brain, here's the best (and shortest) piece of dietary advice you'll ever receive: Eat real food. These include fresh fruits and vegetables, meat, poultry, seafood, eggs, nuts, herbs and spices, and brain-healthy fats like olive oil and coconut oil. Eating unprocessed food as much as possible will go a long way to getting rid of the culprits such as sugar, artificial sweeteners, MSG, artificial colors and other food additives, as these have been shown to negatively impact symptoms of ADHD in youth.

SEROTONIN

Known as our "happy hormone," serotonin is produced in small amounts in the brain, with the remaining 80 percent to 90 percent produced in the gastrointestinal tract.[1] Serotonin provides a healing, nourishing, satisfied feeling to the brain and body.

When serotonin is secreted at optimal levels, your sleep is deep and peaceful, your mood is boosted and you think rationally. Serotonin helps to resynchronize the brain to help you feel fresh and recharged in the morning. This is because serotonin is converted into melatonin in the brain's pineal gland. Low cortisol can hinder the conversion of serotonin to melatonin and cause difficulty sleeping. If cortisol is too high, melatonin levels can drop. Therefore, it is important to keep cortisol and melatonin levels in check for proper serotonin function.

It is also important to spend time outside since the messages we get from the angle of the sun informs our brain of what time of day it is and when to start producing melatonin. Too much time spent exposed to artificial light sources—including our electronic devices—can trick our brain into thinking it is morning when it might be late in the evening. This occurs when you are exposed to excessive blue/green light coming from your laptop and bright light fixtures.

Too much serotonin can cause you to feel nervous, hesitant, distracted, vulnerable to criticism and afraid of judgment.

Meanwhile, serotonin deficiency causes symptoms such as:

- loss of pleasure in hobbies and interests
- feeling of inner rage and anger
- feeling of depression
- difficulty finding joy from life pleasures
- unable to fall into deep restful sleep
- constant craving for carbohydrates
- depression

Serotonin deficiency is most associated with low mood and depression, hence why Selective Serotonin Reuptake Inhibitors (SSRIs) are commonly prescribed to help deal with the negative symptoms of depression. SSRIs ease depression by increasing levels of serotonin in the brain and blocking the reuptake of serotonin so that a good mood lasts longer. Yet, they come with a price. Repressed libido, fatigue, weight gain, apathy, insomnia and headaches are among the most reported side effects.

Monoamine Oxidase Inhibitors (MAOIs) are another older type of antidepressants that are prescribed commonly as well. MAOIs work a little differently. Monoamine oxidase is an enzyme your body makes, which breaks down serotonin, epinephrine and dopamine. MAOIs block the effects of this enzyme, and, as a result, the levels of those neurotransmitters get a boost. Although by looking at one's symptoms, it may seem like these drugs are helping treat depression, they may be causing a bigger problem. People will often develop a tolerance to the drug, which results in higher doses or new drugs being prescribed.

Luckily, there are several ways to boost serotonin production through lifestyle choices. These include balancing hormones, eating tryptophan-rich foods (like shrimp, spinach, or turkey), exercising daily and supplementing with compounds such as 5-HTP and Tryptophan—again, do not take these if you are already on an antidepressant. Other nutrients and botanicals important in serotonin production are P5P (the active form of vitamin B6), niacinamide, magnesium citrate, methyl B12 and folic acid.

It is also very important to minimize blood sugar fluctuations in order to promote healthy levels of serotonin. Why does blood sugar affect the brain and serotonin? Excess insulin reduces the brain's ability to clear out amyloid plaques, the plaques that are the hallmark of Alzheimer's disease. In addition, too little insulin impacts the amount of tryptophan (a precursor of serotonin) that is able to reach the brain, causing a decrease in serotonin production.

It's important to remember that as much as 80 percent of our serotonin is produced in our gut. Therefore, proper gut function is crucial to serotonin production. This is one more reason to keep your good bugs happy so they can help make *you* happy!

In addition to developing lifestyle habits that promote healthy serotonin levels, predisposition needs to be taken into consideration as well. Individual differences in the genetic makeup of the serotonin system have been shown to increase one's vulnerability to depression, anxiety and other psychiatric conditions, particularly if individuals are exposed to stressful events in their lives.

Specifically, the SERT gene, or 5-HTT, is the protein that carries serotonin. Based on one's genetic makeup, this gene can either be expressed as a short or long allele. Studies are showing that people who have the short allele of the serotonin transporter gene have a greater biological reactivity to stressful events, including a larger hormonal response to stress and a greater brain reactivity to threat.

In other words, both the hormonal and brain systems involved in fear and anxiety are more active in response to stress in individuals who have a short allele, as opposed to a long allele. This genetic difference may also account for individual differences in personality. People who have a short allele for the serotonin transporter have been suggested to exhibit more "anxious" personality traits.

This means that this difference in gene function can create a tendency to be more negative, anxious, or stressed. For such individuals, a lifestyle that promotes healthy serotonin production becomes even more crucial as they may already be predisposed to a higher risk for serotonin-deficient conditions like depression. The importance of lifestyle and expression of genes will be discussed in greater detail in **Chapter 47: Epigenetics—You Are What You Think.**

DOPAMINE

Dopamine is produced in many areas of the brain and is released by the hypothalamus (the master controller of our hormones.) Dopamine generates the signals that control voluntary movement, posture, intelligence, abstract thought, goal setting, long-term planning and personality. It has numerous functions in the brain related to motor coordination, motivation and reward. Yet, having too much of this neurotransmitter can also cause impulsivity, an overly active libido and power-seeking behavior.

Dopamine is most commonly known for its association with Parkinson's disease. This is a disease brought on by the destruction of the brain's substantia nigra, one of the several places dopamine is made, and long-term dopamine deficiency.

NEUROTRANSMITTERS   CHAPTER 44   407

People with poor dopamine activity feel symptoms such as:

- an inability to self-motivate
- an inability to start or finish tasks
- feelings of hopelessness and worthlessness
- loss of temper for minor reasons
- anger and aggression while under stress
- the desire to isolate from others
- food cravings
- a low sex drive
- excessive sleep
- balance and motor control problems
- mood swings
- procrastination
- lack of working memory and poor concentration

SOLUTIONS FOR DOPAMINE IMBALANCE

Lifestyle recommendations for balancing dopamine levels include deep breathing exercises, meditation or other relaxation methods, anaerobic exercises such as weightlifting, and a reduction in environmental stimulants and toxins. Nutritional compounds that directly stimulates dopamine synthesis are mucuna pruriens, beta-phenylethylamine, selenium, blueberry extract, alpha-lipoic acid and N-acetylcysteine, which can provide additional support to neurotransmitter production and balance. High phenylalanine foods are meats, eggs, cheeses, oats and chocolates.

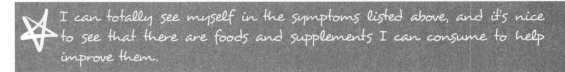

I can totally see myself in the symptoms listed above, and it's nice to see that there are foods and supplements I can consume to help improve them.

On a chemical side, there are some antidepressants that affect dopamine pathways. These are categorized as Dopamine Reuptake Inhibitors, or DRIs. Response to these DRIs is a strong indication that dopamine activity is compromised. DRIs can eventually deplete the body of important co-factors necessary for dopamine synthesis and activity, as well as create resistance to dopamine. Many ADHD drugs and illicit drugs, like amphetamines and cocaine, are dopamine reuptake inhibitors that allow our dopamine to be present for longer periods of time.

GABA (GAMMA-AMINOBUTYRIC ACID)

GABA is made in brain cells from glutamate and functions as an inhibitory neurotransmitter. It provides calmness and even directly affects aspects of personality such as punctuality, levelheadedness, confidence, practicality, objectivity and organization. GABA is also involved in the production of endorphins, the feel-good chemicals released during exercise.

When there is an imbalance in levels of GABA, one may experience symptoms such as:

- feelings of anxiousness or panic
- feelings of dread
- feelings of inner tension and excitability
- feelings of being overwhelmed
- a restless mind
- difficulty getting the mind to turn off
- disorganized attention
- worrying about things you had never thought of before
- hypertension
- depression
- Obsessive Compulsive Disorder (OCD)

Some drugs are designed to make up for GABA deficiency. However, like many other drugs, they may create side effects and other neurotransmitter imbalances. What's more, GABA medication can also lead to tolerance and addiction. Some of the most addictive medications are called benzodiazepines, which are GABA-activating drugs. These include Valium, Klonopin and Xanax—to name just a few. To add to the complexity of things, some people (about 20 percent to 30 percent of the population) have genetic defects (meaning they don't have the right SNPs), so they can't process these types of drugs properly. Only genetic testing can determine whether or not a person possesses these SNPs (more on this in Chapter 47).

With this in mind, what can one do to ensure that their GABA is functioning optimally? For starters, it is important that you get a proper supply of fuel to the brain (glucose or ketones, if you are keto-adapted) and of amino acids for optimal GABA production. Aerobic activity and supplementing with compounds such as L-glutamine, L-theanine, taurine, P5P, magnesium, zinc, manganese, valerian root, lithium orotate and passion flower extract have been shown to improve levels of GABA. When it comes to GABA as a supplement, the jury is still out on its benefits. Some scientists are saying that it is unable to cross the blood-brain barrier in the first place, due to its large molecular size—unless the person has what is referred as leaky blood-brain barrier. So, GABA is often used to test if someone has an altered blood-brain barrier.

Hopefully, your brain is not hurting with all this information on neurotransmitters. As you can see, the brain is complex and we need to do everything in our power to support it. Eating the right food is key to get all the nutrients our brains need to function optimally. As Benjamin Franklin famously said, "An ounce of prevention is better than a pound of cure."

The following diagram shows examples of health habits with corresponding hack levels. To download the *Hack Your Health Habits Worksheet*, visit

www.hackyourhealthhabits.com/worksheets

READY #HEALTHHACKER?
EXAMPLES OF LEVEL 1, 2 AND 3 HACKS FOR THIS CHAPTER

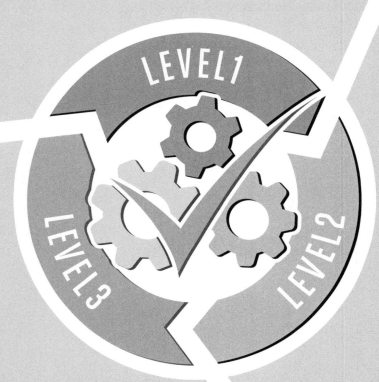

✓ Reading over the symptoms listed in this chapter, can you identify any that you may be experiencing?

✓ If not already on prescription medication, consider taking a daily brain support supplement such as the ones mentioned in the chapter.

✓ Take part in neurotransmitter-boosting activities such as aerobic exercise on a daily basis.

HACK YOUR HEALTH PROGRESS

||||||||||||||||||||||||||||||||||||||||||||||||||||||||||||||||||||||

CHAPTER 44

THE NERVOUS SYSTEM
Is Yours Turned On?

"There is a vast difference between treating effects and adjusting the cause."

— D. D. PALMER

THINK IT OVER

- Do I understand the function and the impact of my nervous system on my overall health?

- Can I explain what a vertebral subluxation is?

- When was the last time I had my spine and nervous system evaluated?

Disclaimer: The author of this book is extremely passionate about the nervous system. As a chiropractor for more than two decades, she has experienced firsthand the powerful impact of an optimally functioning nervous system on overall health and well-being. Readers beware— an optimally functioning nervous system may result in improved digestion, more energy, greater immune function, enhanced focus and increased vitality.

NERVOUS SYSTEM 101

In the previous chapter, we've talked about certain aspects of the nervous system, specifically the brain, and its neurons and neurotransmitters. In this chapter, we will focus more on:

1. the central nervous system, which is made up of the brain and the spinal cord; and

2. the peripheral nervous system, which is made up of the nerve fibers that branch off from the spinal cord and extend to different parts of the body—including the internal organs, neck, arms, torso, legs and skeletal muscles.

The peripheral system, itself, is comprised of two components:

- The somatic nervous system is responsible for sending motor and sensory information both to and from the central nervous system. This system is made up of nerves that connect to the skin, sensory organs and all skeletal muscles. It is also responsible for many voluntary muscle movements. In addition, it is also important in the processing of sensory information that arrives via the senses, including hearing, touch and sight.

- The autonomic nervous system regulates certain body processes such as blood pressure and the rate of breathing that occur without conscious effort. The autonomic nervous system has two branches: the sympathetic nervous system and the parasympathetic nervous system. The sympathetic nervous system is often described as the "fight-or-flight" system, while the parasympathetic nervous system is often referred to as the "rest-and-digest" system.

PROPER NERVOUS SYSTEM COMMUNICATION—HOW CAN THINGS GO WRONG?

The spinal cord has 31 pairs of nerves that exit between the spinal bones. Although the spinal column offers protection to these sensitive nerves, their function can be disrupted, affecting nerve communication between the brain and the body, and resulting in interference.

What can cause this interference? Interference can be caused by what chiropractors call Vertebral Subluxation Complex (VSC). Sound complex? In order to simplify the intricacies of the VSC, chiropractors have used the "bone out of place" model to help patients better understand. However, since our readers have kept up so well with all the facts and science in this book, I'll give the full explanation. The explanation of the VSC has deepened throughout the years, but it first started with a five-component model developed and popularized by Dishman and Lantz but attributed to Faye in the early 1980s. These included spinal kinesiopathology, neuropathology, myopathology, histopathology and biochemical changes.

Lantz has since revised and expanded that model to now include nine components: kinesiology, neurology, myology, connective tissue physiology, angiology, inflammatory response, anatomy, physiology and biochemistry.

✦ I always try to explain to people that chiropractic is much more than just pain relief!

Now, let's make things even more complex and go over a summary of each the three main chiropractic models:

1. **The segmental model.** Subluxation is described in terms of alterations in specific intervertebral motion segments. In segmental approaches, the involved motion segments may be identified by radiographic procedures, which assess intersegmental disrelationships, or by clinical examination procedures such as motion palpation.

2. Postural approaches. In postural approaches, subluxation is seen as a postural distortion. Practitioners of postural approaches assess "global" subluxations using postural analysis and radiographic techniques, which evaluate spinal curves and their relationship to the spine as a whole.

3. Tonal approaches. In 1910, D. D. Palmer wrote, "Life is an expression of tone. Tone is the normal degree of nerve tension. Tone is expressed in function by normal elasticity, strength and excitability... the cause of disease is any variation in tone." Tonal approaches tend to view the spine and nervous system as a functional unit. Tonal approaches emphasize the importance of functional outcomes and acknowledge that clinical objectives may be achieved using a variety of adjusting methods.[1]

WHAT CAN MAKE YOUR PANEL TRIP?

Subluxations occur when the body is stressed beyond its capacity to adapt to its environment—whether physically, bio-chemically or psychologically.

Examples of negative stressors are:

*   **Physical stressors** – like slips, falls, car accidents, collisions in contact sports, a traumatic birth, broken bones, sprains and strains, hours in front of the computer, etc. These do not necessarily have to be recent events. You could be suffering consequences from a fall that happened when you were five years old or the impact of mild whiplash from a car accident when you were in your 20s.

*   **Biochemical stressors** – like the processed foods we eat, the quality of the air we breathe, the water we drink, the chemicals in the products we use, etc.

*   **Psychological stressors** – like financial worries, family issues, being unhappy with your work, taking care of a sick family member, lacking a life purpose, the loss of a loved one, etc.

Subluxations can impair proper functioning of the nervous system by impeding the communication between the brain and the rest of the body. Since we *live* our lives through our nervous system, we need to ensure that it is working at its best to achieve optimal health. Subluxations are the number one cause of interference on the body's innate ability to heal itself and self-regulate through the nervous system.

If you still find the concept of a subluxation elusive, here is an analogy I tell my patients to help them really grasp the concept of a subluxation. What happens when you plug too many items into an electrical outlet? The breaker linked to this specific outlet will trip, right? If you go to the electrical panel and look at all the breakers, you will see that they are all aligned except one – the one you have tripped. A subluxation is just like that—your body tripping because it has been stressed beyond its capacity to adapt.

Now, everybody has a different level at which they will trip their panel. We are all different, depending on our body's capacity to adapt. My patients often think that there has to be a big physical event or activity to cause a subluxation. Not so.

I can't tell you how often I hear, "I am in pain, but have no idea what I did. I don't understand why my neck is sore!" People don't realize the amount of impact even the smallest stressor can have on the body. Any stressors like sitting at a computer all day, sleeping poorly in a hotel bed when traveling, eating poorly, skipping the gym for a couple of weeks or months—or tight work deadlines and a demanding boss—can cause stress on the body, make someone's panel trip, and be the cause of vertebral subluxations. Slips, falls and bungee jumping aren't the only causes. Again, we live our lives through our nervous system. You process and experience that beautiful sunset or that family health crisis through it.

One of my favorite posters, which can be found in every room at my clinic, is a huge map of the autonomic nervous system. This poster maps out the nerves in the body, which communicate information from the brain to our organs. It lists all of the symptoms and dysfunctions that can occur if the spine becomes subluxated.

Thinking back to the fuse-panel tripping analogy, here are some examples of specific subluxations:

- If your T5 vertebrae trips, you might experience stomach issues such as heartburn.
- If your C1 vertebrae trips, you might experience headaches, have trouble concentrating, or experience brain fog.

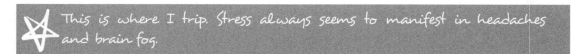

This is where I trip. Stress always seems to manifest in headaches and brain fog.

- If your T9 vertebrae trips, adrenal function will likely decrease, and you may become overwhelmed by stress.
- If your L4 or L5 vertebrae trips, you might experience bowel issues or frequent constipation.

Basically, our nervous system is like our body's control panel. If our spine has proper motion and function, then our nervous system will be powered on and able to carry out its primary function: connecting the brain to the body.

CHIROPRACTIC AND THE NERVOUS SYSTEM

The word "chiropractic" comes from the Greek *chiros* and *praktikos*, meaning "done by hand" and was founded in 1895 by D. D. Palmer. Chiropractic focuses on optimizing the body's own ability to function at its best by removing interference on the nervous system.

Chiropractic is based on 33 healing principles. These principles would be too complex to discuss for the purpose of this book but could be summarized by these key points:

1. The body is a self-healing, self-regulating organism.

2. The nervous system is responsible for coordinating the function of every cell, tissue and organ in the body.

3. Subluxations are the #1 cause of interference with the body's inborn or innate intelligence, which is the ability to self-heal and self-regulate through the nervous system.

4. Chiropractic is the only healing science responsible for locating and correcting subluxations through a chiropractic adjustment, thereby restoring the body's ability to heal itself.[2]

WHAT IS AN ADJUSTMENT?

The method a chiropractor will use to correct a subluxation is called an adjustment. An adjustment involves a gentle and specific application of a force or touch to the spine in order to allow the body to restore normal spinal and nervous system functions.

Several different techniques exist—they all have the same goal, which is to remove the interference on one's nervous system. It's important to find the technique and approach that works for you. Also, keep in mind that you don't need to be in pain to see a chiropractor. The longer you go with a poorly functioning nervous system, the more devastating the effects are to your health and well-being. If you wait for signs and symptoms, detrimental health consequences could already be in progress.

"WE DON'T GUESS, WE TEST"

Most chiropractors use technology that can measure the function of the nervous system. The most commonly used technologies are the:

- **Thermal Scan** – This instrument monitors skin temperature to assess autonomic nervous system function. Temperature indicates where there is dysregulation in the autonomic nervous system and how it can affect organ function. For organs to properly do their job, optimal nerve communication is needed. Determining whether or not there is nerve interference can play an important role in understanding and planning a health strategy.

- **Surface Electromyography (sEMG)** – This highly researched tool evaluates the communication between your nervous system and the muscles that support and move your spine. These muscles are controlled by the nerves alongside them. The test measures how much energy is needed to maintain posture, and the distribution of energy throughout the muscles. A low score can indicate that too much energy is being used because the spine is out of balance. It can also indicate that stress is overworking the muscles. A surface EMG can help measure the progress made after a series of adjustments.

- **Pulse Wave Profiler** – This instrument helps determine your overall ability to adapt to your environmental stressors. It is used to collect Heart Rate Variability (HRV) data, and monitor the balance and activity of the entire autonomic nervous system. A high heart rate variability indicates good adaptability, whereas a constantly low heart rate variability is an indicator of accelerated aging and poor heart health.[3]

When it comes down to it, the less negative stressors you have in your life or the better your body is able to adapt to them, the less chance you have to trip your fuse panel. Unfortunately, stress is everywhere, and if you want to keep your nervous system in tiptop shape, it's best to get checked regularly by a chiropractor to minimize the health effects of vertebral subluxations.

I always tell my patients: "The better your health habits are, like eating right, exercising, decreasing your toxic load and minimizing negative emotional stressors, the less you will need me."

Remember, healing takes place when our mind and body are able to communicate properly via our nervous system and when it is free of interference. It really is amazing what chiropractic can do.

> It's true! Our family gets adjusted regularly and we sure seem to have a much stronger immune system then most other families as we rarely get sick!

The following diagram shows examples of health habits with corresponding hack levels. To download the *Hack Your Health Habits Worksheet*, visit

www.hackyourhealthhabits.com/worksheets

READY #HEALTHHACKER?
EXAMPLES OF LEVEL 1, 2 AND 3 HACKS FOR THIS CHAPTER

✓ Try to minimize your negative physical, biochemical and psychological stressors.
✓ Get checked regularly by a chiropractor.

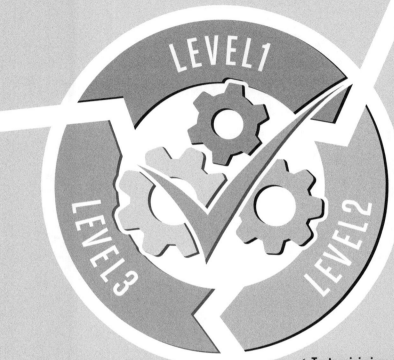

✓ Try to minimize your negative physical, biochemical and psychological stressors.
✓ Get checked regularly by a chiropractor.

✓ Try to minimize your negative physical, biochemical and psychological stressors.
✓ Get checked regularly by a chiropractor.

HACK YOUR HEALTH PROGRESS

Yep, that's correct. The three hack levels are the same!

|||||||||||||||||||||||||||||||||||||||||||||||||||||||||||||||||||||||||||||

CHAPTER 45

46
SHARPENING YOUR BRAIN
How to Mitigate Cognitive Decline

"To live, a man needs food,
water and a sharp mind."

— Louis Zamperini

THINK IT OVER

- Do you perform daily activities to keep your brain sharp?

- What lifestyle factors can help prevent cognitive decline?

- When was the last time you tried something new?

The topic of brain health has become a more popular subject in the last decade, with a noticeable rise in neurodegenerative disorders like dementia and Alzheimer's. Brain health has also become a widely popular topic in the world of sports, where concussions are now recognized to have a significant short- and long-term impact on injured players.

That said, unless you have neurodegenerative disorders in your family or have experienced a concussion, you probably won't start thinking about your brain's health until you start noticing symptoms like brain fog, poor memory and more of those "tip-of-the-tongue" moments. Here's the thing: The longer you wait to do something, the worse the problem will become, so it's best to start thinking about your brain's health today.

Keeping a sharp mind will enable you to make more efficient and wiser decisions as you age. There are so many simple ways to keep your mind sharp, some of which you may already be doing.

You will notice that the information in this chapter repeats many of the messages that you have learned throughout the book as it is said that we need to hear something five times before the information really sinks in. We should all know the importance of exercise, eating well and getting good restful sleep. The question is, are you doing it? Below is a mix of information you know and information you may not know, which can be implemented for better brain health. I challenge you not to just read and say, "I know that," but ask yourself, "Am I doing this daily?" If not, what can you do to incorporate more of it on a daily basis?

- **Exercise daily** – Exercise has a wide array of benefits for your mental and physical health. Endorphins released during exercise work wonders in fending off depression and boosting the immune system. Physical fitness has also been shown to increase mental sharpness as people age. Especially past the age of 40, daily exercise helps maintain acuity in the prefrontal cortex of the brain. In one study, elderly men who were aerobically fit were able to outperform men who were unfit in decision-making tasks.

- **Eat a healthy diet** – Diet can play a key role in keeping your brain sharp. Avoid trans fats, processed sugars and additives in food—which damage brain blood vessels. Be sure your diet includes:

  - healthy fats, such as olive oil and omega-3 fatty acids, found in fish like salmon

  - antioxidants, which contribute to optimal brain functioning

  - plenty of veggies, and the more color, the better

- **Get enough sleep** – The fog of exhaustion will cloud your mental ability. Our brains store daily memories while we sleep, so you need rest in order to remember even mundane details of daily life. You might even consider taking a short nap after learning something new or important, to help store it in your long-term memory. Sleeping less than six hours a night has been shown to decrease mental sharpness even after one night. I am sure, if you have kids, you know exactly what I am talking about!

- **Use your mind instead of a calculator** – Math and problem-solving help strengthen reasoning and problem-solving skills. Many people haven't done math since grade school; give it a try sometime. Next time you are at the grocery store, challenge yourself by keeping a running total of the items in your cart. You don't have to add the exact amount; round each price up to the nearest dollar. When you get to the checkout, you'll find out how close you were.

- **Never stop learning** – A study out of Harvard University found that advanced education is associated with stronger memory as a person ages. Just because you aren't in school doesn't mean you can't keep learning; an old dog can learn new tricks! Read a book. Watch online talks or tutorials. Pick up a new hobby. Take a class at a local community college. The best courses are those that are both mentally and socially demanding, like photography or quilting. These types of courses give you the added benefit of meeting new people and forming new friendships! The point is to constantly have those neurons firing.

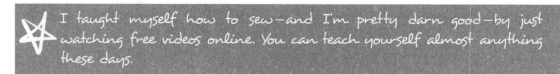

I taught myself how to sew—and I'm pretty darn good—by just watching free videos online. You can teach yourself almost anything these days.

- **Flex your mental muscles** – You can improve your logic, problem-solving, mental orientation and thought process by working on puzzles and doing difficult mental tasks. For instance, start doing crossword puzzles. Studies show that older people who do crossword puzzles have better scores on a variety of cognitive tests than those who don't. To be fair, researchers aren't sure if the puzzles cause better mental ability or if people with better mental ability tend to do more crossword puzzles. Nonetheless, it can't hurt to try. Don't like puzzles? Try memorizing your friends' and family's phone numbers and birthdays.

The other day I did not have my phone with me at work, and I wanted to call my husband. Without my phone's speed dial, I could not believe that I did not know his number by heart.

- **Engage all of your senses** – Using all of your senses activates different parts of your brain, which can help you retain specific memories better. In one study, people were shown images presented with or without a smell and were found to be able to recall the images with a smell better than without. This might mean using mindfulness techniques to notice the sights, smells, tastes, feelings and sounds around you in a given situation, to help recall the event more clearly later. It could also mean playing certain music or engaging your sense of smell while studying or learning something new. An easy way to engage your sense of smell is with essential oils.

  It is important to know that not all essential oils are created equal. When I refer to essential oils, I'm referring to the 100 percent pure, therapeutic grade essences extracted from the flowers, leaves, peel, seeds, etc. of a plant. These are not to be confused with cheaper, man-made synthetic fragrances and perfumes created in a laboratory, which can be toxic and are highly allergenic. Essential oils are a great way to activate your sense of smell at any time during the day. There are great companies out there with all kinds of formulas that can produce calming effects to helping you get focused. For example, the scent of mint has been shown to boost cognition and improve problem-solving and memory.

- **Try using your opposite hand to do everyday things** – Have you ever tried signing your name with your opposite hand? Challenging, isn't it? But, it is a great way to force yourself to concentrate while engaging both sides of your brain. It will probably start out like scrawl, but you will become more aware of your shoulders and gain more control over time. If you are using a computer for a good part of the day, try switching from holding your mouse on one side to the other hand. It might feel awkward at first but it will force your brain to fire differently. As a bonus, it will also give your dominant wrist a break, which can minimize the risk of developing a Repetitive Strain Injuries (RSI).

- **Express yourself creatively** – Creativity has more than one advantage when it comes to keeping your mind sharp and keeping a positive attitude. Creativity forces you to think and flex your mental muscles. The results of creative work have been shown to reinforce self-confidence and help individuals enjoy their daily life. Try your hand at writing poetry, sewing, or playing a musical instrument, gardening, or painting. If you don't feel artistic or creative, baking or writing in a journal are other great ways to express yourself. Try applying creative approaches to daily tasks like shopping on a budget or creating a new recipe with limited ingredients. Keep a positive attitude about your ability to find solutions in everyday situations.

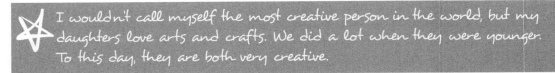

I wouldn't call myself the most creative person in the world, but my daughters love arts and crafts. We did a lot when they were younger. To this day, they are both very creative.

- **Reframe your experiences** – Reframing involves looking at your current situation with a fresh outlook. In many ways, attitude is everything: You can reframe a negative thought or experience to make it positive. For example, you may not be able to recall things as well as you used to, but instead of seeing that as a personal failure, recognize it as a natural effect of a life well lived.

- **Meditate or practice yoga** – By learning to calm your mind and focus your attention, you can improve your mental clarity, which has positive effects on your memory and attention span. In one study, participants who practiced mindfulness for 20-30 minutes daily scored better on standardized memory tests than those who took a nutrition class.

- **Maintain healthy relationships** – Humans are highly social animals. We're not meant to survive, let alone thrive, in isolation. Relationships stimulate our brains. In fact, interacting with others may be the best kind of brain exercise. Research shows that having meaningful friendships and a strong support system are vital not only to emotional health, but also to brain health. In one recent study from the Harvard School of Public Health, researchers found that people with the most active social lives had the slowest rate of memory decline.[1] There are many ways to start taking advantage of the brain and memory-boosting benefits of socializing. Volunteer, join a club, make it a point to see friends more often, or reach out over the phone. And, if a human isn't handy, don't overlook the value of a pet, especially highly social ones like dogs.

- **Keep stress to a minimum** – You knew this one was coming. Everyone talks about the negative effects of stress. Stress is one of the brain's worst enemies. Over time, chronic stress can destroy brain cells and even damage parts of the hippocampus—the region of the brain involved in the formation of new memories and the retrieval of old ones. Studies have also linked prolonged stress to memory loss. It may be inevitable that we will experience stress at one point or another, and a certain amount of stress may even be deemed healthy (i.e. eustress: what motivates us to get work done). However, the point is to try our best to manage situations over which we have control. To minimize daily stress, remember to:

  - set realistic expectations (and be willing to say no)

- take breaks throughout the day

- express your feelings instead of bottling them up

- set a healthy balance between work and leisure time

- focus on one task at a time, rather than trying to multitask

- plan your day and events ahead of time

- **Get out of routine** – Just as too much sitting has proven to be very unhealthy for our bodies, too much of the same day-in, day-out routine isn't too good for our brains, either. Most of us live our lives as a series of fixed routines from morning to night, and there are many good reasons for this. It simplifies life. It limits brain-draining decision making. It lets us perform complex tasks like driving a car with little mental effort. Routines, if you remember, are run by our subconscious and require very little brain energy. Consequently, they provide the brain with very little stimulation. Making a point of shaking up routines and proactively exercising your brain are both keys to a sharper and more vital mind. Some of the reported benefits of brain exercise include faster thinking, improved memory and mood, better vision and hearing, quicker reaction time, and a feeling of increased focus, motivation and productivity.

 So, the spontaneous weekend trips my husband wants us to take every once in a while are actually a good thing.

- **Go Keto!** – Yes, the foods we eat *do* indeed have an impact on our mental and cognitive health as well. As you remember, your brain and body thrive on *ketones* as it is a more sustainable and cleaner source of energy. Knowing this, a keto-adapted individual actually experiences less brain fog, less memory trouble and even gets better sleep. Essentially, a brain running on ketones is more efficient, focused and has a greater ability to perform.

- **BrainTap Technologies** – With the increasing research in neurofeedback technology and brain therapies, Dr. Patrick Porter has put together the ultimate brain-training system: BrainTap Technologies. BrainTap Technologies is a powerfully effective mind-development tool designed to help you overcome the ill effects of the fight-or-flight response while achieving physical, mental and emotional balance. Using guided imagery, acupressure points, binaural sounds and light frequencies to help balance the communication of the right and left brain, BrainTap helps us to relax, reboot and strengthen busy brains. For more on BrainTap technology and how you may benefit from it, visit our resource page at www.hackyourhealthhabits.com/resources

Your brain is an extraordinary machine, and, although there is still a great deal we do not know about it, that shouldn't stop us from wanting to expand its capabilities. Don't blame age for declining cognitive abilities. Test out some of the methods listed above and keep your brain sharp.

The following diagram shows examples of health habits with corresponding hack levels. To download the *Hack Your Health Habits Worksheet*, visit

www.hackyourhealthhabits.com/worksheets

READY #HEALTHHACKER?
EXAMPLES OF LEVEL 1, 2 AND 3 HACKS FOR THIS CHAPTER

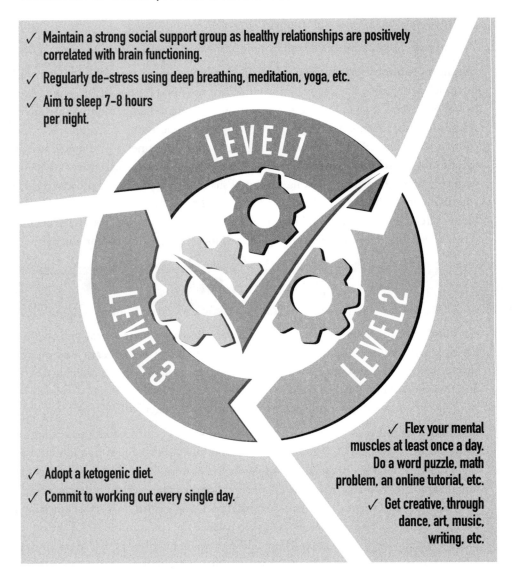

✓ Maintain a strong social support group as healthy relationships are positively correlated with brain functioning.

✓ Regularly de-stress using deep breathing, meditation, yoga, etc.

✓ Aim to sleep 7-8 hours per night.

✓ Adopt a ketogenic diet.

✓ Commit to working out every single day.

✓ Flex your mental muscles at least once a day. Do a word puzzle, math problem, an online tutorial, etc.

✓ Get creative, through dance, art, music, writing, etc.

HACK YOUR HEALTH PROGRESS

||||||||||||||||||||||||||||||||||||||||||||||||||||||||||||||||

CHAPTER 46

EPIGENETICS
You Are What You Think

THINK IT OVER

> "Your genetics load the gun. Your lifestyle pulls the trigger."
>
> — MEHMET OZ

- Are the majority of your daily thoughts feeding the future that you desire?

- Do you know how much of your health is directly related to heredity?

- Do you understand the impact that your lifestyle can have on your DNA?

For years, we have been taught that genes control our destiny. If a certain illness runs in the family, we automatically believe that it's bound to happen to us. The media reinforces this way of thinking, repeatedly suggesting that genes are the root cause of our health conditions and diseases. We have been programmed to think that we are victims of our genetic makeup, that our genes are what influence our health, well-being and personalities.

Just think how many times you have heard someone say: "It's not my fault, I have bad genes. There is nothing I can do about my [insert health condition or disease here]." Well, according to recent research, this is not quite true. We actually have the ability to change the *expression* of our genes at any age and at any time. This emerging field of study is called *epigenetics*.

So, maybe I won't turn into my mother, after all? Lol!

Epigenetics literally means "above" or "on top of" genetics. It refers to external influences on DNA through environmental inputs that can turn genes "on" or "off," so to speak. These modifications do not change the DNA sequence, but instead, affect how cells interpret genes and how they are expressed. Surprisingly, research shows that only about 5 percent of people are actually born with legitimate genetic conditions. That leaves the other 95 percent to lifestyle and behaviors, which means that the majority of our health conditions and diseases can be blamed on our lifestyle choices. Of course, with the exceptions of conditions created by infections, injuries or other uncontrollable causes.

HEALTH AND DNA

In 2003, researchers announced the successful completion of the Human Genome Project (genome refers to our complete set of genes). The goal of the project was to determine the sequence of chemical base pairs that make up human DNA, as well as identify and map all of the genes of the human genome. Surprisingly, the project revealed that there are only 23,688 human genes. Prior to then, the research scientists believed that there would be closer to 140,000 genes, as that is the amount of proteins we have in our body. However, the findings showed that it is the combination of the genes that are turned on at any one time that produces all the different proteins we depend on for life—genes must work together to be expressed (i.e. turned on) or to be suppressed (i.e. turned off). This means that we have way more control over the expression of our health than it was once thought.

To delve a bit deeper into this concept, let's review a little cellular biology. Picture a cell. Hmm, that might be a bit hard to do, so picture a circle—this is the cell membrane. Inside the cell, there is a nucleus, basically a smaller circle in the center of the bigger circle, and inside the nucleus, there are chromosomes, or a bunch of little Xs floating around. Chromosomes are made of genes, which are comprised of 50 percent DNA and 50 percent protein. For years, the scientific world has focused their studies on the DNA component of the cell, essentially ignoring the other 50 percent—which was often referred to as junk DNA. Fortunately, epigenetics has begun to change that focus.

According to epigenetics, our DNA is nothing more than a blueprint. Just like an architect uses a blueprint to build a building, we use DNA to produce protein. According to Dr. Bruce Lipton, author of the book *The Biology of Belief*, our bodies are in fact, protein-producing machines. He argues that *proteins* are the expression of life, *not* genes, which is *great* news. It means we can stop blaming our genes and actually figure out how to produce the *right* protein to create who we *want* to be.

Ask anyone who has taken a biology class (and remembers it) what the "brain" of the cell is, and they will tell you it's the nucleus. However, this isn't true, according to epigenetics. Epigenetic research is telling us that the *membrane* is actually the brain of the cell. This is why signals from outside the cell, from our environment and captured via our skin and senses, are so important, and can literally change the expression of our genes.

Let me illustrate this better. A study done at the Spanish National Cancer Centre in Madrid looked at 40 pairs of identical twins—who, by definition, are born with the exact same DNA. What they discovered is that the young identical twins had very similar epigenetic patterns. However, as these twins aged and accumulated distinctive experiences, their epigenetic states diverged. At the time of the study, the older twins led different lifestyles and spent the majority of their lives living apart. Due to this, their epigenetic patterns were notably different.[1] Essentially, the experiences we live leave a mark on our DNA, and these marks greatly impact how our genes are expressed.

Let's clarify a bit. In his book, *You Are the Placebo*, Dr. Joe Dispenza talks about epigenetic variations using the analogy of a computer. Imagine you buy two identical computers—one for you and one for your spouse. The computers have identical hard drives and the same basic software. You need your computer for work, while your spouse just wants to surf the Internet. You download several programs and your spouse leaves their computer the same. Within no time, the once-identical computers become very different. This is representative of epigenetic variation. Even if a computer (or twin) might start off the same, any new software (or difference in habits, environments, etc.) will affect what the computer (or person) does and what it is able to do.

Ask yourself this question: What software are you downloading on your hard drive? Are you downloading advantageous or disadvantageous software? Every bit of information you feed yourself, whether it is through your food, your thoughts, your activities, your hobbies—even the people you hang around—helps to engineer your cells and health outcomes. If you know you have a family background or predisposition to a negative health outcome, you can take charge of it. Eat well, move, keep stress to a minimum and foster a positive mindset. We control our own destiny way more than we ever thought possible.

MAKING THE RIGHT CHOICES

Our thoughts largely impact our choices. It is said that we think somewhere between 50,000 and 70,000 thoughts every single day, and 90 percent of these thoughts are exactly the same ones we had the day before. Believe it or not, according to Dr. Joe Dispenza, 95 percent of who you are is determined by the time you are 35 years old. By this point, we have internalized our behaviors, skills, emotional reactions, beliefs, perceptions and attitudes. The 95 percent is our subconscious state of being. The other 5 percent is our conscious state of being, where we make conscious decisions. This means we are on autopilot 95 percent of the time.

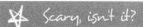 Scary, isn't it?

This explains why we often fail to think positively. The conscious 5 percent of our mind that we use to think positively is in a constant battle with the subconscious 95 percent of our mind that we have programmed to think a certain way. It's no wonder we have trouble changing our habits and behaviors. It is literally like our mind and body are in opposition. According to Dr. Dispenza, in order to create new outcomes, we need to change the way we think. We need to make new choices and adopt new behaviors, in order to create new experiences and feelings. These feelings are what will create our new state of being.

THE POWER OF THOUGHT

To show you the power of thoughts, beliefs and our environment, let's look at another study. Eight men in their 70s and 80s were brought to a monastery for a five-day retreat. The environment was designed to help the men imagine that they were 22 years younger. Music and newspapers from their younger years were placed in the environment, and the TV showed old shows they used to watch, and so on.

For five days, the men reminisced about the old days. The results? There were improvements in their height, weight, gait, grip strength, arthritis and mental cognition. The men did not just feel younger, they physically became younger![2]

Simply put: Our thoughts alone can impact our health. The questions to ask ourselves here are: "What thoughts are we choosing daily? What reality do we choose to live in? Who are we pretending to be?"

As you know, the right and left brain play different and important roles in creating new thoughts, beliefs and feelings. Most people are aware that the left brain is known for being logical and the right brain for being creative. But, according to health experts, it goes far beyond that. The right hemisphere is related to novelties, and the left is related to routine.

Take for example, a musician learning a new piece of music. We think music is generally a creative process, so it must be associated with the right brain, no? When learning the piece, the musician is indeed using the right side of his brain, but as soon as the piece of music is learned, it goes to the left side, as it is now learned and familiar. This can be applied to any new thing we learn: We use our right brain for learning, and once the skill is learned, we use our left brain to execute. Why is this relevant?

When was the last time you learned a new skill or experienced something new? If we want to create new thoughts, beliefs and feelings, we need to create new experiences for ourselves. Think about it. We sleep on the same side of the bed, get up at the same time, go to work, come back home, cook dinner, go to bed and do the same thing the very next day. I challenge you to try something new every single day. Activate your right brain so that you can create the world that you want.

THE MIND-BODY CONNECTION

Let's talk about one last important concept in the field of epigenetics: the mind-body connection. Our bodies have what is called *innate intelligence*—a term originally coined by Daniel David Palmer, the founder of chiropractic. According to Palmer, all life contains innate intelligence. At its core, innate intelligence is the force that is responsible for the organization, maintenance and healing of the body.

The chiropractic philosophy is based on the premise that, by removing interference to the nervous system (via spinal adjustments), innate intelligence is able to do its work and help our body heal. No doctor can cure anything. It is always the body that does the healing. I am blessed to have seen innate intelligence at work in my practice for more than 20 years. Our bodies are truly amazing.

Another great method of harnessing the mind-body connection is through practices such as yoga, meditation, Tai Chi and mindfulness. These practices move our attention away from our outer world (our environment) to our inner world (our thoughts and feelings). This causes us to feel more at peace, and repairs damaged connections and even reprograms new neural pathways. More on the topic of meditation will be discussed in **Chapter 50: Meditation—You Don't Have to Be a Monk.**

Before I end this chapter, I have one more question for you: Who do you want to be? You are not your genes! Just because your father suffers from heart disease or your grandmother suffered from dementia, doesn't mean you will, too. You have the ability to make positive choices and change your outcome. You can create the life you want. Wake up to the possibilities and design something great for yourself. The world could really use *the best* version of *you.*

The following diagram shows examples of health habits with corresponding hack levels. To download the *Hack Your Health Habits Worksheet*, visit

www.hackyourhealthhabits.com/worksheets

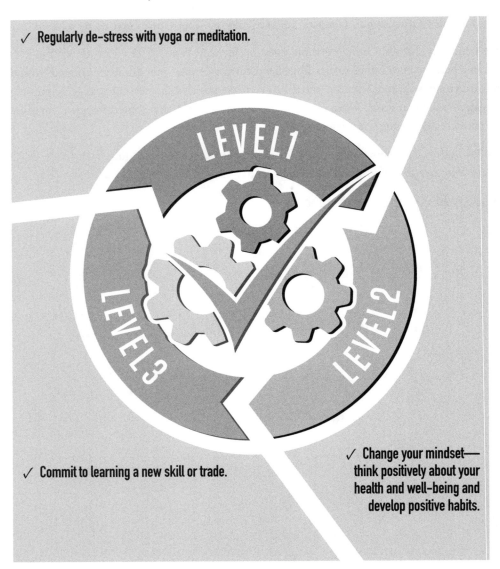

✓ Regularly de-stress with yoga or meditation.

✓ Commit to learning a new skill or trade.

✓ Change your mindset—
think positively about your
health and well-being and
develop positive habits.

HACK YOUR HEALTH PROGRESS

||||||||||||||||||||||||||||||||||||||||||||||||||||

CHAPTER 47

AGING
Slowing the Process

48

"I am not getting older, I am just becoming a classic."

— Unknown

THINK IT OVER

- Do you feel like you're aging before your time?

- Do you know the contributing factors to accelerated aging?

- How can you slow down the aging process?

Joint soreness and stiffness, skin issues like age spots and wrinkles, frailer bones, weaker muscles, hormonal decline, slower metabolism, a decrease in cardiovascular and lung functions, weaker immune system, decreased sexual desire, and a decline in vision and hearing—we are all subject to the effects of aging. But what if I told you that we have the power to slow down the process?

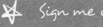 Sign me up, please!

Everyone ages, though some faster than others.

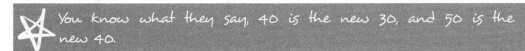 You know what they say, 40 is the new 30, and 50 is the new 40.

Genetics may play a small role in the aging process, but there are things that everyone can do to slow down the effects of aging. This is what this chapter will be exploring.

First and foremost, a healthy lifestyle is imperative. We all know how important a proper diet and exercise is to keep healthy. But, did you know that there are certain natural supplements that you can take to help your body function more efficiently and look and feel younger?

ACCELERATED AGING

Though aging has its perks—wisdom being the biggest—it does have many drawbacks. Baby boomers seem to be the first generation really concerned about aging. They want to stay active and independent for as long as they can. They want to continue to be able to do the things they enjoy most. No one wants to feel unwanted, unimportant, or unvalued by society. And, no one wants to lose their freedom or become a burden on their loved ones.

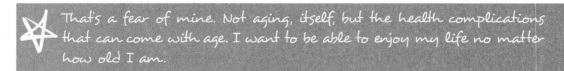

That's a fear of mine. Not aging, itself, but the health complications that can come with age. I want to be able to enjoy my life no matter how old I am.

So, what are the things that make us age faster? And, how can we slow down the process? There is a host of lifestyle and environmental factors that impact our cells and make us age at a more rapid rate. Yes, it can help to have good genes, but there's a lot more to it.

There are three major causes of the aging process. Understanding these three components is key in implementing the right actions to minimize the aging process:

1. **Degradation of our telomeres.** Telomeres are the protective caps at the end of each strand of cellular. Think of them as being similar to the plastic tips at the end of shoelaces that prevent the lace from falling apart. Telomeres are critical to aging, as they prevent DNA degradation. There is a multitude of products on the market promising the eternal fountain of youth, with claims that they stop telomere degrading—or even elongate them. How do telomeres degrade? Every day, a great amount of our cells die, and our bodies replace them with copies. Unfortunately, sometimes these copies are not exactly like the originals. This, in the long run, can lead to a significant decrease in the length of the telomere.

2. **Decreased efficiency of our mitochondria.** Mitochondria are your body's powerhouse and energy supply (through the production of ATP). Our body has approximately 10 million billion mitochondria—yes, you read that right—about 10 percent of our body weight. As we age, the number of mitochondria in our body decreases, leading to a decrease in the body's overall energy output, affecting all systems in the body: heart, lungs, brain, liver, etc.[1]

3. **Free radical and oxidative stress.** By now, you should understand the importance of antioxidants. Antioxidants counterbalance free radicals, also known as oxidants. They ensure that the body is in balance when it comes to oxidation—the body does need some oxidation,

a process named mitohormesis. Too little or too much can cause problems. A good example of oxidation is an apple turning brown after cutting it into slices. This "rusting" also occurs to our cells when they are exposed to things like pollution, strenuous exercise, increased toxic load, etc.

Here is a list of lifestyle factors that affect the rate at which we age:

- **Chronic lack of sleep** – This is shown to significantly shorten our telomeres, therefore negatively impacting our DNA.

- **Chronic stress** – This can impact our cortisol levels and accelerate aging.

- **Over- and under-exercising** – Too much exercise or too much of a sedentary lifestyle can negatively impact aging.

- **Poor nutrition** – A diet that lacks food rich in antioxidants, vitamins and minerals is detrimental to our overall health and well-being.

- **Lack of vitamin D** – Of the approximately 20,000-25,000 genes identified in the human genome, vitamin D deficiency has been shown to influence about 3,000 of them.[2] It influences many diseases, from cancer to heart disease and rheumatoid arthritis, just to name a few.

- **UV rays** – Excessive UV-ray exposure can damage the DNA of our skin cells, increasing the likelihood of wrinkles.

- **Imbalance in omega-3 and omega-6 ratio** – As discussed in previous chapters.

- **Sugars and processed carbs** – Too much sugar and processed carbs will lead to formation of AGEs (Advanced Glycation End-products), which have been shown to affect cellular aging.

- **Obesity** – Excess adipose tissues create more oxidative stress in the body.

- **Alcohol intake** – Alcohol decreases the body's antioxidant count and leads to free radical formation.

- **Genetically modified foods** – These affect our immune functions, speeding the aging process.

- **Drugs** – Over-the-counter or prescribed medication add to the body's toxic load, putting greater stress on the cells themselves by causing inflammation.

- **Pesticides, herbicides and environmental toxins** – These also add to the body's toxic load.

SUPPLEMENTS FOR ANTI-AGING

To combat the causes of aging, proper diet and exercise are needed. Supplements can also play an important role. Certain supplements are able to focus on the health of your telomeres, mitochondria and oxidative stress. Remember that there is no magic pill. An integrative approach is needed to stay healthy and fit as you age.

Listed below are seven key players that will help slow down the aging process:

1. **Glutathione** – Glutathione plays a critical role in the production of DNA and the proteins that make up our body. This antioxidant is involved in creating our skin, hair, nails, muscles, bones, organs, enzymes, hormones and even immune cells. Like many other important biomarkers, glutathione levels decline as we age. This has a profoundly negative effect on the health of nearly every cell in our body. Glutathione is found in many foods, including fruits, vegetables and meats. Some examples include asparagus, spinach, garlic, avocado, squash, zucchini, potatoes, melons, grapefruit, strawberries and peaches. Glutathione can also be taken in supplement form.

2. **Ashwagandha** – While cortisol plays an important role in controlling the impact of stress on the body, increased levels of cortisol coupled with poor sleep are known to accelerate the aging process. Furthermore, it has been shown to increase the degradation of DNA telomeres. Ashwagandha helps counterbalance the negative effects of high cortisol levels. It lowers cortisol, improves sleep, and helps keep your telomeres and cells healthy and youthful. It is an Ayurvedic herb that can be found at your local natural food store.

3. **Coenzyme Q10** – CoQ10 is also a very potent antioxidant and is essential to the health of our mitochondria. Healthy mitochondria mean more energy, better body function and more vitality. CoQ10 is found in organ meats such as liver, kidney and heart. It can also be found in beef, sardines and mackerel. Vegetable sources of CoQ10 include broccoli and cauliflower; supplement sources are also available.

4. **Curcumin** – Curcumin, the active ingredient found in turmeric, is a very potent antioxidant. Curcumin seeks and destroys damaging free radicals, lowers oxidative stress, slows telomere degradation and reduces levels of biomarkers associated with accelerated aging. Turmeric, sometimes called "poor man's saffron," is the best-known source of curcumin. It's a spice often used in curry powders. Fresh turmeric can be added to smoothies for added benefits, and can also be found as a supplement at your local health food store.

> ✦ I add turmeric to just about everything I can. Sprinkling some on some roasted vegetables is a family favorite.

5. **Resveratrol** – Resveratrol reduces inflammation in the body by inhibiting sphingosine kinase and phospholipase D—two molecules known to trigger inflammation. Consuming resveratrol can mimic the effects of exercise—also lowering insulin levels, which is key to fighting disease and staying young. It's also a potent antioxidant that helps prevent the rampant spread of cancer cells, improves blood circulation, and protects your brain from the development of Alzheimer's disease. It prevents neurological disorders such as strokes, ischemia and Huntington's disease. Resveratrol can be found in peanuts, pistachios, grapes, red and white wine, blueberries, cranberries and dark chocolate. Resveratrol can also be taken in the form of a supplement.

6. **N-acetyl-l-cysteine (NAC)** – Playing an important role in heavy metal detoxification, NAC is a derivative of the dietary amino acid l-cysteine. NAC has been known to improve lung health, assisting the lungs through mucolytic and antioxidant action. NAC also enhances

glutathione production, known as the mother of all antioxidants. NAC is found in granola and oat flakes. Vegetables like broccoli, red pepper and onion are also significant sources of NAC. Other plant sources include bananas, garlic, soybeans, linseed and wheat germ. NAC supplements are also worth looking into.

7. **Alpha-Lipoic Acid (ALA)** – Both water- and fat-soluble, alpha lipoic acid is able to function in almost any part of the body. It is a potent antioxidant, which enhances the activity of vitamins C and E. On top of providing protection from free radicals, alpha-lipoic acid supports various metabolic processes. In addition to this, ALA is known to support nerve health, cardiovascular function and glucose metabolism. Alpha lipoic acid is mainly found in organ meats like heart, liver and kidneys. Plant-based sources include broccoli and spinach. ALA is also present in yeast, particularly Brewer's yeast. And, as you may have guessed, it also comes in a supplement.

I know it may sound like a lot, and I am not suggesting that you add *all* of the recommended supplements to your diet. Remember that it's important to eat a variety of foods. It's up to you to decide what is right for you.

For instance, if you don't like the taste of turmeric, a curcumin supplement is a great alternative. Or, if you can never remember to take your vitamins, adding broccoli to your morning smoothie can be a great way to consume CoQ10s and alpha-lipoic acids.

Do what works for you, but remember, there's no magic pill. You're going to have to put in a little bit of work to slow down the aging process. However, you *can* age gracefully by following a nutritious diet, exercising regularly and taking your supplements!

The following diagram shows examples of health habits with corresponding hack levels. To download the *Hack Your Health Habits Worksheet*, visit

www.hackyourhealthhabits.com/worksheets

READY #HEALTHHACKER?
EXAMPLES OF LEVEL 1, 2 AND 3 HACKS FOR THIS CHAPTER

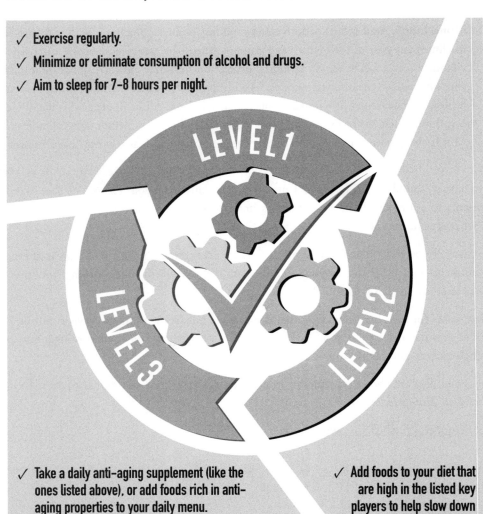

✓ Exercise regularly.
✓ Minimize or eliminate consumption of alcohol and drugs.
✓ Aim to sleep for 7–8 hours per night.

✓ Take a daily anti-aging supplement (like the ones listed above), or add foods rich in anti-aging properties to your daily menu.

✓ Add foods to your diet that are high in the listed key players to help slow down the aging process.

HACK YOUR HEALTH PROGRESS

|||||||||||||||||||||||||||||||||||||||||||||||||||||||

CHAPTER 48

SECTION 10

*Get Rest, Recharge and
Be More Zen*

Are you letting stress get the best of you?
Learning healthy ways to manage your stress is one
of the keys to optimizing overall health.
Section 10 teaches you ways to develop daily habits
that support proper rest and rejuvenation for the
body and mind. You will also discover simple
practices that will promote restful sleep and help
you be more "zen."

SLEEP
More Than Just Beauty Rest

"Sleep is the golden chain that binds health and our bodies together."

— Thomas Dekker

THINK IT OVER

- **Are you sleeping enough?**

- **What are the effects of sleep deprivation on your overall health and brain function?**

- **How can you improve your quality of sleep so that you wake up feeling refreshed in the morning?**

Are you getting enough sleep? We all know that we should be aiming for 7-9 hours of sleep per night, but how feasible is that? A lot of people are surviving on 5-6 and feel just fine. Are you one of those people? I hate to break it to you, but that 5-6 hours will catch up with you one day. Studies show that lack of sleep could have long-term detrimental effects on your brain, immune system, hormones, metabolism and many other vital bodily functions.

An estimated 3.3 million people, or one in every seven Canadians aged 15 and older, have problems getting to sleep or staying asleep at night.[1] Part of the problem is the misconception that sleep does not breed success. A whopping 80 percent of North Americans think that it isn't possible to sleep 7-9 hours per night and be successful at the same time. It probably isn't a coincidence, then, that 75 percent of people experience daytime sleepiness, and 34 percent of people say sleepiness interferes with their daytime activities[2]; that's certainly no way to live.

> *That's terrible! Sleep is such a fundamental aspect of health. Many of the hacks in this book involve getting enough sleep.*

Sleep is important for a multitude of reasons but, above all else, it rebuilds, repairs and recharges your body. When you're asleep, your immune system is most active and repairs what it needs to while your brain recharges. Without sleep, you get sick in both mind and body.

Sleep disorders such as insomnia and sleep apnea are currently on the rise and come with a slew of negative effects on overall health. Sleep apnea, for example, is becoming more and more of an issue as 30 percent of those aged 60 or older experience its symptoms. It is characterized by the cessation of breathing for 10 seconds or longer during sleep, which reduces blood oxygen levels and can be dangerous if not looked after. Some symptoms can include daytime sleepiness, excessive snoring, poor attention, or waking up gasping for air. Insufficient oxygen supply to the brain can later result in early aging, cognitive decline, weight gain, diabetes and even increased blood pressure.

Other Symptoms of Sleep Deficit

- Daytime fatigue
- Poor memory and mental performance
- Depression and apathy
- Morning headaches, waking up feeling unrefreshed
- Heart disease
- Heartburn
- The need to urinate in the middle of the night
- Loud snoring
- Diminished sex drive
- Decreased exercise tolerance
- More than five pounds of weight gain in the past year
- The need for stimulants

Poor sleep can negatively affect almost every aspect of your health. This is due to the fact that sleep deprivation confuses your *circadian rhythm* (the sleep-wake cycle), and, as a consequence, has a major impact on the body. Although most people can still function on 4-6 hours of sleep per night, the impact chronic sleep deprivation has on your adrenal glands is the same as physical stress or chronic illness, which explains why continuous sleeplessness increases your risk for conditions such as high blood pressure, heart disease, hormone imbalances, weight gain, Alzheimer's and cancer.

Lack of sleep can also contribute to a prediabetic state, making you feel hungry even if you've already eaten. Another scary outcome of sleep deprivation is premature aging. Growth hormones are released by your pituitary gland during deep sleep. Lack of sleep interferes with the production of your growth hormones and speeds the aging process, but that's not all.

A system called the glymphatic system was recently discovered in the body. As the name suggests, it is a cross between brain cells and the lymphatic system. Its role is to clear toxins out of the brain. The glymphatic system works predominantly while we sleep. If we don't sleep, we aren't able to clear toxins out of the brain, which greatly impacts our body's ability to detoxify.[3]

THE EFFECTS OF SLEEP DEPRIVATION

Beyond what was just discussed, lack of sleep can contribute to the following:

- **Hormonal disruption** – Lack of sleep affects hormone levels. A disrupted circadian rhythm may create shifts in hormones like melatonin. Melatonin is made in the brain by converting tryptophan into serotonin and then into melatonin, which is released at night by the pineal gland in the brain to induce and maintain sleep. Melatonin is also an antioxidant that helps suppress harmful free radicals in the body and slows the production of estrogens which may activate cancer. Meanwhile, a link between cancer and the disrupted circadian rhythm lies with a hormone called cortisol, which normally reaches peak levels at dawn then declines throughout the day. When you don't get enough sleep, your cortisol levels don't peak as they should. Cortisol is one of many hormones that help regulate immune system activity, including natural killer cells that help the body battle cancer.

- **Heart attack and stroke** – Lack of sleep has been associated with high blood pressure and high cholesterol, both potential risk factors for heart disease and stroke. Your heart will be healthier if you get between seven and nine hours of sleep each night.

- **Stress** – When your body is sleep-deficient, it goes into a state of stress, creating an increase in blood pressure and production of stress hormones. These stress hormones, unfortunately, make it even harder for you to sleep. Since reducing stress will allow your body to get a more restful sleep, learn relaxation techniques to help counter the effects of stress.

- **Inflammation** – When you don't get enough sleep, the level of inflammation in your body also rises. Inflammation is thought to be one of the main causes of the body's deterioration, creating more risk for heart conditions, as well as cancer and diabetes.

- **Energy level** – A good night's sleep makes you energized and alert the next day. Being engaged and active not only feels great, it increases your chances of another good night's sleep. When you wake up feeling refreshed and you use that energy to get out into the daylight and to be active and engaged in your world, you sleep better that night.

- **Memory** – Researchers don't fully understand why we sleep and dream, but a process called "memory consolidation" occurs while we sleep. While your body may be resting, your brain is busy processing your day and making connections between events, sensory input, feelings and memories. Getting a good night's sleep will help you remember and process things better.

So, those all-nighters studying when I was in college didn't help me as much as I thought they did.

- **Weight** – Researchers have found that people who sleep less than seven hours per night are more likely to be overweight or obese.[4] It's believed that the lack of sleep impacts the balance of hormones in the body that affect appetite. The hormones ghrelin and leptin, important for the regulation of appetite, have been found to be disrupted by lack of sleep.

- **Depression** – Sleep impacts many of the chemicals in your body, including serotonin. People with a deficiency in serotonin are more likely to suffer from depression. You can help prevent depression by making sure you are getting the right amount of sleep.

- **Body repair and detoxification** – Sleep is the time when your body repairs damage— everything from a wound to a sunburn. Your cells produce more protein while you're sleeping. Proteins are the building blocks for your cells, and these proteins also enable cells to repair damage from our daily activities. In addition, adequate rest helps the body's detox pathways function more efficiently.

I know, that's a heck of a long list! Now that we know why 7-9 hours of sleep a night is necessary, let's get into the nitty-gritty—how to actually fall asleep and stay asleep.

TIPS FOR FALLING ASLEEP AND STAYING ASLEEP

- **Listen to white noise or relaxing music** – Some people find the sound of white noise, like a fan or nature, sounds to be helpful and soothing for sleep.

- **Avoid before-bed snacks** – Avoid grains and sugar before bed, as these foods will raise blood sugar and can negatively impact your sleep. If you have to snack, choose a high-protein option, such as a whey protein shake. This will provide L-tryptophan, needed to produce serotonin and melatonin, which actually help you sleep.

- **Keep a schedule** – Go to bed and wake up at the same time every day. This will train your body to sleep on a schedule. If you can maintain this schedule for three weeks, you'll probably find yourself falling asleep faster and feeling more refreshed. To achieve this, however, you can't sleep in on weekends or stay up too late, either. Keep in mind that the natural human biorhythm is to sleep between 10 p.m. and 6 a.m.

- **Create a bedtime routine** – Create a nightly routine to tell your body that it's time to sleep. Start about 30 minutes before you lay down to help release stressful thoughts. Your routine could include meditation, deep breathing, or reading. The key is to find something that makes you feel relaxed, then repeat it each night to help you release the day's tensions. Try a warm bath with Epsom salts. Avoid watching TV or reading something too adventurous, though, as this will stimulate your brain and likely have the opposite effect, prompting you to stay up later.

- **Maintain a healthy weight** – Being overweight can increase the risk of sleep apnea, which will prevent a restful night's sleep.

- **Exercise daily** – Daily exercise has been shown to improve your chances of falling asleep quickly and sleeping soundly. Research shows that you get a better sleep with regular exercise. Try to exercise early in the day and avoid exercising within three hours of bedtime. Working out too late in the day can make it difficult for you to fall asleep because exercise is a stimulant.

- **Make your bedroom dark** – As mentioned earlier, you need to produce the hormones serotonin and melatonin in order to sleep deeply. Since even a little bit of light will diminish their efficiency, sleep in a dark room, and don't turn on the lights at any time during the night if you need to get up. Consider getting an eye mask to help you block out any light that might impede your sleep.

- **Get some sunshine** – Sunlight helps regulate your internal clock stimulating your body to produce melatonin, which normalizes your sleep cycle. You need exposure to bright light every day. Morning sunlight exposure can be especially helpful. Be sure to open the drapes every morning to let light in. Spend time outside!

- **Avoid caffeine after noon** – Some people are caffeine-sensitive and can't drink coffee, tea or any other caffeinated beverage up to six hours before bedtime. Some people just can't metabolize caffeine efficiently. If you're having trouble sleeping, try not to consume caffeine past noon.

- **Journaling** – If you often lay in bed and can't quiet your mind, it might be helpful to keep a journal and write down your thoughts before bed. This allows your mind to rest and may even help create solutions in your sleep.

- **Avoid alcohol** – That small glass of wine can actually make it more difficult for you to stay asleep. After an evening drink, you might fall asleep just fine but you will likely wake up in the middle of the night. This effect is caused by a rebound in blood sugar and withdrawal from the alcohol after it has metabolized. Try avoiding alcohol before sleep and see if you sleep more soundly. For every drink you have, give your body at least an hour before trying to fall asleep. Keep in mind that alcohol will also keep you from falling into the deeper stages of sleep when the body does most of its healing.

- **Remove electronics from your bedroom** – Computers, mobile phones, tablets, even your alarm clock have electromagnetic fields that can interfere with your body's recuperative abilities. If you read before bed, ensure you read a physical book as the light from your phone or tablet will stimulate your eyes and brain. If you do decide to use your phone or tablet, there are now some blue-light filters you can either download onto your device or purchase some blue-light filtering glasses that will ensure your sleep is not disturbed.

- **Make preparations for the next day** – Before heading to bed, determine what you'd like to accomplish for the next day so you don't have to think about it while trying to get to sleep.

- **Take power naps** – If you have the opportunity, napping during the day (10-20 minutes) isn't only an effective and refreshing alternative to caffeine, but it also promotes wellness and makes you more productive. Studies show that people who nap several times a week have a lower risk of dying from heart disease. Napping also improves memory, cognitive function and mood.

I've been telling people for years that there should be napping pods at work. Think of how much more productive you'd be if you could take a little snooze during lunchtime!

- **Use natural supplements** – If you have tried all the above tips and still can't get to sleep, you may want to consider taking natural supplements like melatonin, 5-HTP (if you are not on prescription medications like SSRIs), taurine, or magnesium. All of these act like natural sleeping aids. If your adrenals are fatigued, try taking herbs like ashwagandha to rebalance them so you will not wake up in the middle of the night.

Ready for a good night's rest? Off to bed you go!

The following diagram shows examples of health habits with corresponding hack levels. To download the *Hack Your Health Habits Worksheet*, visit

www.hackyourhealthhabits.com/worksheets

READY #HEALTHHACKER?
EXAMPLES OF LEVEL 1, 2 AND 3 HACKS FOR THIS CHAPTER

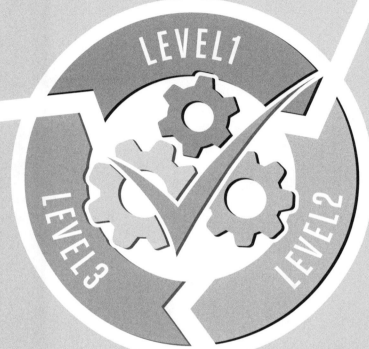

✓ Exercise regularly, but not too close to bedtime.
✓ Aim to go to bed and wake up at the same time every day—yes, even on weekends.

✓ Make your bedroom an electronic-free zone—yes, that means excluding the TV, too.
✓ If you're having issues sleeping, consider taking a natural sleep aid.

✓ Maintain a healthy body weight. If overweight, try to lose the extra pounds.
✓ Avoid caffeine after 12 p.m.

HACK YOUR HEALTH PROGRESS

|||||||||||||||||||||||||||||||||||||||||||||||||||||||||||

CHAPTER 49

MEDITATION
You Don't Have to Be a Monk

"Meditate: because some questions can't be answered by Google."

— Unknown

In today's fast-paced world, it's important to make time for activities that allow you to relax, restore and regenerate—activities like meditation. Now, some of you may be thinking, "Meditate? You mean sit down and not move or think about anything for more than two minutes, yeah, right!" While, at first, meditation can be challenging, I urge you if you have not tried it yet to give it a go.

Meditation has been shown to improve one's state of mind, physical well-being, quality of life and self-awareness. In addition, it can have especially powerful benefits for people with chronic health issues. It has been shown that remaining present and observant under challenging situations can improve your stress response, reducing the negative physical effects that stress has on the body.

Meditation has been around for thousands of years; its benefits are even supported in medical literature, yet not many people practice it. Why is this? While some think it's hokey, most people claim that they don't have the time. Life is busy, and setting aside time to meditate can be challenging—but it's important. Think back to the chapter on "Personal Prime Time." Scheduling time for ourselves to meditate can improve productivity and mood while promoting health. Even in small doses, meditation can change brain waves and improve resilience.

SO, WHAT EXACTLY IS MEDITATION?

Meditation can be defined as focused, contemplative time, and has been practiced by many cultures all over the world. Its goal is to create and sustain a focused, present mental state. Meditation can decrease heart rate, breathing and cortisol responses. Meditation can be done while lying down, sitting, or walking, as long as you can achieve a calm and positive state of mind. Meditation has been shown to:

- reduce pain, anxiety, depression and stress
- strengthen the immune system
- improve concentration and creativity
- decrease pain and blood pressure

Now that we know some of the benefits, let's get into the nitty-gritty. What kinds of meditation are out there, and how does one get started?

TYPES OF MEDITATION

MINDFULNESS MEDITATION

Mindfulness improves emotional and physical health, reduces stress and improves sleep. It can improve quality of life and optimize tissue repair during the day and at night. Awareness of the present leads to mindfulness, which can lead to balance, the place where calm and relaxation are in equilibrium with sleep, active living and optimal wellness. When less time is spent worrying, and focus is redirected from the past or future to the present, a path is opened for improved health and sleep.

Mindfulness meditation is defined as focusing awareness on each moment, including the environment, as well as physical and emotional sensations. Mindfulness can assist with managing social relationships, economic concerns, decision-making, as well as improving mental state.

> "Mindfulness is the aware, balanced acceptance of the present experience. It isn't more complicated than that. It is opening to or receiving the present moment, pleasant or unpleasant, just as it is, without either clinging to it or rejecting it."
>
> — Sylvia Boorstein

This type of meditation often uses either slow, intentional breathing or imagery to help to focus the thoughts. In clinical studies, practicing mindfulness and/or mindfulness meditation before bed can lead to:

- reduced insomnia

- deeper sleep

- fewer episodes of wakefulness during the night

- improved mood and resilience

- greater daytime energy

- less anxiety

 I've never tried mindfulness before. I like that it focuses on giving yourself the space to think and feel instead of trying to keep your mind blank.

MINDFUL BREATHING

Breath is vital. When we are stressed, happy or exercising, our breath will reflect our physical state. It can be either voluntary or involuntary, which means that we can control it. Being conscious and breathing in a particular way can lead to deep relaxation, decreased pain and improved mental state. Abdominal breathing, also called diaphragmatic breathing, changes the oxygenation levels in your body as well as strengthens the diaphragm. Many people feel calmer and more centered afterward, and it may help to reduce negative emotions. Since it can be practiced anytime, anywhere, why not try it today?

GUIDED MEDITATION

Guided meditation can be experienced either in a class with the help of a meditation teacher, or by listening to a guided meditation recording on your own. The idea behind guided meditation is to have a voice walk the participant through a series of mental images, deep-breathing techniques and relaxation. The facilitator typically encourages the participant to become more mindful of their present experience, more self-aware, and to become more aware of their senses. For those who are just starting out, guided meditation may be an effective way of reducing the mental chatter while allowing a professional to guide them through their feelings. There are many recordings that can be downloaded online, as well as many apps that also have guided meditation.

MANTRA MEDITATION

Originating in India, mantra meditation is based on the premise that repeating certain sounds, chants or mantras such as "Ohm" will create vibrations that put our bodies into lower frequencies that are in line with those of the universe. Mantra meditation is said to have substantial therapeutic benefits for lowering stress, blood pressure, anxiety, and inducing greater feelings of relaxation and well-being.

HOW TO GET STARTED WITH MEDITATION

- Select a quiet place where you can relax. Sit, stand, or lie down comfortably.

- Pay attention to your environment. Listen to the sounds. Smell what is around you, and feel the temperature of the room.

- Focus inward. Take several deep breaths, paying attention to how your body feels as you breathe. Let your eyes close as you become more relaxed.

- Scan your body and assess how you feel. Focus your awareness on the parts of your body that are tense or in pain. Breathe deeply and acknowledge the feeling without judging it.

- If desired, you can imagine your body becoming heavier, more anchored to the earth.

- You can also visualize a location that makes you particularly happy. That could be a natural setting, a vacation spot you remember fondly, or a place where something good happened in your life.

- Let the thoughts flow. If you have anxious or worried thoughts, let each occurrence be an opportunity to observe the thought and let it go. Rather than fighting the thoughts, imagine standing still and letting the thoughts go around you. Bring your attention back to your breath.

- If you are concerned about losing track of time, set a timer.

- Practice mindfulness meditation before you get ready for bed. Perhaps meditate before you brush your teeth, after shutting off your phone or computer, or as you lie in bed ready to fall asleep. Make mindfulness meditation part of your routine.

There is nothing mystical about meditation. When we meditate, we are moving from our subconscious mind to our conscious mind. Meditation, mindfulness and breathing help us move our attention away from the outer world (our environment) and into our deepest thoughts and feelings. These techniques allow us to reprogram our old self and create new beliefs, thoughts and habits.

In order to achieve this, we need to reach a heightened state of energy during meditation practice. In other words, we need to have our internal experiences evoke an energy stronger than the external, past experiences that have contributed to the beliefs and perceptions we want to change. This is the energy that changes our biology, our neurocircuitry and our genetic expression. Meditation can take us from survival to creation. Personally, I used to dread meditation. Now, I look forward to it as I get excited about what I can create with the power of my mind. What do you want to create?

The following diagram shows examples of health habits with corresponding hack levels. To download the *Hack Your Health Habits Worksheet*, visit

www.hackyourhealthhabits.com/worksheets

READY #HEALTHHACKER?
EXAMPLES OF LEVEL 1, 2 AND 3 HACKS FOR THIS CHAPTER

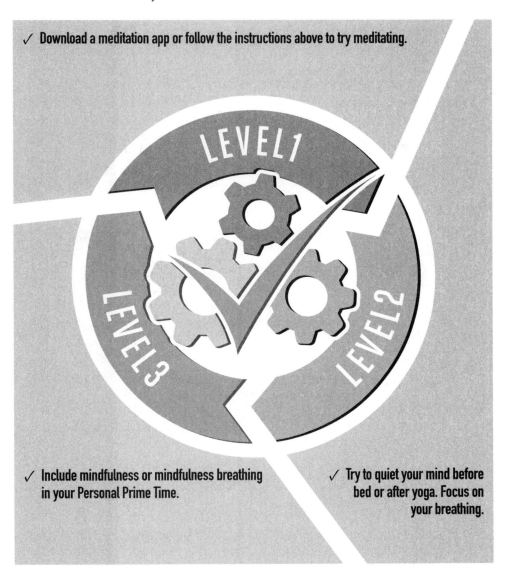

✓ Download a meditation app or follow the instructions above to try meditating.

✓ Include mindfulness or mindfulness breathing in your Personal Prime Time.

✓ Try to quiet your mind before bed or after yoga. Focus on your breathing.

HACK YOUR HEALTH PROGRESS

CHAPTER 50

51

DE-STRESSING
Explore the Tapping Technique

"It's not stress that kills us, it is our reaction to it."

— Hans Selye

THINK IT OVER

- Do you often find yourself feeling anxious or stressed?

- Do you often catch yourself engaging in negative self-talk?

- Have you heard of the emotional freedom technique to decrease stress?

Anxiety, fear, resistance, jealousy, doubts—these are all unpleasant emotions we wish we could avoid. But the truth is, they can often overpower us. Wouldn't it be nice if there was a way to relieve these feelings almost instantly? The answer is at your fingertips, literally. It's called the Emotional Freedom Technique, or EFT for short.

WHAT IS EFT?

EFT has its background in energy psychology. It is a form of psychological acupressure that uses your fingertips to stimulate exact points on the head, chest and upper body while concentrating on the issue at hand and voicing out positive affirmations. It is based on the same energy pathways used in the traditional practice of acupuncture that has been used to help improve physical and emotional ailments for thousands of years. EFT works to aid in resolving emotional difficulties and problems, and restores your mind and body's balance, which is crucial for ultimate health and the management of emotional and physical stressors.

Let's take a look at some of the more specific benefits of incorporating this technique. EFT can:

- relieve emotional disturbances
- abolish anxiety conditions
- reduce food cravings or other addictive behaviors
- eliminate or significantly reduce bodily pain and discomfort
- help reduce daily stress in regulating cortisol secretion
- improve energy and overall sense of well-being[1]

If at this point, you're shaking your head in disbelief, you are not alone in your disbelief. Many people still approach this method warily, along with other restorative electromagnetic energy practices such as earthing or grounding (discussed in **Chapter 53: Earthing—Recharging with Nature**). But, despite your skepticism, I highly recommend you give it a try.

On each of the points, you will be tapping five to seven times. There is no particular order in which the points need to be tapped, as long as each point is covered by the end.

There are two important factors that one must consider when trying EFT:

- finger-tapping location and technique
- voicing of positive affirmations

For each tapping point, feel free to use as many fingers as needed to tap, and choose to either use one hand or two, if you're tapping on both sides of the body.

Here is the sequence of tapping locations:

1. **Top of the head** – at the center of the skull
2. **Eyebrows** – just above and to one side of the nose, at the beginning of the eyebrow
3. **Sides of the eye** – on the bone, bordering the outside of the eye corner
4. **Under the eye** – on the bone under the eye
5. **Bottom of the nose** – between your nostrils and upper lip
6. **Chin** – midway between the point of your chin and the bottom of your lower lip
7. **Collarbone** – where the collarbone and the first rib meet
8. **Under arm** – on the side of the body, about four inches below the armpit
9. **Wrists** – inside of both wrists

Next, we will go through what you should be voicing while you are tapping. Traditional phrases include:

Even though I have _____, I love myself.

Even though my _____ is in pain, I love myself.

Even though I think _____, I love myself.

Even though I crave _____, I love myself.

Even though I fear _____, I love myself.

Even though I dislike _____, I love myself.

Or reversed:

I love myself, even though I have _____ .

I love myself, even though I fear _____ .

I love myself, even though I feel _____ .

I love myself, even though I crave _____ .

This forces you to acknowledge the current problem or condition, followed by an affirmation of self-acceptance. Even if you may not deeply believe the phrases, they need to be said, out loud.

EFT is based around the statement: "The cause of all negative emotions is a disruption in the body's energy system."[2] Negative emotions result from certain internal thoughts, which, in turn, cause your energy system to disrupt. Therefore, saying positive affirmations in a confident voice channels thoughts to change your cognitive patterns. This mimics the self-talk that occurs in our mind, which creates thoughts and beliefs we possess about ourselves. It is essential to focus your energy on these cognitive shifts, as they are crucial for the EFT to work.

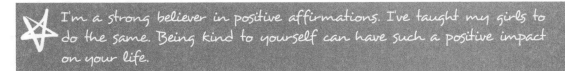

I'm a strong believer in positive affirmations. I've taught my girls to do the same. Being kind to yourself can have such a positive impact on your life.

WHEN SHOULD YOU PRACTICE EFT?

Practice EFT in the morning to start your day on a positive note or right before bed for a sound sleep. Practice it while on an evening walk or on lunch at the office. Ultimately, there's no perfect time to practice EFT. The key is to be persistent, as changing thoughts or beliefs take time. Tapping right before bed allows your mind to internalize your affirmations which become embedded in your subconscious during sleep. The same concept applies when you are trying to learn or memorize, as sleeping will help internalize the information.

In addition, word choice and phrase structure are crucial. Phrases such as "I don't think," and "I never," or "I need to rid myself of," are highly discouraged. Instead, phrases such as "I choose to change," and "I am confident that," or "I know I will," are encouraged, as their positive connotation helps with the cognitive shift in self-image and self-belief.

In conclusion, keep in mind that your thoughts become your reality. Your beliefs and attitudes toward yourself and the world are a reflection of your consistent thought patterns. Your choices of words and thoughts have the subtle, yet powerful, ability to alter or condition your cognitive system. Whatever you choose to focus on creates your reality. Similar to cognitive behavioral therapy in psychology, working on changing your thought processes and channeling your energy to accept yourself and what you can improve yields life-changing results. What do you have to lose? Give it a good try, open your mind and see how it feels!

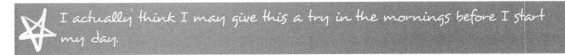

I actually think I may give this a try in the mornings before I start my day.

The following diagram shows examples of health habits with corresponding hack levels. To download the *Hack Your Health Habits Worksheet*, visit

www.hackyourhealthhabits.com/worksheets

READY #HEALTHHACKER?
EXAMPLES OF LEVEL 1, 2 AND 3 HACKS FOR THIS CHAPTER

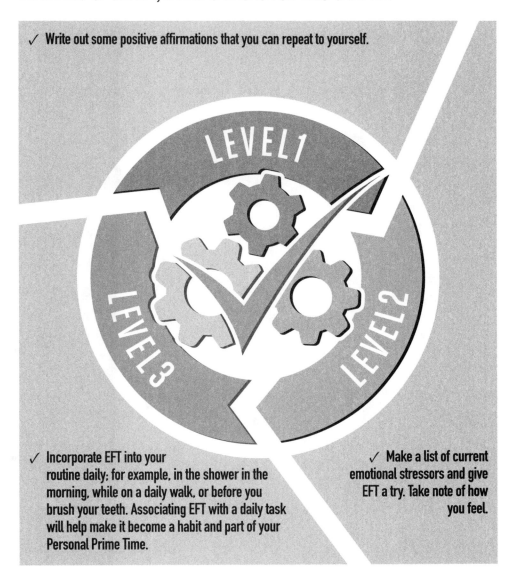

✓ Write out some positive affirmations that you can repeat to yourself.

✓ Incorporate EFT into your routine daily: for example, in the shower in the morning, while on a daily walk, or before you brush your teeth. Associating EFT with a daily task will help make it become a habit and part of your Personal Prime Time.

✓ Make a list of current emotional stressors and give EFT a try. Take note of how you feel.

HACK YOUR HEALTH PROGRESS

||||||||||||||||||||||||||||||||||||||||||||||||||||||||||||||

CHAPTER 51

ELECTROMAGNETIC FIELD
What You Don't See Can Still Hurt You!

"We are magnetic beings. The energy around us can affect us positively or negatively. Choose your surroundings wisely."

— Dr. Nathalie Beauchamp

THINK IT OVER

- Am I doing enough to decrease my family and my own exposure to electromagnetic fields?

- Am I spending long hours in front of a computer screen with no EMF protection?

- Do I experience chronic headaches or other symptoms that may be linked to EMF exposure?

Advancements in technology within recent years have come with many benefits. There is a world of information and entertainment conveniently located at our fingertips. The development of the smartphone, alone, has revolutionized the way we function, consolidating many of our needs and desires into one small device. However, these technological advancements have also come at a cost. For years, health professionals have debated whether Electromagnetic Fields (EMFs) should be of valid health concern. They claim for example that prolonged exposure to radiation from cellphones can lead to the development of cancerous cells.[1] Their studies have shown that EMFs can also alter normal gene expression and prevent proper DNA repair.[2]

Furthermore, studies show that EMFs can prevent nutrients from entering our cells and toxins from leaving them, creating cellular inflammation and chronic diseases.[3] While these claims may be contested by some, only time will really tell us the long-term effects of EMFs exposure. I do realize that we can't control everything around us, but awareness is key to start implementing things over which we do have control.

This is a little scary. I'm glued to my phone between work and the kids.

WHAT ARE EMFs?

Electromagnetic radiation is a term used to describe the energy that comes out of a source. Depending on the source, level of radiation and duration of exposure, radiation can either be beneficial, harmless or extremely dangerous to humans.

There are two primary types of EMFs. The first type is natural, like the sun, and the second type is man-made. Man-made EMFs will either be ionizing (i.e. x-rays) or non-ionizing (thermal or non-thermal). Smart Meters and cellphone towers are examples of non-ionizing, non-thermal EMFs. Cellphones and Wi-Fi are examples of both non-ionizing, thermal and non-thermal EMFs.

It is generally known that thermal EMFs pose the greatest risk to our health. They are the ones "cooking" our cells. However, new research indicates that non-thermal EMFs may also be affecting our cells. While there are polarized views on this, it is believed that non-thermal EMFs can impact cell communication.

It is important to remember that we are electrical beings, and susceptible to disruptions. All types of EMFs can have an impact on our body, big or small. They can disrupt something as small as a sodium-potassium pump (an active cellular transport mechanism) or something as big as our Krebs cycle (which produces energy).

Some sources of man-made electromagnetic fields include:

- Wi-Fi
- cellphones
- wireless devices
- Smart meters

- Bluetooth
- electrical towers
- wearable devices
- antennas

These sources of EMFs have been classified by the WHO and the International Agency for Research on Cancer (IARC) as possibly carcinogenic to humans, based on an increased risk for glioma, a malignant type of brain cancer that is associated with wireless phone use.[4] Despite this classification, no one in the United States or Canada seems to be talking about the risk. And, why would they? Cellphone manufacturers are not required to test their products for EMF safety. To cast doubt on the cancer claims, a few industry-sponsored studies have been conducted and were reportedly inconclusive. This is interesting, considering independent research groups continue to provide evidence that exposure to thermal and non-thermal EMFs are detrimental to human health. Unfortunately, this information is not widely shared. We also lack data regarding the cumulative effects of EMFs, as they have been ramping up in the last few decades.

THE IMPACT OF WEARABLES ON THE HUMAN BODY

Between TVs, laptops, cellphones and Wi-Fi, being exposed to electromagnetic fields is almost inevitable in this day and age. As time progresses, we see devices being made more user-friendly and accessible. However, such advances can come at a higher cost to our health.

A prime example of this is wireless devices. Going wireless may allow us to ditch the much-maligned and ever-tangled cords of conventional earbuds, phones and other technologies, but do we truly understand what it could mean for our health in the long run? Without naming any brand names, and knowing that technology is evolving at the speed of light, here are three things I believe we should keep in mind when using wearable devices.

1. Research shows that wearable devices relying on Bluetooth and Wi-Fi have a less negative effect on our bodies than other devices with 3G/4G data receivers built in.[5] Knowing that, we have to acknowledge the fact that Bluetooth and Wi-Fi *still* are sources of EMFs, and we should try to limit their use as best as we can.

2. Second, although it's handy to have your wearable device transmit information that it collects throughout the day (such as your activity level, calories expended, steps taken, sleep cycles, etc.) directly to your phone, it would be best to download the information onto your mobile device at the end of the day rather than having it connected and syncing to your phone at all times.

3. And, finally, although we like to keep track of the information picked up by these devices, we have to ask ourselves, do we truly know the long-term health effects of these sensors flashing on our skin 24/7?

The bottom line is that, although many people enjoy the convenience of these wearable devices, they do still have to be aware of what they are being exposed to, and the potential effects this exposure could have on their health over the years.

HEALTH IMPACT OF EMFs

Conditions such as persistent headaches, difficulty with concentration, anxiety, depression and other radiation-related issues have a higher risk of occurrence with EMF exposure. As mentioned previously, links are being made between EMF exposure and the accelerated development of tumors—more specifically, brain tumors—due to the constant use of the cellphones. In addition, suppressed melatonin production, heart abnormalities and infertility have also been linked to overexposure to radiation.

Constant exposure to EMFs can wreak havoc on the body. It's important to note that side effects manifest differently in children and adults. How safe is it for a 5-year-old to be using a cellphone? Not very. Children have smaller heads, thinner skulls and more fluid in the brain, allowing them to absorb more radiation than adults. EMF exposure has been linked to hyperactivity, sleep disturbances—due to effects on the pineal gland, which produces melatonin—memory and attention deficits and increased stress levels in children.[6]

> My 13-year-old struggles with anxiety. In talking with other parents, it seems a lot of kids these days struggle with it. So many kids are glued to their phones... I wonder if limiting phone time could help.

Some research has even shown an increase in learning disorders and behavioral problems when kids are exposed to EMFs in the womb.[7] Adults are subject to more extensive side effects when cellular devices are carried near certain body parts. For men who keep their cellphones in their pockets, some research has shown a correlation between radiation and lower sperm count, leading to fertility issues. For women, research has shown the potential risk of ovarian problems when phones or portable devices are constantly kept in their pockets, or even an increased chance of breast cancer when these devices are kept near their chest.[8]

Some adults may also experience a hypersensitivity to EMF exposure. If you often experience these symptoms and are not sure why, you too may be electromagnetic sensitive:

- chronic headaches and migraines
- cognitive problems, impaired learning and poor memory
- chronic infections
- depression
- fatigue and weakness
- joint and muscle pain
- numbness or tingling in the extremities
- respiratory, gastrointestinal and cardiovascular problems

There is no blood test or urine test to test for EMF toxicity but there are some devices that you can buy to see if there are high amounts of EMFs around you. People who are sensitive to EMFs will most likely have noticed that they don't do well in big cities or beside power lines.

EMFs AND CANCER

Although many would still prefer to be in denial, a recent multi-year study funded by the U.S. federal government called "Report of Partial Findings from the National Toxicology Program Carcinogenesis Studies of Cell Phone Radiofrequency Radiation in Hsd: Sprague Dawley SD rats (Whole Body Exposures)" has found that, indeed, cellphone radiation is a contributing factor to various types of cancer.

Scientific American reports:

The findings, which chronicle an unprecedented number of rodents subjected to a lifetime of electromagnetic radiation, present some of the strongest evidence to date that such exposure is associated with the formation of rare cancers in at least two cell types in the brains and hearts of rats.

They also stated:

The researchers found that as the thousands of rats in the new study were exposed to greater intensities of RF radiation, more of them developed rare forms of brain and heart cancer that could not be easily explained away, exhibiting a direct dose-response relationship. Some of the rats had glioma—a tumor of the glial cells in the brain or schwannoma of the heart. Furthering concern about the findings: In prior epidemiological studies of humans and cell phone exposure, both types of tumors have also cropped up as associations. In contrast, none of the control rats—those not exposed to the radiation—developed such tumors.[9]

It is evident that the cellphone industry is not too keen on spending money on research that may reduce their profit. However, they can no longer claim that these kinds of findings are bad science. The research, even if limited and in its early stages, is showing the clear, dose-related link between exposure to radiation emitted from cellphones and the development of brain and heart tumors. It is important to note, however, that different forms of radiation can bring on different symptoms, and individuals themselves can be affected differently.

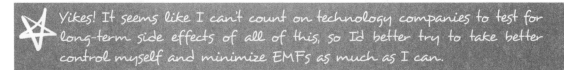

Yikes! It seems like I can't count on technology companies to test for long-term side effects of all of this, so I'd better try to take better control myself and minimize EMFs as much as I can.

HOW TO LIMIT EXPOSURE

It may seem difficult to reduce exposure to radiation, considering we are surrounded by cellphone towers, Wi-Fi hotspots and so on. But, there are lots of things we can do to minimize our personal exposure:

- **Limit your Wi-Fi exposure** – Although inconvenient, turn off your home's Wi-Fi before heading to bed at night to eliminate overnight exposure.

- **Favor a landline over your cellphone** – Use a landline at home or at work whenever possible instead of your cellphone, especially if you are going to be on the phone for a good length of time.

- **Don't wear your cellphone** – Be mindful of where you keep your mobile devices (pockets, bras, etc.). As much as possible, try to not have it on your person.

- **Use cord headphones or a speakerphone** – Whenever possible, use headphones or place your phone on speaker to avoid direct contact between your mobile device and your head.

- **Avoid electronic devices in the bedroom** – Try to avoid having electronics in your bedroom or have them on airplane mode. If you're using your phone as your alarm, make sure it's far away from your bed. Radiation may also interfere with the quality of your sleep. Be aware of sleeping apps that are used to track your sleep, as they will be right by your head, emitting radiation.

- **Reduce usage of other wireless devices** – Be aware of how many wireless devices you use—wireless keyboards, speakers, baby monitors, etc.).

- **Lights Out!** – Light is a form of EMF. Try to limit your exposure to fluorescent lights; although they save energy, they emit radiation that incandescent bulbs do not. In addition, try to limit your blue light exposure (i.e. from smartphones, tablets and laptops). Consider using a blue blocker screen for your computer monitor, or opt for blue-light blocker glasses.

- **Disable your Bluetooth when you are in the car** – I know it's a pain but a car is essentially a cage, and the small space concentrates harmful frequencies.

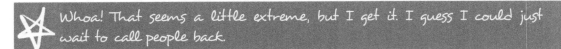

Whoa! That seems a little extreme, but I get it. I guess I could just wait to call people back.

- **Monitor your child's use of electronics** – Limit your child's use of iPads, cellphones, or any device that connects to Wi-Fi or data services. Yes, it does keep them entertained, but that young and fragile developing brain may be negatively affected.

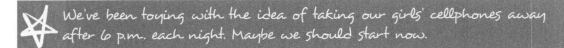

We've been toying with the idea of taking our girls' cellphones away after 6 p.m. each night. Maybe we should start now.

- **Think twice before buying an electrical car** – Yes, electrical cars are awesome for the environment, but are they really safe for us in the long run? Think about it. The electricity generated from an electric or hybrid car can also be a major source of EMF, and constant exposure can potentially cause health implications.

- **Find time to disconnect in nature** – Really take some time to disconnect from the virtual world and engage in an outdoor activity without the use of electronics. Countless studies show that there are many benefits to spending time in nature, as it can have positive effects on our stress management and overall well-being. Remember that old TV commercial catchphrase, "Can you hear me now, can you hear me now?" In the past, we weren't as connected as we are today, but somehow we managed.

- **Buy an "EMF shield"** – EMF shields can protect you from the harmful effects of EMFs by harmonizing radiation and reducing the heating of your mobile phone when it is in use. I purchased one for my cellphone, one that I wear on my body at all times and one for the wall where our Smart Meter is.

The following diagram shows examples of health habits with corresponding hack levels. To download the *Hack Your Health Habits Worksheet*, visit

www.hackyourhealthhabits.com/worksheets

READY #HEALTHHACKER?
EXAMPLES OF LEVEL 1, 2 AND 3 HACKS FOR THIS CHAPTER

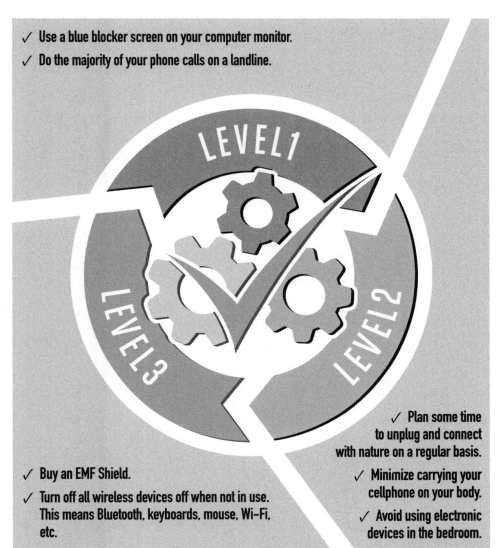

✓ Use a blue blocker screen on your computer monitor.
✓ Do the majority of your phone calls on a landline.

LEVEL 1

LEVEL 2

LEVEL 3

✓ Plan some time to unplug and connect with nature on a regular basis.
✓ Minimize carrying your cellphone on your body.
✓ Avoid using electronic devices in the bedroom.

✓ Buy an EMF Shield.
✓ Turn off all wireless devices off when not in use. This means Bluetooth, keyboards, mouse, Wi-Fi, etc.

HACK YOUR HEALTH PROGRESS

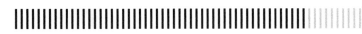

CHAPTER 52

EARTHING

Recharging with Nature

53

"Nature does not hurry, yet everything is accomplished."

— Lao Tzu

THINK IT OVER

- Do you know the benefits of being barefoot outdoors?

- Have you heard of the Earth's electrical charge?

- Do you know how earthing can help reduce the harm caused by EMF exposure?

Do you remember the last time you ran barefoot through a field or laid in the grass to look at the clouds? What about the last time you slipped off your sandals and got sand between your toes? In the health field, this type of activity is known as earthing. Earthing involves placing your bare feet in the sand, grass and even mud. It can be messy, but it feels good and has recently been shown to be beneficial for your overall health.

 There is nothing I love more than the feeling of grass between my toes. I find it so comforting. I didn't realize it had actual health benefits.

THE BENEFITS OF EARTHING

- Improved quality of sleep
- Reduced inflammation and chronic pain
- Regulation of hormones such as cortisol for stress reduction
- Restored balance between the sympathetic and parasympathetic nervous systems
- Improved energy and overall sense of well-being

All that can be done by just kicking off your shoes? Yes! Earthing works by connecting you to the healing energy of the ground, thereby neutralizing free radicals and reducing chronic inflammation in the body. It may sound a bit far-fetched, but it works, and there are a few reasons why.

HOW EARTHING WORKS

The first reason has to do with electrical conductance. As you may know, you wouldn't be alive without electricity. From your cells to your nerves, trillions of electrical impulses are being emitted in your body every minute. All of your movement, thoughts, behaviors and actions are powered by these impulses.

The Earth itself is also electrically charged, meaning when you, a bioelectrical human being, make direct contact with the ground, you are absorbing a steady flow of electrons into your body. These electrons have an antioxidant effect, which helps restore your body's natural balance. Even short periods of time engaging in this activity yield significant health benefits, whether it is on sand, rock, dirt, or grass.

The problem today is that not enough people are benefiting from this simple practice. The biggest reason for this is the clothes and shoes we wear. Shoes inhibit the natural flow of electrons. You see, the Earth's natural elements, along with your body, are very good electrical conductors. However, materials such as rubber, leather, plastic and polyester—which are in the majority of the apparel we wear—are not. This prevents us from having direct contact with the Earth's natural healing properties.

Another important reason to take part in earthing is due to the electromagnetic environment that we are constantly surrounded by, in this day and age. As we discussed in the previous chapter, this includes EMFs from Wi-Fi, cellphones, power towers, satellite TVs and radios, cordless phones, energy efficient light bulbs, and electric heaters and coolers. Essentially, any cable or wire in your household can be hazardous to your health in the long term.

Exposure to electromagnetic pollution or "dirty electricity" can have varying adverse effects on different people. Yet, in the short term, it's most known for disrupting sleep patterns, reducing concentration and disrupting the body's natural electron balance. By attempting to reduce exposure to such fields and by regularly reconnecting with the Earth's own EMF, we may be able to reduce and even reverse these negative effects.

Walking barefoot in the great outdoors also provides the added benefit of reflexology. Reflexology is a technique based on the theory that specific pressure points on the bottoms of our feet relate to specific organs and glands in the body, and stimulating those points promotes health in those organs and glands. By walking on uneven grounds and the changing textures of the earth, these points in our feet are kneaded and stimulated, which in itself has stress-reducing and restorative properties.

Now, to kill two birds with one stone, you can incorporate earthing into your weekly exercise routine by working out outdoors in bare feet—weather permitting. Not only are you getting the benefit of physical activity, but you are also getting vitamin D from the sun and restoring your body's natural electron balance. Think of traditional yoga or Tai Chi, which strongly encourage outdoor practice.

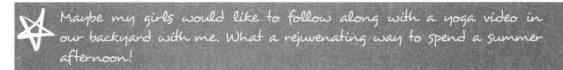

Maybe my girls would like to follow along with a yoga video in our backyard with me. What a rejuvenating way to spend a summer afternoon!

The practice of earthing may be one of the most overlooked factors in holistic health. Despite nourishing our bodies with whole foods and exercising daily, energy still plays a crucial role in our well-being. When energy through earthing is restored, many people report significant improvement in a wide range of ailments. So, kick off your shoes and get to it.

The following diagram shows examples of health habits with corresponding hack levels. To download the *Hack Your Health Habits Worksheet*, visit

www.hackyourhealthhabits.com/worksheets

READY #HEALTHHACKER?
EXAMPLES OF LEVEL 1, 2 AND 3 HACKS FOR THIS CHAPTER

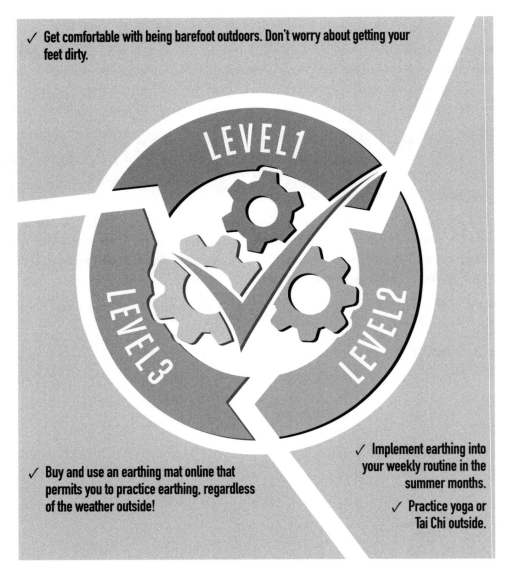

✓ Get comfortable with being barefoot outdoors. Don't worry about getting your feet dirty.

✓ Buy and use an earthing mat online that permits you to practice earthing, regardless of the weather outside!

✓ Implement earthing into your weekly routine in the summer months.

✓ Practice yoga or Tai Chi outside.

LEVEL1

LEVEL2

LEVEL3

HACK YOUR HEALTH PROGRESS

||||||||||||||||||||||||||||||||||||||||||||||||||||||||||||||||||||||

CHAPTER 53

SECTION 11

Get In Control—You and Your Wellness Team

Want to start making healthy changes but simply don't know where to start? Develop your own personal Wellness Team Action Plan and explore the different natural health care options available in Section 11. Learn how to take responsibility, action and accountability towards your own health. That's right, it's time to take control!

54

IT'S YOUR HEALTH
Who Is in Charge?

"Everything in your life is a reflection of a choice you have made. If you want different results, start making different choices."

— UNKNOWN

THINK IT OVER

- What are some things you can do to take responsibility for your health?

- What kind of mindset do you have regarding change?

- How ready are you to commit to bettering yourself?

We have all read a book, watched a documentary, attended a workshop and read tips and tricks online. There is an abundance of information out there, thousands of ideas, solutions and ways to improve our lives. Yet, many of us still find it difficult to change our circumstances. When it comes down to it, it's not information we lack, but the ability to turn that information into action. Why is this? Perhaps it is because we don't want to step outside of our comfort zone; change requires too much effort and persistence. Maybe it is because we lack the necessary steps and support needed to actually make a change. Or, perhaps it is due to fear—fear of what change will mean for ourselves and the people around us.

Throughout this book, you have been introduced to various ways to take control of your health and make changes to improve your overall well-being. From mindset to sleep and everything in between, you have acquired the tools to make important health decisions. The question is, what happens when you close this book? Do you make a change? Or, does all the knowledge you gained get stored in your subconscious, never to be used again? I'm sure that at some points in this book, you thought to yourself, "I'd like to try that, but... I don't have the time... it runs in the family... I don't have the money... it requires extra work... I am not motivated... I lack the resources... I don't know where to start... etc." Here's the thing: These self-limiting beliefs aren't helping you. They are holding you back. In order to become the person you want to be, you need to overcome your excuses and your fears.

It is easy to blame our circumstances on a lack of drive. We tend to do this a lot. We think that we cannot move forward because we do not have the time or motivation to do so. That simply isn't true. In this chapter, I want to introduce a concept that many of us still don't have a full grasp on the concept of *choice.*

A choice is a simple decision to take charge of ourselves, to stop blaming our counterparts, our situation, our age, our genes, our culture, our work, or our lifestyle for the way things are, and to start accepting that we, ourselves, are fully responsible for every outcome we create. At the risk of sounding harsh, the reality is that we can either choose to run our lives or allow our lives to run us. We can choose to take action or make excuses. It is the simple matter of choice that stands between who you are now and who you desire to be.

Of course, there will always be situations that we do not have control over: physical limitations, an illness, a natural disaster, an accident or an unsafe environment. While we may not be able to control these situations, we can control how we respond to them—in terms of our attitude toward them—and that is our greatest power.

In her book, *Mindset,* Dr. Carol Dweck talks about growth mindsets versus fixed mindsets. She explains that, depending on which mindset an individual has, they will react differently to an unforeseeable circumstance.

A fixed-minded individual will point fingers and blame others while victimizing themselves. On the other hand, a growth-minded individual will accept what has happened and will rise to the occasion, making the best of the situation. A growth-minded individual sees a challenge as a means of betterment, is resilient to adversity, and is in constant need of self-improvement. In contrast, a fixed-minded individual accepts where he or she currently is in life as their fate, is afraid of challenges, and does not have the willpower to create positive change in their lives. Ask yourself where you stand. Are you resilient to adversity or afraid of challenges?

In *The Question Behind the Question: Practicing Personal Accountability in Work and in Life,* author John G. Miller pushes readers to change their way of thinking when faced with challenges. Instead of asking, "Why me?" and "Who is there to blame?" Miller suggests asking "What is there to be done?" and "How can I improve this situation?"

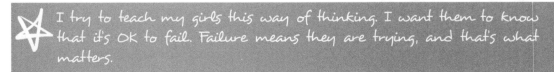

I try to teach my girls this way of thinking. I want them to know that it's OK to fail. Failure means they are trying, and that's what matters.

This simple shift in self-talk changes our perspective from being a victim of circumstances to accepting personal responsibility. It may be difficult to make this shift, especially if you are one who allows exterior forces to hold the reins on your decision-making, but it is this choice to take control of our lifestyle that will ultimately take us to the next level, freeing us to be who we want to be.

We all have the potential to reach our ideal selves, to self-actualize and to lead intentional lives. Take a few minutes to envision your ideal self:

- What does this person look like?

- How does he or she talk and dress?

- What are the habits and rituals of this person?

- Who does he or she spend time with, and what kinds of activities does he or she participate in?

- What does he or she do for work?

- What kind of lifestyle does this person lead?

- How does he or she view himself or herself?

- And, most importantly, what will this person be remembered for?

Once you have a clear image of who this person is, you can reverse-engineer them and start building a new reality based on your ideal. To start this process, focus on the things you do on a daily basis. This brings us back to the notion of habits and our daily actions, and how they ultimately make up who we are.

Our habits demonstrate the amount of control we have in our life. They can show how much we value ourselves, our health, our lifestyle, and whether we are working toward self-betterment. Habits are the sum of our self-motivation. Someone who is in the habit of waking up late and calling in sick to work does not seem as motivated as someone who arrives on time in high spirits. Focusing on our daily habits will allow us to determine where we spend our energy, what we expose ourselves to physically and mentally, and what changes we need to make in order to reach our goals.

So, are you ready? Are you ready to commit yourself to taking control of your choices? Of being in control of your habits? Of accepting that you are personally responsible for your actions, and, ultimately, your health? You are the sum of your choices, and every day, you are given the chance to either take action or make excuses. Choose wisely. I know you've got this.

The following diagram shows examples of health habits with corresponding hack levels. To download the *Hack Your Health Habits Worksheet*, visit

www.hackyourhealthhabits.com/worksheets

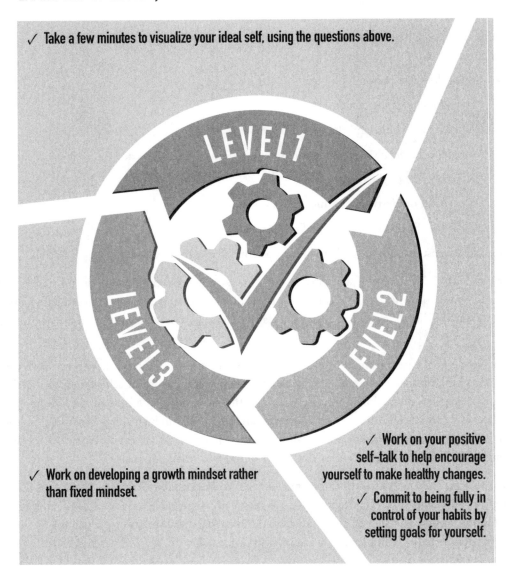

✓ Take a few minutes to visualize your ideal self, using the questions above.

✓ Work on your positive self-talk to help encourage yourself to make healthy changes.

✓ Commit to being fully in control of your habits by setting goals for yourself.

✓ Work on developing a growth mindset rather than fixed mindset.

HACK YOUR HEALTH PROGRESS

||||||||||||||||||||||||||||||||||||||||||||||||||||||||||||||

CHAPTER 54

KNOW YOUR NUMBERS
Understanding Your Tests Results to Take Control of Your Health

"Torture numbers and they
will confess to anything."

— GREGG EASTERBROOK

THINK IT OVER

- Is your annual blood test painting a full picture of your health?

- Looking at your blood test results, would you be able to extract what they mean?

- Are you aware that there are tests that can help you identify genetic alterations, allowing for a personalized approach to optimal health?

BLOODWORK—DOES IT SAY IT ALL?

When it comes to getting regular bloodwork done, it's always reassuring to hear that your tests results came back normal. A regular panel of blood tests done by your doctor is a great place to start when addressing your current state of health. However, one must keep in mind that it is a fairly basic evaluation that doesn't necessarily paint a picture of your whole health.

True. My brother-in-law suffered from a heart attack shortly after receiving a clean bill of health from his yearly physical. When it comes to health, things are never that simple.

Blood panels give a snapshot of how efficiently your body is working at a specific time, by evaluating certain health biomarkers.

One of the important things to understand with basic bloodwork is the difference between *pathological* range and *functional* range of normality. A pathological range is used to diagnose and treat disease, while the functional range is used to assess *risk* for a disease before it develops. The functional range parameters are, therefore, narrower.

Unfortunately, conventional medicine is mainly concerned with the diagnosis and treatment of a disease and less with its prevention. By looking at where your results fall on the functional range, you can address issues by adjusting lifestyle behaviors like nutritional changes and exercise, before your numbers fall into pathological range or a diagnosis is given.

Another concern with routine bloodwork is that it is limited in what it measures. With the advancement of biotechnology, there are a wide range of tests available, yet only a few are commonly used. This is often due to a lack of health care or insurance resources. Oftentimes, when blood test results come back "normal," the patient's symptoms, if they are experiencing any, may be dismissed. Ultimately, it should be the clinician's job to interpret the functioning of *all* symptoms and systems in the body and connect the dots to paint a more holistic picture. We are, after all, the sum of all our parts.

BLOOD TESTS ROADMAP

This chapter is all about providing you with the basic knowledge required to better understand your own test results. It will run through how a blood lab report would ideally be read in terms of logical sequence. It's important to note that this chapter is not meant to tell you what tests to do and which labs or country can do them. It's also important to consider that blood chemistry is focused on discerning patterns that can assess possibilities. With that in mind, interpretation of the results must be done with a full detailed patient history at hand, along with clinical signs and symptoms, and accompanied by a comprehensive physical evaluation. The expertise of your healthcare provider will help you discern which tests are meant for you.

Before we dive in, I know that this chapter may seem a little dry and technical to some. It's hard to make test results sound fun or sexy. However, it is worth reading if you are someone who suffers from symptoms and is frustrated by the lack of answers you've received in the past. Or, if you are already knowledgeable in this area and are looking to dig a little deeper, read on so you can determine what health changes you need to make in order to live as healthy as possible and for as long as possible. I don't know about you, but I still want to be the life of the party at 90 years old! Ready to get started?

LET'S GET SOME OXYGEN!

As human beings, every cell, tissue and organ needs oxygen in order to function. The body carries oxygen to the tissues by means of red blood cells. Hemoglobin is the iron-rich protein in red blood cells that gives the blood its red color—and which enables red blood cells to carry oxygen from the lungs to the body's tissues, and then return carbon dioxide from the tissues back to the lungs. The most oxygen-sensitive organ in the body is the brain. It makes up 2 percent of the body weight and, at times, can use 30 percent of your oxygen.[1]

A complete blood count (CBC), measures the red blood cell count (RBC), white blood count (WBC) and platelets. RBC markers include hemoglobin (HGB), hematocrit (HCT), red cell distribution width (RDW), mean corpuscular volume (MCV) and mean corpuscular hemoglobin. Other common markers related to RBC are serum iron, iron saturation, ferritin, transferrin and total iron-binding capacity (TIBC).

These markers are used to identify various types of anemias. Anemias are conditions marked by a deficiency of red blood cells or of hemoglobin in the blood. Anemias are conditions marked by a deficiency of red blood cells, alteration of the red blood cell characteristics, alterations in the components of the red blood cells or of hemoglobin in the red blood cells. Symptoms of anemia include fatigue, weakness, pale skin, irregular heartbeats, dizziness, cold hands and feet and headaches.

There are many types of anemia that exist, including:

- iron-deficiency anemia – either not getting enough iron, not absorbing it, or losing too much via blood loss

- vitamin-deficiency anemia – B12 and folic acid (B9)

- anemia of a chronic disease – caused by conditions like rheumatoid arthritis, kidney disease and intestinal diseases, which would affect absorption

- aplastic anemia – can be caused by infection, autoimmune diseases and exposure to chemicals

- hemolytic anemia – where red blood cells are destroyed faster than they are produced, something that can be inherited or develop later in life

- anemia associated with bone marrow diseases, such as leukemia

- other anemias such as thalassemia

As you can see, anemias can be very complex. To keep it simple, what we need to watch for is that your body is making and maintaining enough red blood cells, has enough iron that can be readily used, has enough iron in storage (as measured in ferritin levels) for when it is needed, has adequate amounts of vitamin B6-B9 and B12, and has no chronic diseases or genetic disorders that could affect the red blood cells' status.

Side note: We consume two types of iron: heme-iron from animal foods and non-heme iron from plants and supplements. Heme iron is more easily absorbed, whereas non-heme is not absorbed as well. Vegans beware.

Just as oxygen is key to the body, so is iron. Let's make sure we're not anemic.

SUGAR LEVELS—AVOIDING THE UPS AND DOWNS

"Dysglycemia" refers to abnormalities in blood glucose levels. It is a growing problem in industrialized countries and is often caused by a lack of physical exercise and the consumption of high-calorie, high-sugar processed foods. We have discussed the importance of controlling our blood sugar in a previous section, so here we will focus on the tests that can be done to evaluate the efficiency of someone's sugar metabolism.

There are basically two types of functional blood sugar imbalances: The first one is called *functional reactive hypoglycemia*, and the second one is called *insulin resistance*. Both may lead to metabolic syndrome and diabetes.

Many hormones and parameters need to be evaluated when it comes to sugar regulation. Fasting blood glucose is the most common biomarker used to evaluate potential blood sugar imbalances. For this test to be accurate, it is very important that blood be taken in a fasted state. A lipid panel is also very useful to discern insulin elevation from insulin resistance, as insulin resistance impacts lipid metabolism by increasing total cholesterol, low-density lipoprotein (LDL) and triglycerides (TG)—while high-density lipoprotein (HDL) becomes suppressed.

Another test for measuring blood sugar metabolism is the C-Peptide test. C-Peptide is a protein that is produced in the body with insulin. It is used as a stable marker to identify pancreatic cells' capacity to produce insulin. Clinically, it is used to help differentiate Type 1 diabetes (autoimmune diabetes) from Type 2 (acquired due to lifestyle).

Hemoglobin A1c, also called *glycated hemoglobin*, is another important marker. In 2010, the American Diabetes Association recommended the use of the HbA1c test to diagnose diabetes with a threshold equal or greater than 6.5 percent.[2] The test uses the average plasma glucose concentration over a period of four to eight weeks. Autoimmune tests are also available to measure antibodies to related sugar metabolism parameters like Glutamic Acid Decarboxylase (GAD), A1c and pancreatic islet cells.

Adrenal function should also be checked as elevated glucose levels can be associated with adrenal hyperfunction (i.e. high cortisol levels). Meanwhile, low glucose levels can be associated with adrenal hypofunction (i.e. low cortisol levels).

Some of you may be scratching your head right now. Don't worry, next time you get blood results, all of this information will start coming together, I promise.

CARDIOVASCULAR PROFILE

We can't talk about sugar metabolism without talking about lipid profiles. As mentioned above, dysglycemia can lead to an abnormal lipid profile. But, before we look at what a lipid profile measures, let's first talk about cholesterol, as it has gotten a bad rap in past years.

Cholesterol is a white waxy substance found in all body cells. Optimal levels of it are vital for heart health, cognitive function and hormone production.

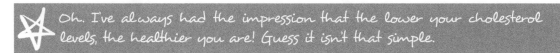

Oh. I've always had the impression that the lower your cholesterol levels, the healthier you are! Guess it isn't that simple.

It is also necessary for the production of hormones, cell membranes, vitamin D and bile acids—to name a few of its functions. Approximately 75 percent of our cholesterol is made by the body, and only 25 percent comes from the foods we eat. In addition, 25 percent of the body's cholesterol is found in the brain—kind of important, don't you think? The reality is, we do need cholesterol, despite the efforts of conventional medicine to tell us otherwise. In addition, "good" and "bad" cholesterol is not as black and white as it may seem.

CARDIOVASCULAR MARKERS

Components that should be present in a standard lipid profile:

- Total cholesterol
- Triglycerides (TG)
- High-density lipoprotein (HDL) Cholesterol
- Low-density lipoprotein (LDL) Cholesterol
- Very low-density lipoprotein (VLDL) Cholesterol
- Total cholesterol-to-HDL ratio
- LDL/HDL ratio

Special tests that can provide more information:

- Homocysteine – an amino acid that can damage the cell wall that lines the arteries
- C-reactive protein – a protein produced by the liver that increases during whole-body inflammation
- Lipoprotein (LP) phenotype profile
- Plasminogen activator Inhibitors-1
- Fibrinogen activity
- Prothrombin time

An overall lipid panel showing an increase in cholesterol, LDL and TG but decreased HDL can be indicative of dysglycemia or insulin resistance, thyroid hypofunction, a fatty liver, hereditary conditions, or improper diet and insufficient exercise. An overall lipid panel showing a decrease in cholesterol,

LDL and HDL, can be indicative of gastrointestinal malabsorption, a vegetarian diet, or inflammatory conditions.

LIVER PROFILE

Your liver, which is one of the main organs involved in your body's detoxification process, can become overburdened from diet and lifestyle choices. It is your liver's job to distinguish between the nutrients you need to absorb (like vitamins and minerals), and the dangerous or unnecessary substances that must be filtered out of your bloodstream (like harmful toxins).

Unfortunately, maintaining the health of your liver is easier said than done, especially in this day and age. Pollution, processed foods, medications, and alcohol clog and overwhelm your liver, making it difficult for it to process the nutrients and fats your body needs. This causes a buildup of toxins in the body that drastically affects your overall health and well-being. It is for this reason that monitoring liver function is important.

High liver enzymes can indicate abnormal liver function and toxicity. A liver panel typically checks for alanine transaminase (ALT), aspartate transaminase (AST) and gamma glutamyl transpeptidase (GGT).

When looking at liver function, it is also important to take into account tests that can also detect gallbladder dysfunction, infections, or muscle damage. It is important to know that liver enzymes' levels can come back within range and yet the liver may not be working optimally, as its ability to biotransform endogenous compounds (i.e. metabolic waste) and exogenous compounds (i.e. waste from environmental inputs) may be compromised.

THE THYROID GLAND—A KEY PLAYER

The thyroid gland plays an important role not only with the function that the thyroid plays on its own, but also in the effect it has on bone metabolism, male hormones, gallbladder and liver function, growth hormones, body composition, glucose metabolism, estrogen and cortisol metabolism and liver detoxification, to name a few.

In order to diagnose hypothyroidism, TSH (thyroid stimulating hormone) levels have to be—depending on the laboratory ranges—between 0.5 and 6 milli-international units per liter with or without abnormalities of T3 or T4. Oftentimes, only a partial thyroid panel is performed. This partial panel may be within normal range; however, this does not necessarily mean the thyroid is functioning optimally.

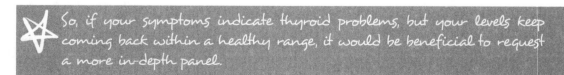

So, if your symptoms indicate thyroid problems, but your levels keep coming back within a healthy range, it would be beneficial to request a more in-depth panel.

Sometimes, the problem is with the thyroid gland's ability to produce the thyroid hormone, otherwise known as thyroxine, or T4. Other times, the issue is related to what happens to the T4 after it has been produced—if it isn't being converted efficiently into T3, its active form.

In many cases, further thyroid tests are needed to determine why the thyroid or thyroid hormones are not working as they should. In conjunction with TSH, markers like T4, T3 uptake, free thyroxine index (FTI), T3, Free T3, Reverse T3 and Free T4 should be tested in order to fully understand where, in its process, the thyroid may be going wrong. It is also important to test for thyroid antibodies, as the most common cause of hypothyroidism (85 percent to 90 percent) is Hashimoto's disease[3], an autoimmune condition. In order to diagnose Hashimoto's, thyroid peroxidase antibody (TPO) and thyroglobulin antibodies tests should be performed. If either of the two or both are elevated, that confirms the presence of Hashimoto's autoimmune reaction is occurring, leaving your thyroid vulnerable to further attack by your immune system.

Other tests may also be necessary when hypothyroidism is present to rule out contributing conditions like hypochlorhydria, B12, iron deficiency, pernicious anemias, leaky gut syndrome, systemic inflammation, impaired degradation of lipids, abnormal liver functions and thyroxine-binding globulin (TBG), to name just a few.

The point here is that if you think you have thyroid symptoms, get more than your TSH tested. And, if you have hypothyroidism, find out what else may be affected. A full picture of what is going on is necessary because of the impact the thyroid has on many physiological functions.

IS THE IMMUNE SYSTEM COMPROMISED?

White blood cells are a crucial part of the immune system. They originate in the bone marrow and circulate throughout the bloodstream, as these cells help fight infections by attacking bacteria, viruses and germs that can invade the body. There are five major types of white blood cells: neutrophil, lymphocytes, monocytes, eosinophils and basophils.

A low white blood cell count can be an indication of a chronically compromised immune state, while a high white blood count can be indicative of an acutely compromised immune state. Generally speaking, an increase in neutrophils and a decrease in lymphocytes can be a sign of bacterial immune challenge, while an elevation in lymphocytes and decrease in neutrophil would reflect a viral challenge. Elevated monocytes are often present with a recent immune challenge or an inflammatory process. Elevated eosinophils and/or basophils are associated with parasites and/or allergies. Elevated basophils are associated with inflammation.

A healthcare provider may request that a patient test their antinuclear antibodies (ANA) as part of an evaluation for possible autoimmune disease. ANA are proteins that are made as part of an immune response. Normally, the immune system responds to an infection by producing large numbers of antibodies to fight the foreign invaders. However, when a person has an autoimmune disease, the immune system directs antibodies to mistakenly attack one's own body. These self-directed antibodies are called autoantibodies. Autoantibody-mediated inflammation and cell destruction may, in turn, affect blood cells, the skin, joints, kidneys, lungs, the nervous system and other organs of the body.

A negative ANA result usually means that a patient's symptoms are not caused by an autoimmune disease. However, in the case that an immune disorder is still suspected, there are other more specific tests that can be done. These tests can evaluate antibodies to various proteins in our body, from myocardial peptide and myelin basic protein, to platelet glycoproteins and arthritic peptide.

It is important to know that these tests cannot diagnose autoimmune diseases. Their purpose is to identify an immune reaction to a specific tissue, signaling the potential for autoimmune disease. Sadly, autoimmune disease cannot be diagnosed until specific tissues are destroyed.

INFLAMMATION—MARKERS OF A BODY ON FIRE

By this point in the book, the negative effects of inflammation should be well known. As a little recap, the body reacts to both acute and chronic inflammation. Inflammation can be caused by infection, trauma, cancer, tissue destruction, surgery, or burns. But, it can also be caused by the food we eat, the environment we live in and by emotional stressors. There are several proteins that are modified during inflammation, and these proteins are laboratory biomarkers in either routine blood tests or used to evaluate systemic inflammation. When it comes to inflammation, it is also specifically key to measure liver and gallbladder function, in addition to cardiovascular risks.

The most common inflammatory markers are: erythrocyte sedimentation rate (ESR), C-reactive protein, plasma viscosity, HDL, total cholesterol, fibrinogen activity, ferritin, albumin, globulin, WBC count, lymphocytes, LDH and platelets.

DEFICIENCIES AND OVERLOAD

It's no surprise that having too little or too much of something like electrolytes, hormones and vitamins can cause significant health problems. That's why it's important to rule out a deficiency or surplus when looking at the bigger picture.

Here are some important things to look at.

KIDNEY FUNCTION PROFILE

The kidneys are two bean-shaped organs that extract waste from the blood through urine, balancing bodily fluids and aiding in other important bodily functions. They reside against the back muscles in the upper abdominal cavity. The kidneys are involved in many physiological mechanisms needed for homeostasis, such as regulating acid-base balance, electrolyte concentration, extracellular fluid volume and blood pressure.

Kidney issues can lead to chronic hypertension, diabetes, autoimmunity and inflammatory conditions.

The following biomarkers are commonly tested for kidney function:

- **Glomerular filtration rate (GFR)** measures how well the kidneys are working.

- **Blood Urea Nitrogen (BUN)** measures the amount of nitrogen in blood that comes from the waste product area, a by-product of protein metabolism.

- **Creatinine** is a chemical waste product produced by muscles.

- **Electrolytes** include sodium, potassium, chloride, calcium, phosphorus and magnesium.

HORMONE FUNCTION PROFILE

We talked at great length about hormones in the hormone section, especially about the dried urine test for comprehensive hormone (or DUTCH test). This measures metabolites of estrogen, progesterone, testosterone, cortisol and DHEA. Other hormones that may be important to measure are growth hormones and thyroid hormones, which were discussed earlier in this chapter.

FUNCTIONAL VITAMIN AND MINERAL STATUS

Comprehensive nutritional evaluations are available to identify clinical imbalances that may inhibit optimal health. These advanced diagnostic tools can help people with chronic conditions make lifestyle changes more efficiently. These tests can evaluate, among several other biomarkers, vitamins and minerals, such as:

- antioxidants like vitamins A, E and C

- B Vitamins (B1, B2, B3, B6, B7, B9 and B12)

- the minerals manganese, molybdenum, magnesium and zinc

VITAMIN D LEVELS

Getting vitamin D levels tested is important. For instance, if someone is deficient or on the low side of the optimal range, supplementing with the daily recommended dosage of 1,000 international units (IU) per day may be far from sufficient—especially if you live far from the equator.

Here's a reminder from **Chapter 25: Vitamin D—Are You Operating on Low?** of the ranges from severe deficiency to high levels:

- severe deficiency: below 25 nmol/L (nanomoles per liter)

- mild to moderate deficiency: 25-80 nmol/L

- optimal: 80-200 nmol/L

- high: 200-250 nmol/L

Notice that even within the optimal spectrum, levels vary between 80 and 200 nmol/L. That's a pretty big gap. Oftentimes, someone will fall near the 80 mark and be told that their levels are optimal despite being very close to deficient. It's important to find out exactly where on the scale you fall.

NUTRITIONAL GENOMICS—THE ULTIMATE NUTRITIONAL PERSONALIZATION

Nutritional genomics studies the relationship between human genome, nutrition and health. It can be divided into two categories:

1. Nutrigenomics: studies of the effects of nutrients on health through altering the genome, proteome, metabolome and the resulting changes in physiology.

2. Nutrigenetics: studies of the effects of genetic variations on the interaction between diet and nutrition and health, with implications for susceptible subgroups.[4]

SINGLE-NUCLEOTIDE POLYMORPHISMS (SNPS) PROFILE

Single nucleotide polymorphisms (SNPs, pronounced "snips") are the most common type of genetic variation among people. Each SNP represents a difference in a single DNA building block called a nucleotide.

With advancements in biotechnology, there are now tools available that can use the raw data collected in tests, like those done by 23andMe, and analyze specific SNPs. These can include SNPs related to the cardiovascular system, detoxification system, estrogen metabolism process, immune system, inflammation and neurological and methylation processes, among others.

These interpretations not only go into more detail, but also provide a clear plan of action in terms of the functional lifestyle changes and supplementation that one should take, based on their results.

The idea here is that, if you know your genetic flaws, you can take a more personalized and integrative approach to health, one that supports your body's natural processes, which, in turn, can prevent future health complications from developing.

ENVIRONMENTAL POLLUTANTS PROFILE

MELISA stands for Memory Lymphocyte Immunostimulation Assay, and it can test for metal hypersensitivity, phthalates, BPA, parabens, chlorinated pesticides, volatile solvents, organophosphates, etc. Patients with metal hypersensitivity may have various symptoms associated with an over-activated immune system, including chronic fatigue, joint and muscle pain, cognitive impairment, depression, headaches and fibromyalgia.

MELISA is a clinically validated blood test that finds delayed hypersensitivity (type-IV hypersensitivity) to heavy metals such as mercury, nickel and titanium. MELISA works by analyzing the patient's white blood cells against a panel of suspected allergens, based specifically on the patient's past medical and dental history. The report then shows the strength of the reaction and lists common sources of exposure.[5]

A FINAL WORD

No matter how big or small your symptoms are, you shouldn't have to spend your whole life dealing with them. They are, after all, your body's way of telling you that something is wrong. There are a variety of tests like the ones mentioned in this chapter that take a more in-depth, comprehensive approach to wellness tests, which can get to the root cause of your symptoms.

Keep in mind that the more you know, the more you can do. The proper tests can help you personalize your lifestyle and nutrition to optimize your health and longevity. Remember also that symptoms aren't always present when there's a problem. Even if your body seems to be functioning optimally, routine tests should be done—as well as a detailed health questionnaire and physical exams.

The bottom line is that these numbers represent our health. They represent the inner chemistry of what makes us who we are. Just as we are measured in other areas in life—such as how fast we can run a marathon, how high our grades are and how good our credit score is—I believe we should equally focus on our health test result numbers to ensure that we are performing well from the inside out.

Wouldn't it be great if instead of breaking the ice with someone by mentioning the weather, one would ask how their numbers are doing? Remember the old Star Trek Tricorder scanning the crew on board of the *Enterprise* telling Dr. Crusher what was wrong with them? We're not that far away!

The following diagram shows examples of health habits with corresponding hack levels. To download the *Hack Your Health Habits Worksheet*, visit

www.hackyourhealthhabits.com/worksheets

READY #HEALTHHACKER?
EXAMPLES OF LEVEL 1, 2 AND 3 HACKS FOR THIS CHAPTER

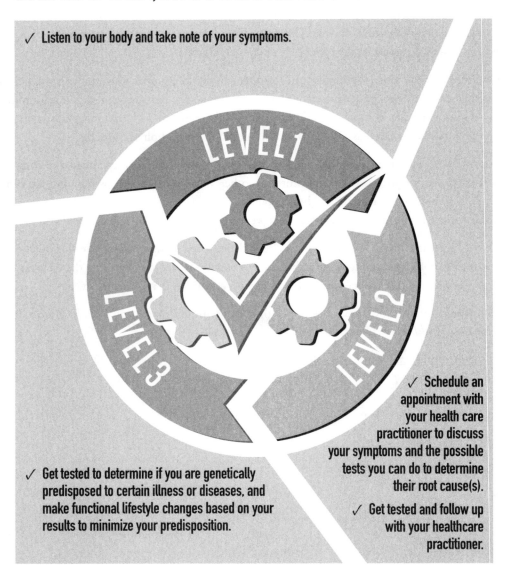

✓ Listen to your body and take note of your symptoms.

LEVEL1

LEVEL2

LEVEL3

✓ Schedule an appointment with your health care practitioner to discuss your symptoms and the possible tests you can do to determine their root cause(s).

✓ Get tested and follow up with your healthcare practitioner.

✓ Get tested to determine if you are genetically predisposed to certain illness or diseases, and make functional lifestyle changes based on your results to minimize your predisposition.

HACK YOUR HEALTH PROGRESS

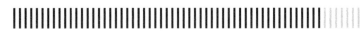

CHAPTER 55

YOUR WELLNESS TEAM

You Don't Have to Do It Alone

> "The doctor of the future will give no medicine but will interest his patient in the human frame, in diet and in the cause and prevention of disease."

— THOMAS EDISON

THINK IT OVER

- Are you aware of what kind of practitioners can help you implement healthy changes in your life?

- What are some of the differences between conventional and alternative healthcare professionals?

- Is your annual physical checkup enough?

By this point in the book, I hope you have discovered areas of your health that you can improve upon and that you are now eager to get started working on them. But, let's face it, just like any major change, it can be a little intimidating at first to tackle this very important job.

When multiple areas of our lives can use some fine-tuning, it may be difficult to know where to begin. Luckily, you don't have to go on this journey alone. In fact, there are many natural health care professionals out there who can help you better understand and apply healthy changes to your current lifestyle. You may be asking yourself, "I see my family doctor annually, and everything seems to be fine—why do I need a natural healthcare practitioner?"

Believe it or not, your regular medical checkup may not be comprehensive enough to cover all the bases of your well-being. Why is that? Well, despite all the advances in medicine over the past few decades, conventional medicine still falls short in one important aspect of health—prevention.

When it comes to acute medical conditions or emergencies such as broken bones, heart attacks, strokes, as well as joint replacements and early diagnoses of certain diseases, traditional western medicine is very competent, and does a great job of taking immediate care of its patients, and very often, it helps save lives.

However, when it comes to chronic conditions, prevention and lifestyle changes are the key to health and the prevention of illness. The majority of the time, these lifestyle factors are our personal responsibility, and it is up to us to make conscious decisions about how we treat our minds and bodies.

As mentioned earlier, there are various types of practitioners who can help you get to the root causes of your current health conditions, and even give the necessary lifestyle recommendations that will aid in preventing chronic illnesses from occurring in the first place. Conditions such as chronic fatigue, adrenal exhaustion, hyper and hypothyroid, GERD, IBS, fibromyalgia, arthritis, SIBO, Crohn's disease, diabetes, high blood pressure, high cholesterol, liver toxicity, depression, anxiety, autoimmune conditions, and so much more can often be prevented and better controlled with positive lifestyle changes suggested by natural healthcare practitioners.

Having someone keep track of your progress ensures that you are on the right path, meaning you are doing the right things for *your* body. Natural health care professionals can even help keep you accountable and make the right decisions based on your unique health needs. For example, a functional health practitioner may advise an individual with adrenal fatigue against running a marathon, or a personal trainer may help an individual stay motivated to keep going to the gym. Someone like a life coach can help you break past barriers you have set for yourself and make changes that are otherwise too difficult to make on your own.

To get you well-acquainted with the types of practitioners out there, I have put together a brief description of those who are most commonly used. It is by no means a complete list, as the repertoire of different natural health professionals has expanded tremendously in the last decade. Here are a few of the most common natural healthcare practitioners you may benefit from:

CHIROPRACTIC

Chiropractic care focuses on optimizing the body's own ability to function at its full potential. It achieves this by removing interference on the nervous system, which controls every cell, tissue and organ in the body. Chiropractic care is a non-invasive and drug-free approach to health. Better yet, you don't need to be in pain to see a chiropractor; many people get checked and adjusted regularly to make sure their spine and nervous system are in tip-top shape. Athletes and high performers use chiropractic care to stay at the top of their games. An optimal spine and nervous system can make the difference between first and second place in a race, or a perfect golf swing—just ask Usain Bolt or Rory McIlroy.

NATUROPATHIC MEDICINE

Naturopathic Medicine is a unique system of primary health care, which focuses on the core causes of various illnesses. It uses the following natural therapies for treatment: traditional Chinese medicine

(TCM), botanical medicine, physical medicine (massage, hydrotherapy, etc.), nutrition, homeopathic medicine and lifestyle counseling. Lifestyle counseling is especially important because it allows you to isolate the negative factors that contribute to health and eliminate them from your routine.

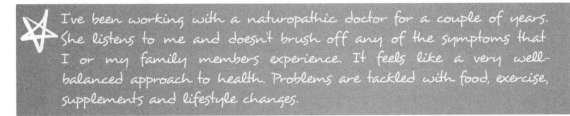

I've been working with a naturopathic doctor for a couple of years. She listens to me and doesn't brush off any of the symptoms that I or my family members experience. It feels like a very well-balanced approach to health. Problems are tackled with food, exercise, supplements and lifestyle changes.

HOMEOPATHY

Similarly, homeopathic medicine is a system of medicines based on three principles: finding cures based specifically on symptoms, taking remedies in extremely diluted forms and targeting multiple symptoms with a single remedy. Homeopathy is the second-most widely used system of medicine in the world and is valued for its holistic, natural and safe methods. Furthermore, homeopathy uses what is referred to as the "law of susceptibility," which implies that a negative state of mind can attract and produce disease and illness.

HOLISTIC NUTRITION

Holistic nutrition focuses on a natural approach to a healthy diet and considers the individual as a whole, including all aspects of his or her lifestyle. A holistic nutritionist can help clients with specific food needs, allergies, or health conditions to maintain their health. They also provide nutritional coaching to guide their clients in making the necessary lifestyle changes that suit their health goals and needs.

PHYSIOTHERAPY

Physiotherapy assists people to restore, maintain and maximize their strength, function, movement and overall well-being. Specifically, physiotherapists can help you with:

- preventing injury and disability
- managing acute and chronic conditions, activity limitations and participation restrictions
- improving and maintaining optimal mobility, independence and physical performance
- rehabilitating injuries and the effects of disease or disability with therapeutic exercise programs and other interventions
- educating and planning maintenance and support programs to prevent re-occurrence of injury, or functional decline

MASSAGE THERAPY

Massage therapy is a hands-on manipulation of the soft tissues of the body focusing specifically on the muscles, connective tissue, tendons, ligaments and joints. Massage therapy treatment has a therapeutic effect on the body and improves health and well-being by acting on the muscular, nervous and circulatory systems. Physical function can be developed, maintained and improved on. Physical dysfunction and pain can be relieved or prevented through the use of massage therapy.

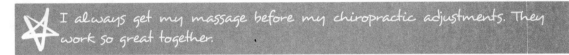

I always get my massage before my chiropractic adjustments. They work so great together.

ACUPUNCTURE

Acupuncture is an ancient Chinese medical technique that is said to adjust and alter the body's flow of energy, and treat a variety of illnesses and health conditions. During the process, numerous thin, solid, metallic needles are inserted into areas of the body in order to reduce pain or induce anesthesia. Acupuncture is said to greatly relieve conditions such as headaches, migraines and chronic pains by stimulating the body's natural healing abilities.

PERSONAL TRAINING

A personal trainer is a professionally trained guide with expertise in fitness, nutrition and healthy living. They can assist clients in creating and tailoring fitness plans to match their goals and lifestyle. They offer instruction in various fitness routines and are available to clients through local fitness facilities or by private appointment. They will help keep you accountable and motivated.

ORGANIC DENTISTRY

Organic dentists, also known as holistic, or environmental, dentists operate on the belief system that your teeth are an integral part of your body, and hence, your overall health. They also recognize that your oral and dental health can have a major influence on other disease processes in your body. The primary aim of holistic dentistry is to resolve your dental problems while working in harmony with the rest of your body. They work without the use of mercury fillings, root canals, or fluoride.

LIFE COACHING

A life coach is an individual trained to help clients identify and achieve personal goals. One must remember, however, that life coaches are not therapists. A life coach will help you look at the various parts of your life: health, relationships, finances and environment. They will work with you to discover the best answers and actions to achieve your goals.

HEALTH COACH

A health coach is a trained and certified individual who is able to take a holistic perspective on your health, to co-create a wellness plan that fits your personal health needs and goals. Health coaches can guide you when it comes to nutrition, exercise, sleep, stress management and detoxification. Health coaches can also work with individuals with chronic illness to help manage symptoms. Their role is not to diagnose disease, but rather guide the patient to prevent problems or cope with existing health challenges.

REFLEXOLOGY

Reflexology is a therapeutic method of pain and stress relief through the application of pressure on points on the feet, hands and ears. The theory behind the practice is that pressure points on these parts of the body correspond to organs and certain systems of the body. Manipulation of their corresponding pressure points are said to relieve symptoms of stress, injury and illness of these organs and systems. Reflexology encourages the flow of blood, minimizing the sensation of pain as well as relieving it.

FUNCTIONAL MEDICINE PRACTITIONERS

Functional medicine is a systems biology approach that focuses on the "why" of symptoms and illnesses. By shifting the traditional disease-centered focus of medical practice to a more patient-centered approach, functional medicine addresses the whole person, not just an isolated set of symptoms. Functional Medicine practitioners spend time with their patients, listening to their history, looking at the interactions between genetic, environmental and lifestyle factors that can influence long-term health, including chronic diseases. In this way, Functional Medicine supports the unique expression of health and vitality for each individual.

Want to improve your state of health on your own? There are also plenty of books and online resources available to inform you on what the right path is for your needs. But, buyer beware. Just because you find information on the Internet or in a book, it does not mean that it is true or suitable for your personal needs. So be your own health advocate!

The following diagram shows examples of health habits with corresponding hack levels. To download the *Hack Your Health Habits Worksheet*, visit

www.hackyourhealthhabits.com/worksheets

READY #HEALTHHACKER?
EXAMPLES OF LEVEL 1, 2 AND 3 HACKS FOR THIS CHAPTER

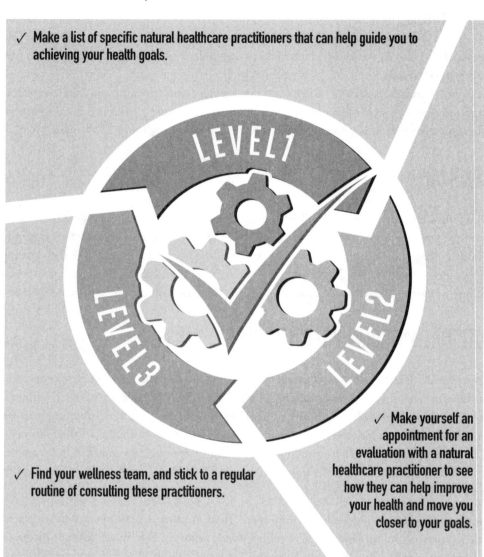

✓ Make a list of specific natural healthcare practitioners that can help guide you to achieving your health goals.

LEVEL 1

LEVEL 2

LEVEL 3

✓ Make yourself an appointment for an evaluation with a natural healthcare practitioner to see how they can help improve your health and move you closer to your goals.

✓ Find your wellness team, and stick to a regular routine of consulting these practitioners.

HACK YOUR HEALTH PROGRESS

||||||||||||||||||||||||||||||||||||||||||||||||||||||||||||||||||||||||||

CHAPTER 56

ACCOUNTABILITY
Who Is Helping You Grow?

"Accountability breeds
response-ability."

— Stephen Covey

THINK IT OVER

- Are you surrounded by strong social support?

- How can an accountability group help you achieve your goals?

- Can you think of a few like-minded people that you would like to spend time with or create an accountability group with?

As you are reading *Hack Your Health Habits*, you're hopefully becoming more ready to take control of your health. You are enthusiastic and committed, and you're sure that this time you will stay on track. You buy what you need, plan your month and start implementing. The first week goes great, but the second week not so much. However, you can pick up where you left off, right? The next week goes by, and you seem to be doing well until a hint of temptation drives your attention away or you get busy. After that, you can't seem to get back into the groove.

What is happening here? You promised you would be committed. You took all the right measures, so why is it that you're still not sticking to your plan? No matter how motivated we are at the start, it's hard to change a behavior for good. Old habits are hard to break, and failure often occurs. How does lasting change take place? If you remember from Section 1, we made the point that motivation doesn't often last, but habits do. Your "why" is your strongest motivating factor, because it creates the discipline and habits needed to actualize your goals.

This is where the role of accountability gains importance. You are more likely to stay on course if you have an equally committed individual, or group of individuals, who share your goal and values. These people can help keep you accountable.

Humans are social creatures and group dynamics make us do fascinating things. Having peers with a similar "why" gives us a space to talk openly, share experiences, challenge each other and provide feedback. A peer group can also provide mutual support, assist in personal growth, and help identify each other's strengths and weaknesses. This allows us to develop a deeper sense of self-awareness, self-compassion and authenticity, as we navigate through areas of life and work.

A truly remarkable example of this is the True North Group developed by Harvard Business School professor Bill George and corporate executive Doug Baker. Through their True North programs, they help individuals develop into leaders by creating accountability groups consisting of like-minded people who meet periodically to discuss various areas of success and failure, and ultimately, to build each other up to attain their goals. This idea originated when a group of businessmen who called themselves the True North Group spoke on a weekly basis for years. Their progress and success were measured, to show that each group member achieved far more than what they would have on their own.

So, how does all of this relate to developing habits? Humans are social animals, and no matter how much self-discipline we possess, the challenges we face can be better dealt with the support of others. To truly be pushed to our self-actualizing limits, we cannot rely entirely on ourselves to help us stay on track.

A small group of people with whom we can have in-depth discussions and share intimately about the most important things in our lives—our happiness and sadness, our hopes and fears, our beliefs and convictions—not only helps build emotional rapport, but also motivates us to achieve more in our personal endeavors. The need or urgency to change and improve ourselves is simply not there, if you are comfortable where you are. Without a doubt, we are inclined to strive higher when our efforts are made in comparison to those of others, and that our ideas flourish in a collectivist setting that encourages our growth.

Now, let's get practical. Think of the goals you want to accomplish in the next year and the habits that you want to implement to get there. What are the actions you will take that will ensure that you stay on track? If it is losing weight, join a weight loss group that is congruent with how you want to go about losing weight. If it is being able to walk or run a 5k, join a walking or running group, or get a dog. If it is learning to play a musical instrument, hire a teacher who will hold you accountable for practicing. If it is learning another language, join a local group so you can learn with others, practice and have fun in the process. If it is to be able to meditate daily, join a local meditation group. You get my point.

I would also suggest, depending on what the goals and desired habits include, that you do an inventory of your friends and see who has succeeded already at what you are wanting to achieve. For weight loss, how about the friend you always admired because he or she has had a steady weight for 20 years and is eating healthy? For walking or running, how about the friend who has been doing it for years and would be more than happy to go with you? For languages, how about your friends that speak the language you want to learn? They will be more than happy to practice their mother tongue with you. For meditation, is it your friend who has been practicing meditation for years and has tools and insight to help you? Maybe you could go to a meditation retreat with her or him.

I have found through the years that people are more than happy to help you with the things that they are already good at, as it is most likely something that they are passionate about and will love sharing. How about other friends that you know who have the same goals as you? Why not pair up with them to reach your goals and keep yourselves accountable?

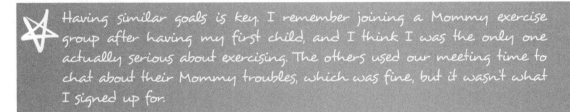

Having similar goals is key. I remember joining a Mommy exercise group after having my first child, and I think I was the only one actually serious about exercising. The others used our meeting time to chat about their Mommy troubles, which was fine, but it wasn't what I signed up for.

CREATE YOUR OWN ACCOUNTABILITY GROUP

Oftentimes, accountability groups are actually subgroups of a larger organization. This can be a college, a club, or a religious organization where like-minded individuals of this common umbrella join forces to discuss individual goals and keep each other accountable. If you aren't part of an organization, that's just fine. Finding people with similar goals and interests is one sure way to keep you more accountable.

What about other people who may have different goals but are committed to getting them done and to personally growing? Can you think of four to five people you enjoy talking to, feel comfortable with, respect and would like to spend more time with who might be interested? You may have to take the lead on this. Just ask! You may be surprised by how many people might be interested.

Change is a process. It has its ups and downs, and you will discover some strengths and weaknesses that you didn't think you possessed through this process. Whether you are just becoming more self-aware and starting your journey to a better you, or if you have plateaued at a certain level, being kept accountable by a strong mutual group may be the key to pushing through.

There will be challenges you will want to take on your own and others that you would rather do with the support of others. The purpose of your accountability group is to develop this safety net that keeps you from falling through with your goals. They can also offer different perspectives on issues that need more thought, while providing a "tough love" environment that keeps you expecting more out of yourself.

ACCOUNTABILITY BUILDS TRUST

Perhaps the most important result of accountability group is *trust*, which is essential in any relationship. Your accountability group will likely consist of individuals with the same core values and similar goals, and thus an interdependence within group members will develop in order to keep each other on track.

Being accountable to something means that you are willing to make commitments to yourself and be responsible for your own actions. You trust others to live up to these standards, and you trust yourself to keep up with your own demands.

ACCOUNTABILITY IMPROVES PERFORMANCE

Accountability will help reduce the amount of time and effort you spend on meaningless activities and other unproductive habits. As we know, many people have the tendency to get distracted easily, especially with the number of available interruptions one can encounter in a day. By building a culture of accountability from the onset, you decrease ineffective behavior and develop an almost competitive, yet encouraging, nature to continuously do better and help your peers do so, as well. When people know that you're actually listening and concerned about their performance, they're more likely to step up and do their best.

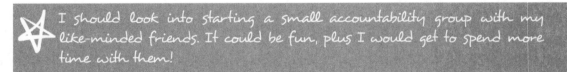

I should look into starting a small accountability group with my like-minded friends. It could be fun, plus I would get to spend more time with them!

MY PERSONAL EXPERIENCE WITH AN ACCOUNTABILITY GROUP

I have been fortunate to be part of an accountability group for the past eight years. On a weekly basis, on the same day, and at the same time, we talk to each other, keeping each other accountable to our short-term, long-term and Big, Bold, Audacious goals. I value their input and credit a lot of my personal and business growth to having such a group. Their friendship, wisdom and willingness to call it like it is consistently brings enormous value to me.

We are a group of four individuals with similar life values who have committed to getting on a call every week to keep each other updated in areas such as business, family and personal development—and to provide encouragement and feedback to one another. We also have committed to meeting two or three times a year in person as we live in different cities of the United States and Canada. On these trips, we work deeper in different areas of our lives (like yearly and long-term goals, finances and legacy planning), but we also create experiences and memories together. We don't always agree with each other or share the same perspectives, but that is part of the beauty of having such a group. We have developed close-knit relationships that provides a safe space for us to share our struggles and our accomplishments. We're committed to ensuring that everyone stays on course with their personal goals. I am very thankful to have an amazing accountability group of people who have become like family to me.

HOW TO GET YOUR OWN ACCOUNTABILITY GROUP STARTED

Before you can start recruiting, you need to be clear on what your own expectations from yourself are. What are your values? What is it that you want to accomplish? What kind of people do you want to surround yourself with? Being sure of yourself and what you hope to achieve out of your accountability group sets the tone for the type of members that you hope to get on your team.

Gathering a compatible group, which has good chemistry and a strong ability to relate to one another, may be a difficult process. Some prior screening of members' values, goals and commitment level may have to be done to ensure your group's success. Once your group has formed, it is important to get a rhythm going. How often and when will you speak? How often will you meet in person? Are there any ground rules for the group?

Another key aspect of forming a group includes understanding each individual's unique communication style and personality, and their attitude toward change and habit formation. Getting to know your group members allows for better communication, while helping them choose goals and strategies that best suit their needs.

In her book, *Better Than Before*, Gretchen Ruben describes four tendencies that people seem to have toward expectation. The first she describes are the upholders, who meet outer expectations, while also meeting inner expectations. These are people who respond well to being told what to do, but are also able to meet expectations they set for themselves, as well. Second, are the obligers, who respond well to outer expectations, but not so well to inner ones. These are people who constantly need someone to hold them accountable in order to stay the course.

Next, she describes the questioners. These people resist outer expectation but meet inner ones. They are wary of others' opinions and beliefs, and do not like following instruction without first conducting their own research on the matter. They may come off as skeptical or stubborn, but essentially, they want to accomplish something because they chose to, not because they were told to. And, finally, there are the rebels, who resist both inner and outer expectations, meaning they chose to make their own rules and abide by them when they feel like it. Rebels resist habits and enjoy exercising their freedom to choose their actions daily.

Understanding each individual's tendencies and communication styles doesn't only create smoother meetings, it also helps us avoid imposing our own way of thinking onto others. Ultimately, we are there to help the other person grow and feel accepted, not to pressure them to make decisions that we believe are right for them.

There are exercises that may help your group members get well-acquainted, such as the lifeline exercise, in which you map out major events that have occurred over your lifetime. It is a sure way to get to know each other quickly on a deeper level. Another great tool to keep each other accountable and help each other set goals is the EOS "Personal Plan," which can be found on the EOS website. (It can be accessed in "tools" when you opt in on www.eosworldwide.com).

Here are some key things to remember to ensure that your group will be around for a long time:

- **Maintain respect and confidentiality** – Depending on the level of intimacy of the group, some pretty touchy subjects or personal information may be shared. It is crucial to maintain your group members' respect and trust by keeping this information to yourself and respecting opposing opinions, even if it may seem like a minor detail. Remember, this group was formed on the basis of trust, and you do not want to compromise that. What is said in a meeting stays in the meeting.

- **Keep your ego in check** – Sometimes in such settings, weekly calls can turn into a boasting match on who has achieved more. This does not serve the purpose of an accountability group. Although some feeling of competition may be healthy, this group has formed to help each other develop—not just one person.

- **Things may change over time** – Goals change, priorities change and often people change. Sometimes a group member no longer fits in with the goals and values of the group. This individual may even be you, and you must be strong enough to realize when to pull out of the group.

- **Stay dedicated** – The reason why certain groups fall apart sometimes is due to the lack of dedication to participation. Vacations, sick days and neglecting the group's routine are all contributing factors. Make an effort to stay accountable to your accountability group. Remember, they are there to help you grow.

Given these statements, it's important that you come in with a collaborative mindset from the start. The whole concept of accountability groups may sound very business-like and productivity-driven—and I've always said that if we conducted our personal lives more like businesses, we would indeed be more successful. But, it does not have to be that way.

What personal goals do you have that may be shared with others? This could include things like eating better, being more present for your family, making more financially wise decisions, sticking to a workout routine, or trying things you never have before.

Remember that accountability is building a culture of trust and not fear. Your goal is not to judge and look for errors and mistakes. Instead, you seek to provide feedback, fill in gaps, improve on solutions, reward productive behavior and remove unproductive ones.

Ultimately, accountability is just another tool to help you develop the right habits and be more motivated to be your best self. If you're more of a tech-oriented person, there are apps that allow you to connect to others virtually and strategize your goals together. Yes, there really is an app for everything these days!

The following diagram shows examples of health habits with corresponding hack levels. To download the *Hack Your Health Habits Worksheet*, visit

www.hackyourhealthhabits.com/worksheets

READY #HEALTHHACKER?
EXAMPLES OF LEVEL 1, 2 AND 3 HACKS FOR THIS CHAPTER

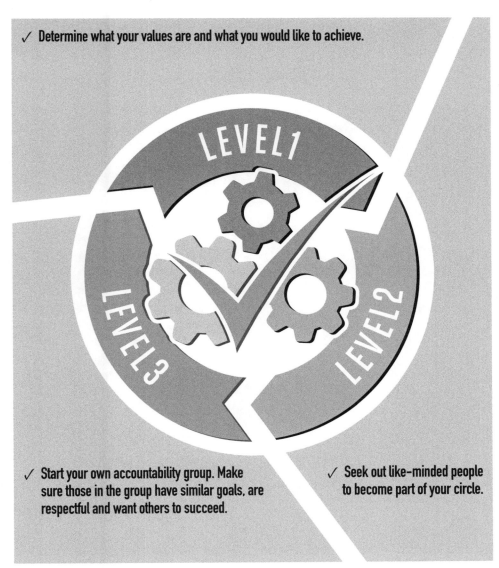

✓ Determine what your values are and what you would like to achieve.

✓ Start your own accountability group. Make sure those in the group have similar goals, are respectful and want others to succeed.

✓ Seek out like-minded people to become part of your circle.

HACK YOUR HEALTH PROGRESS

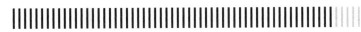

CHAPTER 57

SECTION 12

Get on Purpose—Designing the Life You Want

Have you found your life's purpose? Are you remaining congruent to your values and outlook? Section 12 shares a design for planning, goal setting and learning to master thoughts that empower your health and lifestyle. Here, you will create your own vision of success, learn how to harness your strengths and gain inspiration through the stories of others.

58

LIFE PURPOSE
Are You Living Yours?

> "If you don't know your purpose, follow your passion and it will lead you to your purpose."
>
> — T.D. Jakes

THINK IT OVER

- Are you living a life that is congruent with your ideal self?

- Are you currently living your life's purpose?

- Do you have a personal manifesto? What is it?

Purpose is an intention, objective, or reason for existing—the drive that allows us to do what we are meant to do in order to feel fulfilled. Do you know your purpose in life? Not many people do, and this can lead to a lifetime of poor decisions.

I am fortunate to have found my purpose early on in my life. Although I am not defined by my profession, it has been an amazing vehicle to express my life's purpose. I know my life's purpose is to educate and empower people to take control of their health and their lives. I am not saying that my life is perfect by any means, and I face challenges on a regular basis. But, for the most part, I feel satisfied and fulfilled by the life I have created.

Sadly, I realize that this isn't the case for everyone. In my 20+ years of practice, I have seen countless patients who are unsatisfied with their lives. They often have settled for comfort, either unsure of their purpose or not confident enough to go after it. This is typically evident in the career choices they make.

So many people suffer from what is often referred to as "golden handcuff syndrome." They lack passion for their job but stay in it for the stability, income and pension, counting down the days until their retirement. What does this have to do with wellness, you ask? Everything! Living a life with purpose brings balance, meaning and happiness to our lives. Without it, we are not living to our fullest potential.

> ✦ I can only hope my girls find their life purpose. I've been fortunate to find mine. I love my job, love my family, and genuinely enjoy the life I'm leading. My husband and I encourage the girls to do different things and to enjoy and learn from their experiences. We also fully support their personal growth. We want them to be happy and fulfilled.

Unfortunately, many of us go through adult life on autopilot. We wake up, go to work, count the minutes until we can go home, pick up the kids from school, make dinner, clean up, go to bed and repeat the same cycle the very next day. We are busy: our job, family and other responsibilities take up time. It's easy to get caught up in the rat race and lose sight of our individuality, what makes us who we are.

Our passions, interests and strengths often go to waste. Some of us are stuck in old patterns. Others lack the confidence to pursue goals or are too afraid of failure. We need to realize that our life is a reflection of our choices—our choices lead to actions that ultimately create our reality. We all have control over our immediate behaviors, and we have the power to create the lifestyle we desire.

Sit back and evaluate where you are in life right now. Is this where you imagined you would be, as a younger person? What accomplishments do you feel happy about? How much have you evolved over the last few years? What do you have to look forward to?

Our lives should be in a constant state of change and development. In my opinion, we should always be in search of improvement. When we settle and our lives become stagnant, we become numb to our surroundings and stop putting effort into personal growth. We settle for comfort and routine. We do the same things year after year, without questioning if we are truly satisfied. Life is not a dress rehearsal; we get only one shot to design a life that we can be proud of!

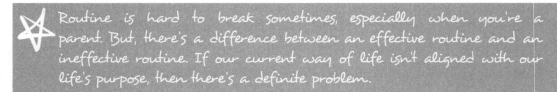

> ✦ Routine is hard to break sometimes, especially when you're a parent. But, there's a difference between an effective routine and an ineffective routine. If our current way of life isn't aligned with our life's purpose, then there's a definite problem.

WHAT IS YOUR LIFE PURPOSE?

In order for us to identify our life's purpose, it is important to know our core values and understand our personal philosophy. What beliefs and attitudes do we have regarding our conduct and what we stand for? When we act in accordance with our beliefs, we stay congruent with our core values. Just as a business develops a mission and vision statement for their company as their guiding system, we should have one for ourselves. A mission outlines what our purpose and intentions for our actions are, and a vision outlines our desired future state.

If our behavior differs from our beliefs, we are likely to experience an inner conflict known as cognitive dissonance. In order to feel fulfilled and satisfied, we must act on our beliefs, do as we think, and stay true to our values and aspirations. However, this is one thing many of us neglect in our work, relationships and lifestyle. Many of us are led by what we think others want us to do, instead of what *we* want to do. In order to keep up with the Joneses and stick to societal norms, we sacrifice our true desires. We may rush into getting married, buying an expensive house, or having kids. We settle into less-than-desirable relationships or jobs. These decisions do not allow us to fulfill our ideals and can leave us feeling unhappy and dissatisfied.

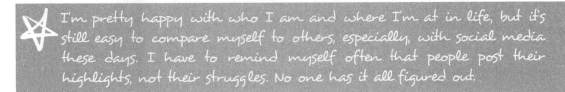

I'm pretty happy with who I am and where I'm at in life, but it's still easy to compare myself to others, especially with social media these days. I have to remind myself often that people post their highlights, not their struggles. No one has it all figured out.

To define our purpose sometimes we need to decide what it is we *don't* want, in an effort to uncover what it is we *do* want. What are we not looking for in our careers, relationships and habits? What type of characteristics or personality traits do we think we lack? Once those are ruled out, we can begin mapping out what it is we truly desire and how we will get there.

A helpful exercise is making a list of things that bring happiness to our lives and provide us with a sense of fulfillment. For example:

I feel my life is at its best when I am_____.
Doing _____ makes me lose track of time.
When I engage in _____, I am at my happiest.
I feel by _____, I bring value to my life and the life of others.
If I could _____ without getting paid, I would.

These are all good ways to identify what our true interests, strengths and passions are. Once these are identified, we can then determine how to integrate them into our lives.

WHAT IS A TRUE PURPOSE?

What is your true purpose? Think about what you are good at, what you are paid for, what you love to do and what the world needs. Your purpose is at the intersection of your passion (what you love doing and what you are good at), your mission (what you love doing and what the world needs), your profession (what you are great at and what you are paid for), and finally, your vocation (what you are paid for and what the world needs).

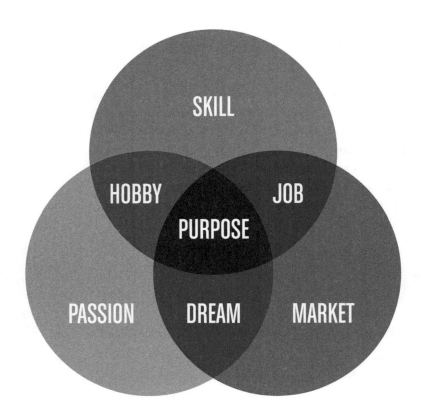

When these elements come together, that's when you know you're living your life's purpose. The good news is that this process isn't as complicated as you think. And, you don't have to do it all at once. Just take baby steps to identify these areas of your life, then add a piece of the puzzle from every area over time. Soon, you'll notice how much happier and satisfied you feel as you introduce more of your passion into your life.

Now I understand that not everyone will decide to build a career out of their passion, and I also realize that everyone's purpose may be different. But, there is no reason someone cannot integrate aspects of their passion into their daily life. Living a life of fulfillment is about doing more of what is important to *you*, and doing more of what makes you happy.

I believe that everything worth achieving in life involves some sort of sacrifice. Everything includes some sort of cost. Nothing is pleasurable or uplifting all of the time. So, the question becomes, "What struggle or sacrifice are you willing to tolerate?" Ultimately, our ability to handle the rough patches and ride out the inevitable rotten days determines our ability to stick with something we care about.

Ask yourself, "Is what I'm doing on a day-to-day basis congruent with my beliefs and values?"

Think about it. If money wasn't at stake, and you knew you could not fail, what would you be doing? How would you be spending your days? What makes you forget time? What do you want people to remember about you? These are just some questions to ask yourself when engaging in your journey to live out your passion.

With this in mind, you can create a personal manifesto: an affirmation of your core values and beliefs, what you represent and how you plan to live your life. By identifying your values, beliefs and your conceptions of what gives meaning to your life, you can create statements that describe your identity, and, in turn, help clarify your purpose.

A personal manifesto can contain affirmations, along with calls to action. It can serve as a frame for your life, as a means for focusing your mind on what truly matters. It can serve as a source of motivation, as a reminder to remain congruent to your values, as a foundation on which you create your sense of self, and as an inspiration to live your purpose to its fullest.

To create a personal manifesto, start by asking yourself questions like these:

- What are my values?
- What do I stand for?
- What are my strongest beliefs?
- How do I want to live my life?
- How do I choose to define myself?
- What changes do I need to make so that I can live my best life?
- What words do I want to live my life by?
- How do I face hardship?
- What attitude do I have toward life?
- How will I treat my body?
- How will I treat other people?
- What will my relationships represent?
- How will I spend my time?
- What path will I choose to unleash my full potential?

Here are great examples of affirmations and calls to action that clearly define who we are and what we stand for:

- I trust myself and listen to my intuition.
- I improve myself daily in some way, whether it's by dropping a negative belief, adding to my knowledge, or any number of other small actions.
- I give myself permission to be myself. I'm authentic. I live my life on my own terms while respecting others.
- I talk health, happiness and prosperity to every person I meet.
- I create opportunities. I don't wait for opportunities to find me.
- I persevere until I reach my goals, in spite of any challenges or setbacks.
- I see mistakes as feedback; I adjust my aim and take another shot.

- I monitor my energy levels and do more of the things that give me energy and less of the things that take it away.

- I treat my time like the precious commodity that it is as I understand its value.

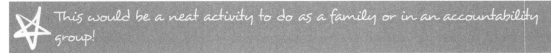

This would be a neat activity to do as a family or in an accountability group!

In your manifesto, you can address personal issues such as your fears, weaknesses, desires, strengths and ideals. Ultimately, the goal is to have a greater grasp on whom you identify as, and what you want your life to represent. A personal manifesto is subject to evolution over time as we pass through different stages in life, and it should grow with us as we age and shift perspectives.

Positive Psychology pioneer Martin Seligman said that a pleasant life is appreciating basic pleasure such as companionship and our basic needs, that a good life is achieved through discovering our unique virtues and strengths and applying them to our lives, and that a meaningful life is achieved by employing our unique strengths for a purpose greater than ourselves.

The following diagram shows examples of health habits with corresponding hack levels. To download the *Hack Your Health Habits Worksheet*, visit

www.hackyourhealthhabits.com/worksheets

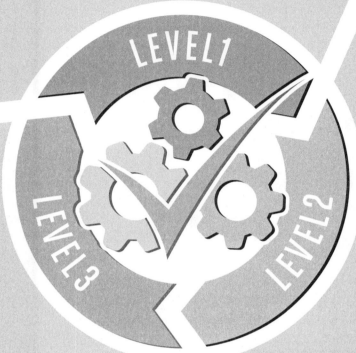

✓ Determine your core values.
✓ Figure out the things you don't want in order to determine the things you do want.

✓ Create your own Personal Manifesto—and live by it!

✓ Determine the intersection point between your passion, mission, profession and vocation to gain clarity on your life purpose.

HACK YOUR HEALTH PROGRESS

|||||||||||||||||||||||||||||||||||||||||||||||||||||||||||||||

CHAPTER 58

59
STRENGTHS FINDER
How to Find and Develop Yours

"Be yourself. Everybody else is taken."

— Unknown

THINK IT OVER

- Do you know what your character strengths are?

- Are you using your character strengths in your daily routine?

- What are some tools to help you find your strengths?

Take a moment to reflect on what you want most out of life. Think about what activities, pursuits and people bring you joy. Write down what lights you up, then determine what you want to bring more of into your life. Some people want lasting love and good relationships. They want better health for themselves. They want to achieve certain things, maybe get a certain degree or rise up in a particular position at their work.

Many people want their children to be happy and healthy. Some say they want to leave the environment a better place than it was when they first came into the world. Others feel they want to be part of something bigger, like connecting with an organization dedicated to empowering youth or helping people with disabilities. Everyone is drawn to different things. The key to remember is to decide what you want, not what anyone around you wants or what you *think* others want for you. Because, at the end of the day, you are the only one living your life!

So, the next step is to ask yourself if you're already working hard toward these goals, but you're not achieving the results you want. If so, then maybe it's time to ask different questions.

Are you focusing on the right things, or is your energy and focus divided? Do you work to your strengths or focus on your weaknesses? One of the many lessons I have learned over the years is that focusing on too many things at once does not produce the best results. I have also learned the importance of focusing on the things that I do best. I've found that working to my strengths—or my character strengths to be exact—allows me to achieve the best results.

What are character strengths? Believe it or not, people tend to think of character in a fairly narrow way. They tend to think of it as either all or nothing, like you either have it or you don't, but that is not necessarily true. Character strengths are the positive parts of your personality that impact how you think, feel and behave. Essentially, character strengths reflect the real you—who you are at your core. And, just like many of our other qualities, the more we use them, the stronger they get.

In his book *StrengthsFinder*, Tom Rath debunks the notion that "you can be anything you want to be, if you just try hard enough." He argues that successful people do not waste their time mastering everything. Instead, they focus their time and energy on their innate strengths, developing them even further. He states that if we spend too much time bettering our weaknesses and working on what we are *not* good at, we lose the opportunity to improve the skills we already have. He proposes that: "You can't be anything you want to be, but you can be a better version of who you already are."

> And, yet our children are forced to work tirelessly on their weaknesses in school. I wonder what would happen if education focused on nurturing a child's strengths?

There are many theories on the importance of using character strengths for achieving ultimate life satisfaction. One theory is found in the work of Martin Seligman. In his book, *Authentic Happiness*, Seligman outlines three orientations of subjective well-being. In other words, he explains happiness as a three-legged stool, with each of the three "legs" contributing to the mental well-being of an individual. These three legs are pleasure, engagement and meaning.

Seligman defines pleasure as maximizing positive emotions through peak experiences—using our innate talents, and decreasing negative emotions by doing so. Engagement involves activities that put one in a state of flow, which occurs most frequently when we concentrate our undivided attention on activities that are moderately challenging to us, and require skill and interest to accomplish. When you are flowing, it may seem like time stops and your sense of self vanishes.

Lastly, a deep sense of meaning is needed. An individual leading a life of meaning belongs to and serves something that is bigger than himself or herself. This can include being part of a team, participating in activities that have meaning to the individual, and even pursuing a goal that contributes to a greater cause and that betters the world. Multiple studies showed that the fulfillment of each "leg" correlates with life satisfaction, while the lack of them predicts low life satisfaction. What's more, Seligman also says that for a person to be truly happy and live a meaningful life, that person must recognize their personal strengths and use these strengths for the greater good.

If we are to take Seligman's advice, we should spend time trying to figure out our personal strengths and not waste our valuable time and life doing jobs that take us away from what we were made to do. With this said, it isn't realistic to ignore all of our weaknesses or quit something just because it isn't completely in line with our strengths. We still need to devote time to developing our basic skills like writing, speaking and teamwork. Developing these types of skills will help us thrive in school, our careers and society, in general.

We must also recognize that there is a difference between spending time on a difficult skill that we enjoy versus one that we despise. An example of this would be a music lover deciding to learn how to play guitar versus a child lacking musicality being forced to learn the clarinet. When someone invests time into something they enjoy and have a knack for, they are more likely to be successful. Tom Rath proposes the following formula: "Talent x Investment = Strength." This suggests that taking a talent or natural skill, and investing time and effort into developing it further, will result in delivering a near-perfect performance in that area.

The Pareto Principle (or the 80/20 rule) is widely recognized as a principle that holds true in many facets of life. It shows how filtering what you focus on can help propel you toward more success. For example, sales executives use it to identify their important customers. They know that 20 percent of their customers give them 80 percent of their revenue. Clever salespeople focus their attention on this 20 percent as a way of achieving their sales goals more quickly and effectively. You don't have to be a sales executive to use the Pareto Principle. What habits can you implement in your life that would give you the best return on your efforts?

Focusing on strengths at work or in leisure will lead to a higher level of satisfaction than when focusing on weaknesses. This may explain why, when we're on the job, we often feel disengaged, face higher levels of stress, or feel disconnected from our true selves. When we are able to use our natural strengths, our work seems less intimidating, we feel a higher sense of accomplishment and we are more productive. This relates to the purpose diagram we talked about in the previous chapter.

When we can develop our skills in an area that we're passionate about and can apply to our daily lives, we are able to experience a state of flow and a higher sense of purpose. Now, we can agree that not everyone can build entire careers on their natural talents, but there are many areas in life that our strengths can be applied. Think it over. Where can you leverage your natural strengths? Your musical talents may not have made you a star, but they can still make an impact.

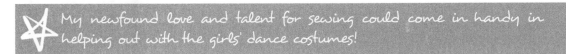

My newfound love and talent for sewing could come in handy in helping out with the girls' dance costumes!

HOW CAN I DISCOVER MY CHARACTER STRENGTHS?

Sometimes our strengths are not as obvious as we think. I am sure you are well aware of certain abilities of yours that are strengths, but what qualities do you possess that you are not aware of? What strengths can you be exercising that you currently are not? Thankfully, many standardized assessments exist that can help you identify these strengths and implement them in your daily life.

One such assessment is the VIA (Values in Action) Strengths Survey. The VIA Classification of Character Strengths is comprised of 24 character strengths that fall under six broad virtue categories: wisdom, courage, humility, justice, temperance and transcendence. They are morally and universally valued, encompass our capacities for helping ourselves and others, and produce positive effects when we express them. Another assessment is the StrengthsFinder Survey, based on Tom Rath's *StrengthsFinder*, which can be purchased online as well.

Not sure what your strengths are? Spend some time figuring them out. Everyone has inborn qualities that, when used, can improve the way they interact, work and feel. When you figure out what your top five strengths are, focus on them and plug them into your life as often as you can. This not only develops your capacity to be more efficient, creative and productive, but you'll be happier and more successful in the long run. Imagine how much more mental and emotional freedom you'll have once you stop focusing on the things you don't like.

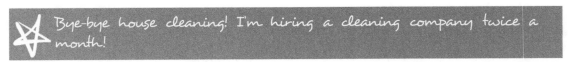

Bye-bye house cleaning! I'm hiring a cleaning company twice a month!

The following diagram shows examples of health habits with corresponding hack levels. To download the *Hack Your Health Habits Worksheet*, visit

www.hackyourhealthhabits.com/worksheets

READY #HEALTHHACKER?
EXAMPLES OF LEVEL 1, 2 AND 3 HACKS FOR THIS CHAPTER

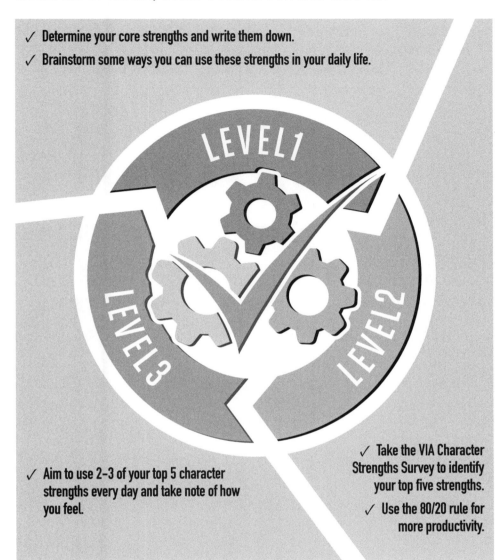

✓ Determine your core strengths and write them down.
✓ Brainstorm some ways you can use these strengths in your daily life.

✓ Aim to use 2–3 of your top 5 character strengths every day and take note of how you feel.

✓ Take the VIA Character Strengths Survey to identify your top five strengths.
✓ Use the 80/20 rule for more productivity.

HACK YOUR HEALTH PROGRESS

|||||||||||||||||||||||||||||||||||||||||||||||||||||||||||||

CHAPTER 59

10X YOUR LIFE

Are You Thinking Big Enough?

"What we think, we become."

— Buddha

What I am about to share with you is a new state of mind, an expanded way of thinking, a mindset that challenges you to reach for more, play a bigger game and move beyond your comfort level. Before we get into it, ask yourself these questions:

- Do I feel challenged, or do I live life from my comfort zone?

- Do I feel like what I do makes a difference in the world, or do I feel like what I do is purposeless?

- Am I excited about life or just going through the motions?

It's important to ask ourselves these kinds of questions every now and again. It allows us to assess whether we are living a purposeful, invigorating life or if we have settled for comfort—meaning we've sacrificed our true potential. Each of us has interests that we are passionate about, elements of ourselves to improve and things we want to learn about and experience. I believe that we need to act on these passions and ideas, not just think about them, and to actually do something! To do so, we need to apply 10X thinking.

What does 10X mean? 10x means just that. Not improving something just a little, but making it 10X bigger, 10X better, 10X more than what it is. Why 10X? Because small improvements don't ignite new thinking, innovation, or transformation. Because gradual changes tend to lack excitement and may not render the same results. And, because it lets us see a whole new world of possibilities.

If I ask you, "Are you meant for more?" then what reaction does it elicit internally? Does this question make you sit up straight and say "Yes! I know that I am meant for more than what I am doing now?" If so, this chapter is for you! [Insert infomercial voice here].

WHAT IS 10X THINKING?

Still not sure what 10X means? Here are some examples of well-known individuals who have applied 10X thinking:

- In 1961, John F. Kennedy stated, *"We will put a man on the moon and return him safely to earth by the end of the decade."* Do you think that he knew then how to make it happen? Nope! He applied 10X thinking. Think of all the advances made in space travel since then.

- Oprah Winfrey set a goal of having her own TV show and network when nobody knew who she was. Did she know how she was going to achieve that? Nope! She applied 10X thinking. Now, look at how many people Oprah has guided and inspired.

- Another example is Roger Bannister, the first man to run a mile in under four minutes. He accomplished this amazing feat in 1954. Everyone told him it was physically impossible. Did that stop him? Nope! He applied 10X thinking. His record lasted only 46 days because he removed the *limitation* that other athletes were putting on themselves. Many others have surpassed his record since then.

Now, you may be thinking, "I am not John F. Kennedy, Oprah Winfrey, or Roger Bannister." But you need to understand that anyone and everyone has the ability, *right now*, to apply the 10X principle to some aspect of their life.

What could you 10X? How about 10X more freedom—being able to go where you want, when you want and with whom you want? Or 10X more money, and not have to worry about money all the time? What about 10X more involvement within your community, being able to give back and affect more people? Or, 10X more fulfillment in your relationships—having relationships that bring you more joy than you ever thought possible? Finally, what about 10X in your career—performing a job that you love or having a business that brings you great satisfaction every day?

In order to figure out what your 10X could be, ask yourself these questions: What excites me? What do I love doing in my free time? What makes me happy? What did I love to do when I was a child? What seems effortless? What do people tell me I'm good at? What makes time fly by when I do it? What problem do I wish there was a solution to?

I want you to find your 10X idea right now! While reading this book, what ideas have popped into your head? What "Aha!" moments have you experienced? You may not find a passion per se, but I believe you will feel strongly about something you can improve in yourself or your surroundings. Maybe you've had a dream for a long time that you didn't believe was possible. Don't wait forever to take action and bring that dream to life! Take an idea that you may have woken up with this morning and put on your 10X thinking cap. What will you no longer accept as status quo? What do you want to solve? What do you want to someday look back on with pride?

HOW TO APPLY 10X THINKING

Here are some situations where you may want to apply 10X thinking:

- You don't like the education system as it is; find ways to change it.

- You have trouble gathering resources in a particular area of interest and wish someone would put together better resources; be that someone.

- You don't like your work, wish you could work for yourself and run your own business; figure out what you need to do to get started.

- You're unhappy with the way you look and feel; decide to transform your body and your health.

- You disagree with some of your local political policies; get involved and work to change them.

Asking these questions and discovering the answers can be scary. We often avoid thinking about the things in our lives that we know we should resolve. Digging deep may mean change, and we often fear change. But this is where the magic happens. This is where you begin to find what you're really about... where you find your essence.

Rethink what is possible for *you*. Create something. It might sound crazy right now, but embrace your idea and start thinking with a 10X mindset, and see what happens. See what you attract in your life to get you there.

Now, of course, the caveat here is that no success comes without sacrifice. Analyze your current circumstances and evaluate what activities, commitments, or relationships are holding you back from unleashing your potential. Letting go of whatever is *not your essence* opens a new door of opportunity for growth and achievement. The 10X mindset means stepping out of your comfort zone and working hard to make things happen.

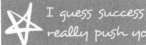 I guess success really doesn't happen overnight. You need to work and really push yourself to make real change.

Whatever you do, don't let excuses stop you from achieving your 10X! What limiting beliefs are you imposing on yourself? You know what I mean! We all have that little voice inside our heads telling us we're too old or too young, too afraid, or don't have the time or money. You know, the one that says it's a crazy idea and will never work, that you're too busy, can't risk it, or you're just not smart enough...and on and on.

Tell that voice of uncertainty to back off! And, imagine your life as one of those who have gone ahead and applied the 10X principle. Think of the great sense of accomplishment you will get when you 10X it and the difference you will make around you if you 10X it. Think of how great you will look and feel when you are at your optimal weight and fitness level if you 10X it. Think of the inspiration you will be to others and of the people you will impact if you 10X it. Think of how happy and fulfilled you can be in your career if you 10X it. Think of the legacy you can leave if you 10X it.

I know you can do it!
10X your beliefs!
10X your ideas!
10X your thoughts!
10X your life!

The following diagram shows examples of health habits with corresponding hack levels. To download the *Hack Your Health Habits Worksheet*, visit

www.hackyourhealthhabits.com/worksheets

READY #HEALTHHACKER?
EXAMPLES OF LEVEL 1, 2 AND 3 HACKS FOR THIS CHAPTER

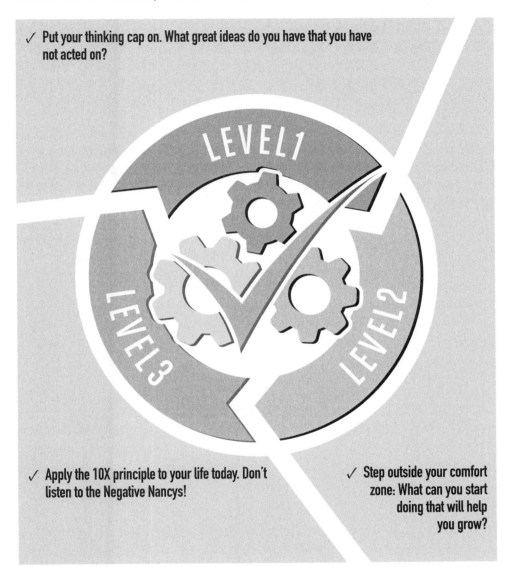

✓ Put your thinking cap on. What great ideas do you have that you have not acted on?

✓ Apply the 10X principle to your life today. Don't listen to the Negative Nancys!

✓ Step outside your comfort zone: What can you start doing that will help you grow?

HACK YOUR HEALTH PROGRESS

||||||||||||||||||||||||||||||||||||||||||||||||||||||||

CHAPTER 60

61

PHILOSOPHY
We All Need It

"It is not a question of whether man chooses to be guided by [philosophy]: he is not equipped to live without it."

— AYN RAND

THINK IT OVER

- Are you clear on your life's philosophy?

- Do you conduct your life in congruence with that philosophy?

- How can you apply Aristotle's five branches of philosophy to develop your own?

If there is anything I want you to take away from this book, it is what we are about to discuss in this chapter. The ideas we are about to look at may not only shift your perspective on how you make decisions in your life but will also give you deeper insight into the underlying factors that control your day-to-day actions. These include the subconscious premises that either drive you or prevent you from reaching your best self.

You may be thinking, "How does philosophy fit into the context of a health book?" It fits in quite nicely, actually. As a matter of fact, it may even be the *foundation* of health. And, I'll tell you why.

When thinking of the word philosophy, what comes to mind? Ancient philosophers such as Aristotle, Socrates, Plato? Or, other old men in corduroy jackets with plaid elbow patches sitting around contemplating some of the world's greatest questions: "What is time?", "What is the nature of the universe?", "What is truth?", "What is reality?", "Is there free will?", "What is the meaning of life?".

This is how the world perceives academic philosophy, and it can leave us with a headache. What if I told you, though, that we apply a personal philosophy in our everyday lives? It is the driver of our thoughts, actions and behaviors. And, many of us don't even know we have a philosophy.

Whether we realize it or not, we all have an ideology that is expressed through our actions. It is the inner voice that guides us between what we feel is right or wrong. It is the force that makes us take a step forward or back, and it is so strong that it creates the circumstances that ultimately shape our reality. As it is subconsciously derived (or maybe usually subconsciously driven), many of us fail to realize that this philosophy is the product of our values, perspectives and outlook. And, in fact, it can be consciously controlled by reason. The long evolutions of philosophy, psychology and neuroscience all seem to point toward a common theme of unlocking true human potential—and that is our capability to leverage reason behind our decisions, to make a conscious effort to live our lives on our own terms.

OUR PERSONAL PHILOSOPHY

Where does this personal philosophy come from? It starts with the values we acquire from things we were taught during our upbringing, from the experiences we have acquired, and the obstacles we have overcome or failed to overcome. These values then manifest themselves in the manner we deal with our peers, family, finances, work, hobbies—and, ultimately, they create the blueprint to how we carry ourselves through life.

The problem is, oftentimes these values or subconscious rules are not vividly mapped out in our minds. So, we find ourselves leading a life of contradiction, meaning we act in a way that is not congruent with who we truly are or who we aspire to be. In other words, the person we perceive ourselves to be and the person we desire to be do not line up, and this is from where most of our anxiety and cognitive dissonance stems.

If you do not have a clear sense of your values, a sense of who you are—if you have contradictions between what you say and what you do—you can never move forward. The sometimes-subconscious reasons for these behaviors are ultimately what prevents you from doing more or propel you to move forward. Developing a conscious philosophy allows you to check whether your actions are congruent with your values, and re-align where it is necessary. And, if a conscious effort isn't put into developing a strong philosophy, then a life of dissatisfaction and contradiction will continue. You become a slave to impulse and distraction, causing you to slowly lose trust in yourself—and along with it, losing your confidence, self-esteem and zest for life.

True enlightenment comes when we realize that our state of mind is simply choosing one thought over the other and that happiness and satisfaction in life is, indeed, a choice. We can also choose behaviors and actions that create desirable outcomes. In this way, we can choose a life philosophy that represents our values, that connects us to a deep sense of who we are, that brings the greatest source of vibrancy and fulfillment in every major decision. This requires some effort on our part, some soul searching— finding our core values, creating boundaries, identifying what we stand for, envisioning our best selves, creating goals and aspirations, defining a purpose, establishing the right habits, and lastly, implementing them into our day-to-day lives.

This idea of a personal philosophy links back to one of our first chapters on motivation. What pushes people to think what they think or do what they do? What is that force that drives a certain person to want to think, act and do more? It all boils down to our "why factor": What makes some search for constant novelty, growth and stimulation, while others stay in their comfort zone?

A reason and a purpose are what drives this, and this takes time and effort to develop. We do not suddenly wake up with a purpose one day. A purpose develops from working toward a common goal, putting energy into something that has meaning and something that aligns itself with our true selves. Issues arise when the various aspects of our lives are not lined up with a common purpose or goal—if our hobbies, our work, our social circle and choices do not reflect our values, or what we want to be known for. We then feel that our identity is torn between multiple directions, none of which represents our true selves. This is the origin of self-destructive behavior; when we lose the sense of who we are, and live a life that isn't on our terms.

LET'S GET PRACTICAL: THE BRANCHES OF PHILOSOPHY

Philosophy, in a sense, is a field devoted to arguing about language and reality, so to expect any consensus over what philosophy, itself, is… would be magical thinking. However, according to Aristotle, there are five branches of philosophical teachings that define what the field entails. Although these branches may seem abstract, they hold practical value that we can learn to apply to our daily habits.

The first branch of philosophy is metaphysics, the study of existence. What is out there, what is reality. The second branch of philosophy is epistemology, the study of knowledge. When you define what reality is, how do you know it? The next branch is ethics, the study of action. Once you define what your reality is and how you know this reality exists, this branch allows you to think about what you do about it with this knowledge. The fourth branch is politics, the study of force. What actions are permissible to alter or maintain this reality? And the last branch of philosophy is esthetics, the study of art. What can life be like?

Philosophy literally means "love of wisdom" and originally was supposed to be a deep but practical examination of how we should live. What philosophy ultimately creates is the ability to question, to ponder and reflect. So, many of us go through life without taking the time to actually think or wonder. Is the way we are living truly a reflection of who we are? Are we currently working toward our greatest potential? And, if not, why?

 I think that's one of the best parts of this book. It's really getting me to think…not just about my health, but about my life as a whole. I sure have some deep thinking to do.

What limitations are we imposing on ourselves, and what changes are we resisting? Some of us might even be gathering the right information by reading books and following people who inspire us, yet when it comes to the application of this inspiration, we fall short. What prevents us from acting? In a very real sense, the five branches of philosophy can be applied to every habit and decision that we make. They lay the groundwork, upon which we can develop a personal philosophy. They allow us to contemplate our current style of living and access which areas can be altered and improved.

Let's look at an example. A common issue among people in the workforce is being unhappy with their work. Although the construct of this model is not as simple as the following, for the purposes of practicality, let's look at how one may implement the five branches of philosophy to this real-life scenario. How would a hypothetical unhappy worker potentially apply the five branches?

1. **Metaphysics: What is the reality?** I currently work in an area that is not a passion of mine, nor do I feel my efforts are appreciated by my colleagues and superiors. I get frustrated at how others who are performing less well get paid the same amount as I am.

2. **Epistemology: How do I know this?** I don't look forward to going to work every morning—in fact, I kind of dread it. I feel like I'm living for the weekends and my holidays.

3. **Ethics: What should I do about it?** Despite everything, I can still have a positive attitude about having security, stability and a full pension. There are still ways I can contribute to the development of my current projects and put my best foot forward in everything that I do. In addition, I can always express my passions outside of work with hobbies, or even a side business. Not to mention, I can always ask for a transfer to a different project and team.

4. **Politics: What actions are permissible?** I am not going to be disrespectful to my colleagues or superiors, or let my productivity slip. I want to maintain high work standards and good relationships with my co-workers. I can always take a few hours each week to work on personal projects outside of work.

5. **Esthetics: What can life be like?** By embracing a positive attitude toward my work, I can change my mindset. I can do my best every day and be proud of the work I do. In my spare time, I can focus on activities that replenish my energy.

If a person has established their personal work philosophy, they will be less frustrated. They will be able to remain within this philosophy and feel fulfilled. It will become clear how to remain within this philosophy to be fulfilled. If they move out of alignment with their personal philosophy, they will quickly recognize it, and take action to re-align. For example, they wouldn't stay in a job they hate for years.

In the end, our philosophy gives us life. It provides us with the blueprint to make our decisions, and every aspect of our lives should align with it. From the way we speak to ourselves, to the way we act, to how we carry ourselves, to the habits we acquire, to what we do for work, to what we do for leisure—every behavior that we adopt must be a reflection of the person that we want to be.

We must constantly be asking ourselves, "What would my ideal self do?" Our sense of purpose stems from this philosophy. In most cases, people who have not found their own purpose just need to revisit their premises and see if all their actions and attitudes are congruent with their true selves. Often, these premises hide in our daily habits, the behaviors we repeatedly do without thinking, which shape our reality. This emphasizes the importance of putting active effort into creating the right habits and implementing actions that will develop the characteristics we want to see in ourselves.

Developing a philosophy is subjective. How to define happiness and success in your own life is unique to your own needs. Some philosophies may not resonate with your own, but that's not the point. As long as someone feels as though they are working toward their best self and are happy with the way they are doing it, then that is *their* purpose. The point is to have a philosophy to live by, as the lack of one causes a lifetime of trivial living until you define your identity.

As one of my colleague and mentors, Dr. Patrick Gentempo, put it in his TED Talk, "Humans are the only species that can choose to have a purpose. If a dog had a choice to have a purpose, it probably wouldn't live with you. If a cow could choose to have a purpose, there would be no such thing as MacDonald's." Animals live by pain, pleasure and survival, and a human being with no sense of purpose does the same. When your purpose is survival, survival is all you will get. We want to live a life where we thrive, not just survive. As Ayn Rand, author of the book *Atlas Shrugged*, once said:

"Man's life, as required by his nature, is not the life of a mindless brute, of a looting thug or a mooching mystic, but the life of a thinking being—not life by means of force or fraud, but life by means of achievement—not survival at any price, since there's only one price that pays for man's survival: reason."

The following diagram shows examples of health habits with corresponding hack levels. To download the *Hack Your Health Habits Worksheet*, visit

www.hackyourhealthhabits.com/worksheets

READY #HEALTHHACKER?
EXAMPLES OF LEVEL 1, 2 AND 3 HACKS FOR THIS CHAPTER

✓ Do a personal inventory of what your core values are. This is the basis for the development of a personal philosophy.

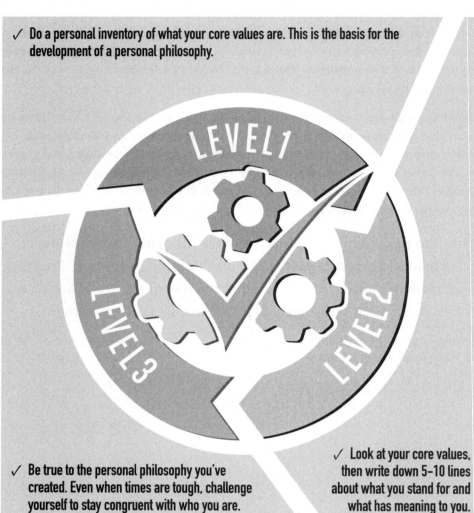

✓ Be true to the personal philosophy you've created. Even when times are tough, challenge yourself to stay congruent with who you are.

✓ Look at your core values, then write down 5–10 lines about what you stand for and what has meaning to you.

HACK YOUR HEALTH PROGRESS

CHAPTER 61

62

YOUR STORY

Is Yours Holding You Back or Driving You Forward?

"If you change the way you look at things, the things you look at change."

— DR. WAYNE DYER

We, as humans, love stories, more specifically, stories about other people. We love listening to how someone overcame major hardship, how they changed, evolved, and the nitty gritty little details of what makes them who they are. Stories help us relate to one another; they can be used to inspire and to motivate, to serve as an example and to help understand each other's behaviors and attitudes. It is moving hearing how well-known people came from almost nothing to achieve worldwide success, such as Walt Disney, Ralph Lauren, Sylvester Stallone, Tony Robbins and Steve Jobs.

But, what about our own stories? What do we have to tell about ourselves? We all have our personal stories based on our upbringing, struggles, obstacles, goals and development. These stories are crucial to how we understand ourselves and the development of our identity. They are avenues we use to express our uniqueness.

Now, think hard about what your story entails. Bring into your awareness what you express about yourself to others: What traits do others recognize in you? Are these positively or negatively reflecting upon your desired self? If we want our stories to inspire, motivate and define our positive character traits, we need to make sure that they mirror our growth and self-improvement.

Two common issues can affect our personal story. The first is that we rely too heavily on past accomplishments to maintain our image. Don't get me wrong, an obstacle or triumph can definitely shape who we are. But it does not necessarily represent what we are doing presently to further our progress. The story of a successful person does not stop at their first victory. Success isn't one thing or moment; it is an ongoing process of improvement.

The second issue is that people accept their current circumstances as their fate and do not actively put any effort into changing it. This can occur with a bad relationship, poor job satisfaction, an illness and much more.

We can allow ourselves to feel helpless, playing victim to our circumstances and feeling less and less satisfied with our lifestyles. It's important to realize that no matter our situation, we have a choice. We can choose to be stuck, or we can choose to be resilient. It's in our choices that our story emerges. This is sometimes easier said than done. Unfortunately, not every story has a happy ending, but we can still choose how we react to it.

Now, take a moment to think. Is your story serving you right? Is it holding you back or propelling you into further success? Is it how you want others to remember you? Think about what character traits you admire and wish to see in yourself: How can you implement these in your life?

POWERFUL STORIES

To help inspire you, I reached out to five women in my life whom I deeply admire and asked them if they would each share their story in this book. To be honest, I think they were surprised when I reached out. After all, they are not celebrities or billionaires, just regular people who are doing great things for themselves and the people around them.

As you will see in a moment, each of their circumstances is different. But, in a similar way, they refused to let their situation limit their lives. These five women were able to move past their circumstances with a positive frame of mind. Each credit their past hardships for where they are today. It is their positive outlook on life and perseverance that I find so admirable. I hope their stories will encourage you to write your own.

Here are their stories.

MARIA'S STORY:

RAISING TWO BEAUTIFUL, WHEELCHAIR-BOUND AND DISABLED BOYS

Meet Maria

Maria is a 58-year-old mother of two who operates a small business with her husband. She also runs a bookkeeping business on the side.

What is the significant event or situation that changed your life?

There are two main events that changed my life. The first was finding out that my sons were born with cerebral palsy, and the second was my divorce.

My sons' condition changed my life in the sense that, even today, I work and take my holidays around their needs, despite them being in their 30s. As long as they, or I, are in this world, I will have to plan my life around theirs.

My divorce changed my life in the sense that it forced me to take charge of myself and of my boys. I became a less naïve person and realized that it was OK to ask for help. It also helped boost my self-esteem, and I became a stronger, more determined person, surmounting my fears of talking to people.

How did you decide to use this event, not to be a victim, but to grow from the situation?

I never saw myself as a victim. It was, and still is, a situation that I deal with every single day with a positive attitude. I've always been a positive person. It is my positive attitude and my natural willingness to help others that have aided me in many difficult situations.

What are the tools that you use and the habits (mental or physical) you created to thrive?

I would say that the tools that I have carried all my life are my positive attitude, my smile and my willingness to help others. I have always tried to eat healthy, to listen to my body and to take care of it. While it's not always easy, I don't beat myself up and try to accept and change my shortcomings.

Looking back at the situation now, is there anything you would have done differently?

Not at all! My boys' situation might have changed my life, but it did not change me. My divorce was the best thing that ever happened to me. I now have the best partner in the world (going on almost a quarter of a century) and am living the best times of my life.

If you had to give one lesson to someone going through a similar situation, what would it be?

Do your best every single day. Do not go to bed with any regrets.

Constantly evaluate your life's situations and make the necessary changes and adjustments needed. Do not wait. If you wait, acknowledge and accept the consequences with a smile, and move on.

How has this event shaped you into who you are today?

I believe that I shaped the events in my life and not the other way around. It is because of my positive attitude that I made, and still make, the best times of my life. No regrets. The events and situations did not change me, they only changed the way I live my life. Would I have done anything differently? No, not at all. Now, had my boys been so-called "normal," not multiply disabled, would my life be different? Probably! Would I still be living where I live? Probably not! But you can't dwell on what could have been.

NATALIE'S STORY:
MOVING FORWARD AFTER TRAGEDY

Meet Natalie

Natalie is a 38-year-old organizational development consultant and community television host. She recently became a new mother.

What is the significant event or situation that changed your life?

In 2011, my husband of almost two years passed away in a truck accident. In that moment, I felt like I had lost my best friend, my future and my opportunity to have a family. Through my healing process, I realized that Phil's death was not something that happened to me, but rather to him. He is the one who won't get to experience all of the things I am able to experience just by being alive. A fatal accident is so final and unchangeable. You can't predict it, and there's no way it can be altered. It changes your life.

How did you decide to use this event, not to be a victim, but to grow from the situation?

I'm someone who naturally grows from situations. It's a fundamental part of who I am. When Victim Services came to my house and announced that Phil had died, the first thing I said to them was, "I'm not a victim, and you should change your title. I'm not opposed to your support, I'm not opposed to your help, but I'm not a victim." I did not want to call myself a widow. I was frustrated when I had to use the term on legal or financial documents. I was someone who was married but lost her husband. Widow didn't sound right to me.

I chose to frame the situation differently. Because Phil couldn't live every day like I did, I decided the moment he died that I would lead an exquisite life. It was a choice, and I've been on that path ever since. Sometimes it's difficult, but I'm always on that path.

What are the tools that you use and the habits (mental or physical) you created to thrive?

There are many. I used a lot of physical tools: walks in nature, yoga—I actually went to Hawaii to do my yoga teacher training—and a lot of meditation. I joined multiple meditation groups, worked with various spiritual healers and sought help from psychologists. I reached out to a wide variety of people in different fields. I leaned on my family and friends and continued to be active and engaged in my community. I made sure to finish my executive MBA and made the decision to go back to work quickly. I took psychic-development courses so that I could tap into my intuition and be more open and aware of everything life had to offer. In terms of habits, I joined the "Morning Club," where you start each day with self-care, identifying your needs for the day and expressing what you are grateful for. All of these tools helped me in their own ways.

Looking back at the situation now, is there anything you would have done differently?

No. I needed to go through what I needed to go through. It wasn't always easy. It took me three years to feel normal again. For a long time, I felt conflicted. I remember attending my friend's baby shower and being very happy for her, but very sad for myself. I remember thinking, "How can I be happy and sad at the same time? Am I a hypocrite?" Eventually, I learned to just observe and accept whatever was in front of me—whatever emotions were in front of me—be it grief, fear, or happiness. I learned to listen to my gut and do what I felt needed to be done to feel better. At times, I would go through 3-5 days of sadness before I felt happy again. Learning to accept my feelings was a big step. I guess there is one thing I would change: I could've been a little more patient with myself during my healing process.

If you had to give one lesson to someone going through a similar situation, what would it be?

Someone gave me this advice, and it helped me immensely: In the first year after someone close to you passes, don't make any big life decisions—give yourself time to grieve. That means no big moves, no new relationships—unless circumstances are out of your control. Give yourself time to grieve, and go through the motions. Losing a husband, wife, child—someone that is in your everyday life—impacts you greatly. You need time to relearn how to live without them there.

How has this event shaped you into who you are today?

I feel like I'm 85 years old. This has given me a life's worth of wisdom and an ability to appreciate life in a completely different way. I have found love again, and I love Jonathan with every fiber in my body. And, my dreams are coming true. We are expecting our first child. I still love Phil and always will. My heart is so full, and I feel so blessed. By being present… that really matters, on living an exquisite life in honor of Phil—he wanted me to be happy—I have healed and found my happy again. We all can do that with some deep work on ourselves. It's truly possible.

MAUREEN'S STORY:
BECOMING A SINGLE MOTHER OF 4 KIDS

Meet Mo

Mo is a 54-year-old cashier and warehouse worker and a single mother to four children.

What is the significant event or situation that changed your life?

When I was 35, my husband decided to leave me and our four children. We had been together for 12 years, married for 10 years. At the point he decided to leave, we had an eight-year-old daughter, a five-year-old son, a three-year-old daughter and a one-year-old son, and I was a full-time stay-at-home mom.

Like any marriage, there were moments where life was challenging, and there were moments when life seemed spectacular. When we met, he was a successful construction millwright. He shared with me that his dream was to be a truck driver. I gave him the money to go and get his AZ license. He did, and we started building our lives together soon after. In the first years, money was tight, but we made it work. Ironically, he started making great money around the same time he decided to leave.

Though he told me his decision to leave was so he could "experience life," I later found out it was largely driven by another woman in the picture. I was devastated. I loved the man with all my heart and soul, and him leaving me hurt like a son of a gun, but I was most upset for my kids. I was scared for them. He left. He made the money. How was I going to be able to do this on my own?

I asked him to stay, work and keep our home so the kids could have a good life. But, he said no. He said he would pay me money, but didn't want to stay. He visited the kids on weekends for six months after he left. After that, he was never seen or heard from again. He lived 20 minutes away, and I remained in our home for the next few years, but he never made any attempt to contact, see, or console our four children. To this day, he still has provided hardly any financial help.

How did you decide to use this event, not to be a victim, but to grow from the situation?

I have had a great deal of feelings to deal with: survival, mistrust, anger, low self-esteem, worthiness, to name a few. Did I become a victim? I believe I did. Subconsciously and consciously, I needed people to help me take care of my children. But, ultimately, I knew that no matter what help I would receive, it was up to me to succeed and help my children develop into the best people possible.

What I told my children (among many pieces of advice) was that they had the decision to live life or sit and feel sorry for themselves because their father had left and wasn't going to be part of their lives. I said that "Although I am sad for what has happened, I am choosing to live life. I want to be able to laugh and cry and experience many different things." They have the same choice. But, if they choose to sit and feel sorry for themselves and do not want to go out, I will respect that. Because their life is their own to live. I am here to help, support and encourage. But, I hope they choose life.

If you had to give one lesson to someone going through a similar situation, what would it be?

My advice to another going through a similar situation is to not become bitter. This is easier said than done, but it is crucial for you and your children's well-being. Whatever your religious beliefs, surrender to God, your guardian angels, or simply the universe to allow you to do the best you can, and keep your children protected and safe.

How has this event shaped you into who you are today?

I would say this has made me stronger as a woman and as a human being. Because of the many challenges I've faced and sacrifices I've made, and the experience of having to be dependent on others, I have learned gratitude, humility and compassion. I also have gratitude for my children being healthy, as well as myself; humility for having to receive, and hopefully doing it with grace; and compassion for others, in what they go through. Mentally, I feel that I learned how easy it is to become an alcoholic, drug addict, sex addict, or any kind of addict.

As I am constantly being pushed to the limit, I understand the desire to want to feel free from the pressures. I love being a mom, but when you don't have money to take care of your kids (even to afford basic needs), you may have the tendency to feel like a failure. The need to escape becomes great. So, if you can focus on all the little accomplishments and not feed into the negative, each day brings you one step closer to success. Do not give up!

LINDA'S STORY:
DEALING WITH A NEUROLOGICAL DISEASE

Meet Linda

Linda is a 47-year-old mother of two daughters. She works as a school teacher and holistic nutritionist, and she is an avid marathon runner.

What is the significant event or situation that changed your life?

In February 2000, I woke up one morning to my daughter's cry, but when I went to greet her, my words didn't come out properly. It was like I had marbles in my mouth. I rushed to the mirror, and the right side of my face was paralyzed. *Oh my God, I had a stroke!* I immediately called my GP and rushed to see her with my daughter. After her examination and confirmation that it actually wasn't a stroke, she referred me to the University of Western Ontario Hospital. She also called my husband and instructed him to meet me there. I was admitted at 10 a.m., and, after numerous scans, probes, neurological tests, bloodwork and then an MRI, at 10 p.m., the intern walked into my room and said: "You have MS."

The first thought that entered my mind was the image of a wheelchair. Why? Because when I was in Grade 3, our school participated in a read-a-thon to raise money for MS. The lady who came to talk to us was in a wheelchair.

How did you decide to use this event, not to be a victim, but to grow from the situation?

At the time of my diagnosis, I was training for my first marathon. I had completed my first 19km. I was so proud of myself, but now this—now MS. I wasn't too sure what to do. Should I continue or should I stop? On the one hand, research was suggesting that strenuous activities should be avoided because it could cause a relapse and make my condition worse. But, then I thought of my hero, Terry Fox. He never quit. Despite his cancer, he ran a marathon a day for 143 days through Canada's Atlantic Provinces, Quebec and Ontario. Sure, I could've chosen to remain a victim to my illness, but I chose to do whatever it took to overcome it.

Completing my first marathon in May 2001 on Mother's Day was a life-changing event for me. It gave the strength I needed to prove to myself that I can get through this, that my body can do it despite my chronic illness.

What are the tools that you use and the mindset that you created to thrive?

In order to achieve the best optimal health for me, I invest a lot of time in myself and use different health modalities. I am very committed to investing in my health. My health comes first, although this is sometimes difficult for people to understand because I look fine on the outside. I wish I could share with them that I look fine on the outside, but the MS ghost is always there harassing me.

Positive affirmations…first and foremost, I thank my body every day, every morning upon waking, for being healthy and for allowing me to be able to exercise. I also nourish myself with healing foods every day that satisfy and totally heal my mind and body. And, I love to run. Many people say that running is exhausting, but for me, running is energizing. It gives me life, and it gives me hope that I will get through this one day at a time.

When I was initially diagnosed, I was told that if I didn't take any medications, after 10 years I would be walking with a cane, and after 15 years, I would be in a wheelchair. Now it has been almost 20 years, and I set my mind to do 20 marathons within 20 years; I have just completed my 18th marathon in September 2016.

I practice yoga, I do daily meditations and I read an affirmation card every morning to find inner strength.

Looking back at the situation now, is there anything you would have done differently?

No, I don't think so. MS has actually taught me many life lessons. The most important is the importance of loving yourself. I strongly believe that I would not be in the state of health that I am now had I not taken my health into my own hands by loving myself, eating healing foods, moving, loving, thinking happy thoughts and doing anything and everything possible to reduce my stress level. I live by the quote, "Take care of your body. It's the only place you have to live," by Jim Rohn.

If you had one lesson to give to someone else with MS, what would it be?

I strongly believe in Hippocrates' wisdom: *"Let food be thy medicine and medicine be thy food."* We need to follow Hippocrates' advice and remember the critical role of food in managing chronic illnesses.

How has this event shaped you into who you are today?

I discovered that we have the power to heal and that our thoughts are just as powerful as the food we put in our bodies. I am a marathoner. I'm not sure I would have had the drive to run all those kilometers without having MS. I appreciate life every day, knowing that tomorrow could be different. I try to appreciate every little moment I spend with my daughters and my husband. I have learned the importance of loving myself. I used to run away from food because I feared getting fat. I now run toward food and embrace it, knowing that it nourishes my body at the cellular level. I now help people living with MS to develop healthier eating habits to better manage their disease.

When I was first diagnosed with MS, my mother-in-law gave me a window pendant that said, *"Things happen for a reason. You just have to believe."* I believe that I continue to live a healthy life—despite living with the challenges of MS—to inspire others living with MS.

CHRISTINE'S STORY:

THRIVING AFTER A CAR ACCIDENT AND MANAGING CHRONIC PAIN

Meet Christine

Christine is a 50-year-old public servant. She is also a certified Reiki master and fitness enthusiast.

What is the significant event or situation that changed your life?

In 2008, I was involved in a car accident. I suffered from serious whiplash and back injuries. My injuries resulted in much more than pain and discomfort. Unable to really move, I gained more than 30 lbs. and continued to gain weight until I reached 221 lbs within three months. I spent years trying to regain my mobility and dealing with constant pain. Little by little, things improved, but the weight never came off. One day in 2013, I told my mom that I wasn't feeling well. I was experiencing chest pains and acid reflux. That night, we talked about how amazing we had both felt the last time we were at a healthier weight.

At that moment, it dawned on me that my biggest fear was to find myself being led down the same path my parents took—both had open-heart surgery due to poor lifestyle choices. Deep down I knew I had to do something—but what? The next morning, as I walked into my kitchen, I had an epiphany and said out loud, "I want to eat healthy!" This is when my journey began, and I have not looked back since.

How did you decide to use this event, not to be a victim, but to grow from the situation?

When you find yourself not feeling well and wondering how much longer you have to live, it puts a different perspective on your life. Facing my fears with sheer determination is what pushed me on my journey. Changing my lifestyle and adapting to a whole new way of eating was not easy, but as the weight came off, I gained confidence in the new person I was becoming. This motivated me to continue and persist in being successful. With renewed energy, I started setting new goals for myself. I started running obstacle races and smaller local races. I even signed up for two half-marathons. Crazy, right? There was no stopping me. I was determined to be fit and as healthy as I could be.

What are the tools that you use and the mindset that you created to thrive?

Well, I began searching online for anything that could help me. Without really knowing what I was looking for, I found the movies *The Secret* and *I am, That I Am*. They both helped me understand that I need to change my mindset and have a positive approach to life.

Continuing my search online, I found all types of information that brought me to self-love, getting rid of negative self-talk, using positive affirmations and creating healthy habits—in terms of both nutrition and exercise. The website cleaneating.com became my bible for eating healthy. I would choose two or three recipes, make them on the weekend, and those where my meals for the rest of the week. Meal preparation became very important. I also found a ton of fitness sites online that helped keep me motivated.

Looking back at the situation now, is there anything you would have done differently?

Absolutely not—what happened to me changed me to who I am today. It was my wake-up call to do something about my life. This car accident, believe it or not, saved my life! It stopped me in my tracks and made me learn more about myself. It has shown me that anything is possible if you set your mind to it. You can pursue any dreams you want. I knew I was already surrounded by an amazing circle of family and friends, but I have also met the most wonderful new people—who I am now proud to call friends. They all supported and helped me to continue on my journey. I guess you can say that I am rich in friendship.

The realization that I did not feel well led me to pursue a journey I never thought possible. Within no time, I was running races, half-marathons and finding myself booking friends for runs and other types of physical activities. How amazing is that? The way I view food now is entirely different. I used to eat my emotions. Now, I eat to provide my body with the energy it needs and eat until I'm full.

If you had to give one lesson to someone going through a similar situation, what would it be?

Believe in yourself. Do not despair or give up. If I can do this, so can you, as I've spent most of my adult life overweight. Everything is a process, and it's about dealing with one issue at a time. This experience led me to discover more about myself than I ever thought possible—but mostly to find out the reason why I was overweight and what kept me overweight all my life.

As I started to change into a more positive person, my perspective on life changed, and I viewed the world in a wholly different way. Being healthy and getting fit became a priority. I searched the Internet for any information I could find.

Let go of the past and look at what a bright future is ahead of you. I'm not saying it's going to be easy. For me, it was really hard at times, especially the psychological aspect of being afraid of regaining the weight back. Taking baby steps is what gave me the courage to take on this journey. As I learned and adapted to a new lifestyle, I grew into a new, healthier version of me.

Set goals for yourself and reach each milestone with renewed determination. Believe in yourself and your ability to succeed. You got this!

How has this event shaped you into who you are today?

Today, I am on top of the world! It's amazing what repurposing your life, making goals and enjoying precious moments can do to a person. This new me now plans outings with the purpose of exercising, without making it look like exercise. Transitioning into newly formed habits has completely changed my life. For once in my life, I can actually say that I am truly happy and blessed.

I no longer eat foods that will make me feel unhealthy. It's amazing how you feel when you eat healthy foods that provide the energy you need to enjoy your day. In the past, I used to dream of running races and being an athlete. Now I know that whatever I set my mind to, I can achieve. The funny thing is that I feel better today than I did in my 30s. Hitting the big 50 this year made me realize that life is meant to be lived and enjoyed to the best of my abilities. When you feed your body healthy foods and ensure your body is in motion, you are guaranteeing many more years of happy living. The question is, aren't you worth it?

Today I am determined to be healthy and am definitely more health-conscious about what it takes to succeed. I now understand the importance and need to eat healthy and exercise. Watch out, this girl is on fire!

INSPIRED YET?

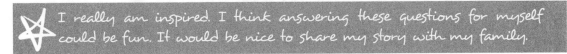

I really am inspired. I think answering these questions for myself could be fun. It would be nice to share my story with my family.

Though each of these stories is different, all share a similar message: Though you may not be able to change your situation, you can change the way you react to it. You are in control of your future. You can decide to be a victim, or you can commit to moving forward. There may be bad days, but that's OK. Be patient with yourself. Show yourself the same love and compassion you would show a friend going through a similar situation.

Each of the ladies interviewed chose to *live*. For every sad moment in their lives, there was a happy one. This collection of moments brought them closer to who they are today. Not one of the women would choose a different path. Given the opportunity, would you?

Now's the time to write your story. Always remember that your story is what you make of it. You are the author of your own life!

The following diagram shows examples of health habits with corresponding hack levels. To download the *Hack Your Health Habits Worksheet*, visit

www.hackyourhealthhabits.com/worksheets

READY #HEALTHHACKER?
EXAMPLES OF LEVEL 1, 2 AND 3 HACKS FOR THIS CHAPTER

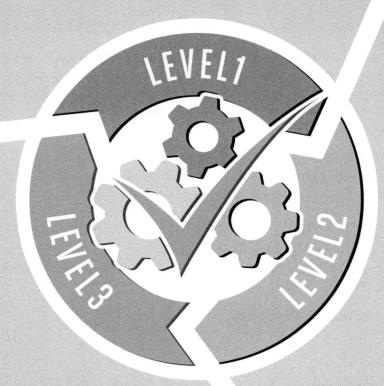

✓ Make a list of significant events that have occurred in your life—whether good or bad—and make note as to how they shaped you into who you are now.

✓ Operate with the belief that you are in control of your life. Write your own story and choose to change your mindset toward challenge and adversity in the future.

✓ Like the five women did, write down your own story. Does your story empower you or disempower you?

HACK YOUR HEALTH PROGRESS

||||||||||||||||||||||||||||||||||||||||||||||||||||||||||||||||||||||||||||

CHAPTER 62

CONCLUSION

Congratulations, you did it! You made it through the 12 sections of the book and are now better equipped to get hacking; a pretty big achievement, if you ask me. It doesn't matter if you read the book in one big sweep or waited to implement the *HACK* exercises later. Either way, you may feel a little overwhelmed after all that we covered. Remember, as the expression goes: *"Rome wasn't built in one day."* Yes, anything worth doing in life, indeed, takes time.

This book was meant to put together an all-in-one resource that simplifies more than 30 years of my own knowledge and experience in my quest to be the healthiest version of myself and help my patients in the process. My aim was to create awareness on health topics that may not currently be mainstream or that are up and coming. Once aware, you can now make the decision to see if you need to dig deeper in the areas that are relevant to you and your health. It is said that knowledge is power, but I have to say that I would add to that statement that the application of knowledge is power. That is why the entire book revolves around the health hacks. I wanted this book to be about information, but also about the execution of that information.

I want to close off the book by bringing to your attention a few fundamental key points for you to reflect on as you implement the different levels of hacks and improve your health habits.

First, it is important to envision the bigger picture when it comes to health. Health and wellbeing are a sum of your daily habits, and it reaches further than just the physical. Health and wellbeing refers to the cohesion of the physical, mental, emotional and spiritual states of a person being in alignment. Everything, from the foods you eat, the thoughts you think, what you choose to expose yourself to, the amount of rest and rejuvenation you choose to give to yourself—they all reflect the relationship you choose to have with yourself. We cannot pay attention to only one aspect of health and expect to feel whole. My entire philosophy with this book was to emphasize the importance of looking at an individual in his or her entirety.

To continue that thought, I would like to emphasize that, in great part, *health is a choice*—yes, there are always exceptions. But, at the end of the day, you choose what foods will fuel your body, what exercises will keep you fit, and what activities will keep your mind sharp. You have the power to lead a healthy and vibrant life, no matter where you are on your health journey. These choices can sometimes be difficult to make, as it can be hard to break free of old habits, even if we know the new ones are for our greater good.

I would like to remind you that, when hacking your health habits, it's OK to start small. No individual is in the same place, physically or mentally. You may be doing great in one area of your life and not so great in another area. Do what feels right for you. Whether this book helps you take better control of your health by implementing two habits or two hundred, I'm rooting for you. Small steps lead to big changes. Have fun hacking your habits, experiment and don't be scared to try new things!

Next, it's important to remember that health isn't a destination, it's a journey. It's something that you have to persistently strive toward. No matter how hard you try, you may encounter a few roadblocks along the way. It's important to not let this deter you from continuing on a healthier path. The goal is not perfection, it's progress. If you stray from your goal, brush yourself off and keep going. We can all be making some changes to lead healthier lives. Think of what your life could be in one year from now, in five years, or twenty years, if you implement the changes you set out to do?

"Once you have mastered time, you will understand how true it is that most people overestimate what they can accomplish in a year, and underestimate what they can achieve in a decade."

—TONY ROBBINS

And, lastly, science and research are constantly evolving. Think back to what your parents thought was healthy, and what we now know—it's leaps-and-bounds different! While I'm very confident in the information I've shared throughout the book, the science surrounding it may, and most likely will one day evolve. I believe that with any piece of information you encounter, it's always important to do your own research and come to your own conclusions, especially in relation to your health. As I've said many times throughout the book, there is no "one-size-fits-all" solution. Take what you have learned, and figure out and decide what's best for you.

If you are not sure where to start or need a helping hand, I've created an online membership site based on *Hack Your Health Habits* that will support you in transforming your health. The program provides a practical approach to the topics we discussed in the book and is filled with tips and tricks to help you succeed on your health journey. For more information on the *Hack Your Health Habits Mastery Program*, visit: www.hackyourhealthhabits.com/masteryprogram

I wish you all the best in your journey to better health and well-being.

Let's get hacking!

Dr. Nathalie

CATHERINE'S CONCLUDING THOUGHTS

I may be finished with the book, but I feel like my journey has just begun. Health is important to me. I value and cherish it, largely because I want to be around for my family as long as possible. More than that, I want to instill healthy habits in my daughters now, so that they can also lead vibrant lives for years to come.

After reading Hack Your Health Habits, I feel like I have a better handle on my health, overall... like, I can make better choices for myself and for my family. It was nice to see that there are a lot of things that I've been doing right. That being said, there is still so much I can do to take my health to the next level. I've used the hack worksheets to note down the hacks that I want to tackle from each chapter and am ready to start putting them into action! I'm going to

> take my time and implement them week by week so that these hacks become permanent lifestyle changes. I won't lie, I'm both nervous and excited; but I know that the effort will be well worth it in the end.

And one last thing, don't forget to take the Health Currency Questionnaire once again! I am willing to bet that you will be "worth" a *lot* more now that you have read and implemented what you have learned in this book!

To complete the Health Currency Questionnaire again, please go to

www.hackyourhealthhabits.com/healthcurrencyquiz

THE HEALTH HACKER MANIFESTO

I am a Health Hacker.

I define my own destiny.

I am in control of my health and take full responsibility for my actions.

I focus on prevention, not on reaction.

I dig deep to find the cause of my problems, rather than solely mask "symptoms."

I am constantly learning and trying new things to improve my mind, body and soul.

I strive to make the best decisions for myself and my family and encourage those around me to become the best versions of themselves possible.

I use critical thinking to assess what I am being fed by mainstream media and trust my inner voice over popular opinion.

I enjoy life.

I choose happiness now, not someday.

I live life by design and not by default.

I create my future.

I am a Health Hacker.

ABOUT THE AUTHOR

Dr. Nathalie Beauchamp B.Sc., D.C. IFMCP, strives to lead through educating, and helping people empower themselves to live their best, most healthy and fulfilling life. She believes that everyone has the potential to live a life of vitality—which is why she is dedicated to educating her patients and followers on the power of natural health solutions. Having overcome a serious eating disorder in her teenage years, she recognizes the importance of a healthy lifestyle as an absolute necessity for success in both our personal and professional lives.

Born in Montebello, Quebec, Dr. Nathalie's professional expertise in the area of fitness, nutrition, lifestyle and wellness began in 1996 when she graduated from the Canadian Memorial Chiropractic College in Toronto as a Doctor of Chiropractic. Prior to this, she completed a Bachelor of Science Degree in the field of Human Kinetics at the University of Ottawa. Recently, she also became certified as a Functional Medicine Practitioner through the Institute of Functional Medicine.

Beyond all of this, she is a former professional natural bodybuilder/figure competitor, wellness consultant and lecturer, business mentor, television and radio personality, international motivational speaker and co-author of the published book—Wellness On The Go: Take the Plunge - It's Your Life!

Dr. Nathalie has been in private practice for over 20 years as owner and operator of Santé Chiropractic and Wellness Centre, a multidisciplinary clinic in Ottawa, Canada that is truly a one-stop-shop for health. Santé offers a wide variety of services including chiropractic care, acupuncture, registered massage therapy, holistic nutrition, functional nutrition and lifestyle coaching, high-quality nutraceuticals and physiotherapy. The mission of this integrative clinic is to provide community members with everything they need to lead a healthy and fulfilling life. Dr. Nathalie aims to deliver outstanding natural wellness care and provide the most cutting-edge knowledge and resources to help guide her patients on their quest for greater health.

Looking forward, Dr. Nathalie aims to have her knowledge and expertise in the areas of health, lifestyle and leadership extend across multiple platforms and in turn have greater impact on the lives of people globally. In addition, she hopes to help lead a movement of collaborative healthcare practitioners that will improve the current state of our healthcare system. Ultimately, true success in enhancing healthcare will be obtained when both doctors and patients are empowered and work in partnership.

NOTES

SECTION 1: GET MOTIVATED, ORGANIZED AND PRODUCTIVE TO TAKE YOUR HEALTH HABITS TO THE NEXT LEVEL

Chapter 1: Habits—You Are What You Do—The Key to Unlocking Your Health Habits

General References:

- Duhigg, C. (2015). *The Power of Habit: Why We Do What We Do in Life and Business*. Cork: IDreamBooks Inc.
- Parts of the Brain - Memory & the Brain - The Human Memory. (n.d.). Retrieved June 26, 2016, from http://www.human-memory.net/brain_parts.html
- Davison, G. C. (2006). *Abnormal psychology, 10th edition*. Hoboken, NJ: Wiley.
- Powell, R. A., Honey, P. L., & Symbaluk, D. G. (n.d.). *Introduction To Learning and Behavior* (5th ed.).
- Barnes, J. (2014). *Mental toughness for peak performance, leadership development, and success: how to maximize your focus, motivation, confidence, self-discipline, willpower, and mind power in sports, business, or health*. Personal Potential Books.
- Cohen, P. (2012). *Habit Busting*. Luton: Andrews UK.

Chapter 2: Motivation—Are You Falling Short?

General References:

- Barnes, J. (2014). *Mental toughness for peak performance, leadership development, and success: how to maximize your focus, motivation, confidence, self-discipline, willpower, and mind power in sports, business, or health*. Personal Potential Books.
- Deckers, L. (2016). *Motivation: biological, psychological, and environmental*. London: Routledge.
- Sinek, S. (2013). *Start with why: how great leaders inspire everyone to take action*. London: Portfolio/Penguin.

Chapter 3: Productivity and Energy Management—Are You Productive or Just Busy?

In-text citations:

1. Bailey, C. (2016). *The productivity project*. London: Piatkus, Little, Brown Book Group.

General References:

- Szabo, S., Tache, Y., & Somogyi, A. (2012). The legacy of Hans Selye and the origins of stress research: A retrospective 75 years after his landmark brief "Letter" to the Editor of Nature. *Stress,15(5)*, 472-478. doi:10.3109/10253890.2012.710919
- 80% of Smartphone Users Check Their Phones Before Brushing Their Teeth … And Other Hot Topics. (2014, December 15). Retrieved June 19, 2017, from https://blogs.constantcontact.com/smartphone-usage-statistics/
- ATUS News Releases. (n.d.). Retrieved July 15, 2016, from https://www.bls.gov/tus/
- Loehr, J., & Tony, S. (2009). *The Power of Full Engagement*. Shubhi Publications.
- Tracy, B., & Ismail, L. U. (2013). *Eat that frog*. Batu Caves, Selangor: PTS Professional.
- Myers , D. G. (2007). *Psychology* (10 ed.). Holland , Michigan: Hope College.
- Selye, Hans. *Stress Without Distress*. New York: Lippencott, 1974

Chapter 4: Personal Prime Time—Are You Setting the Stage for Your Day?

In-text citations:

1. Lee, K. (2016, February 01). The Best Time to Write and Get Ideas, According to Science. Retrieved August 05, 2017, from https://blog.bufferapp.com/the-best-time-to-write-and-get-ideas

General References:

- Bartram, Sean, and Matt Bowen. *High intensity interval training for women: burn more fat in less time with HIIT workouts you can do anywhere*. London: Dorling Kindersley Limited, 2015. Print.
- Kahneman, D., Diener, E., & Schwarz, N. (1999). *Well-being: the foundations of hedonic psychology*. New York: Russell Sage Foundation.

SECTION 2: GET BACK TO BASICS—UNDERSTAND THE FOODS TO CONSUME TO KEEP YOUR BODY PERFORMING AT ITS BEST

Chapter 5: Fats—They're Not All Bad!

In-text citations:

1. https://www.ncbi.nlm.nih.gov/pubmed/12442909
2. Kolata, G. (2016, April 03). Dashing Hopes, Study Shows a Cholesterol Drug Had No Effect on Heart Health. Retrieved September 09, 2017, from https://www.nytimes.com/2016/04/04/health/dashing-hopes-study-shows-cholesterol-drug-has-no-benefits.html

General References:

- Hyman, M. (2016). *Eat fat, get thin: why the fat we eat is the key to sustained weight loss and vibrant health*. New York: Little, Brown and Company.
- Bubbs, M. (2015). *The Paleo Project: the 21st century guide to looking leaner, getting stronger and living longer*. Victoria, BC: Friesen Press.
- Naughton , T. (Director). (2009). *Fat Head* [Video file]. United States. Retrieved October 30, 2014.
- Cholesterol Myths You Need to Stop Believing. (n.d.). Retrieved May 5, 2016, from http://articles.mercola.com/sites/articles/archive/2016/04/20/cholesterol-myths.aspx
- Medscape Log In. (n.d.). Retrieved February 26, 2017, from http://www.medscape.com/viewarticle/832841
- Grapeseed Oil: Is It Healthy Or Not? (2015, November 15). Retrieved June 6, 2016, from https://draxe.com/grapeseed-oil/
- Statin side effects: Weigh the benefits and risks. (n.d.). Retrieved February 26, 2017, from http://www.mayoclinic.org/diseases-conditions/high-blood-cholesterol/in-depth/statin-side-effects/art-20046013

- Wood, J., Enser, M., Fisher, A., Nute, G., Sheard, P., Richardson, R., . . . Whittington, F. (2008). Fat deposition, fatty acid composition and meat quality: A review. *Meat Science,78*(4), 343-358. doi:10.1016/j.meatsci.2007.07.019
- Inflammation Affects Every Aspect of Your Health. (n.d.). Retrieved February 26, 2017, from http://articles.mercola.com/sites/articles/archive/2013/03/07/inflammation-triggers-disease-symptoms.aspx

Chapter 6: Carbohydrates—What's The Deal?

In-text citations:

1. Bubbs, M. (2015). *The Paleo Project: the 21st century guide to looking leaner, getting stronger and living longer.* Victoria, BC: Friesen Press.
2. Management of type 2 diabetes. (2002). *Changing Therapies in Type 2 Diabetes,* 1-24. doi:10.1201/b14327-2
3. Boyd, D. B. (2003, December). Insulin and cancer. Retrieved September 09, 2017, from https://www.ncbi.nlm.nih.gov/pubmed/14713323
4. Increasing Fiber Intake. (n.d.). Retrieved September 09, 2017, from https://www.ucsfhealth.org/education/increasing_fiber_intake/
5. Wescott, T. (2016, February 03). Carb Cycling For Fat Loss. Retrieved November 8, 2016, from http://www.bodybuilding.com/fun/wescott4.htm

General References:

- Glycemic Index Deception Finally Understood. (n.d.). Retrieved September 09, 2017, from http://articles.mercola.com/sites/articles/archive/2006/03/23/glycemic-index-deception-finally-understood.aspx
- B. (2016, May 26). Hormonal Regulation of Metabolism - Boundless Open Textbook. Retrieved September 09, 2017, from https://www.boundless.com/biology/textbooks/boundless-biology-textbook/the-endocrine-system-37/regulation-of-body-processes-212/hormonal-regulation-of-metabolism-799-12035/
- Can Cutting Carbohydrates Out of Your Diet Increase Lifespan? (n.d.). Retrieved August 14, 2016, from http://articles.mercola.com/sites/articles/archive/2010/12/06/cutting-carbohydrates-from-your-diet-can-make-you-live-longer.aspx
- Dietary fiber: Essential for a healthy diet. (n.d.). Retrieved November 26, 2016, from http://www.mayoclinic.org/healthy-lifestyle/nutrition-and-healthy-eating/in-depth/fiber/art-20043983
- Hyman, M. (2016). *Eat fat, get thin: why the fat we eat is the key to sustained weight loss and vibrant health.* New York: Little, Brown and Company.
- Martinez, E. (2015, January 28). Nutrients Found in Foods With Complex Carbohydrates. Retrieved November 26, 2016, from http://www.livestrong.com/article/527610-nutrients-found-in-foods-with-complex-carbohydrates/

Chapter 7: Protein—You Do Need Some!

In-text citations:

1. Bubbs, M. (2015). *The Paleo Project: the 21st century guide to looking leaner, getting stronger and living longer.* Victoria, BC: Friesen Press.
2. Are You Sabotaging Your Health by Excessive Protein Intake? (n.d.). Retrieved August 28, 2016, from http://articles.mercola.com/sites/articles/archive/2015/12/21/excessive-protein-intake.aspx
3. Making The World Safe From Superbugs - Consumer Reports. (n.d.). Retrieved February 26, 2017, from http://www.consumerreports.org/cro/health/making-the-world-safe-from-superbugs/index.htm?utm_source=hootsuite
4. Why Grass-Fed Beef Costs More - Consumer Reports. (n.d.). Retrieved May 13, 2016, from http://www.consumerreports.org/cro/magazine/2015/08/why-grass-fed-beef-costs-more/index.htm
5. 9 Things You Should Know About Farmed Fish. (n.d.). Retrieved February 22, 2017, from http://articles.mercola.com/sites/articles/archive/2013/12/21/9-farmed-fish-facts.aspx

General References:

- Brown, B., & Hussey, R. (2016, July 07). Plant-Based Protein Supplements vs Whey (Infographic). Retrieved August 26, 2016, from http://www.artofwellbeing.com/2015/10/04/plant-based-protein-supplements/
- The Dirty Underbelly of the US Dairy Industry. (n.d.). Retrieved October 23, 2016, from http://articles.mercola.com/sites/articles/archive/2016/09/06/dairy-industry.aspx?utm_source=dnl&utm_medium=email&utm_content=art1&utm_campaign=20160906Z1_C&et_cid=DM115936&et_rid=1652871470#_edn1
- Fergusson, K. (2016, April 20). Organic vs. Free Range vs. Cage Free Eggs. Retrieved February 23, 2017, from https://delishably.com/dairy/Organic-Eggs-vs-Free-Range-and-Cage-Free-Alternatives
- What You Need to Know About Farmed Fish. (n.d.). Retrieved February 22, 2017, from http://articles.mercola.com/sites/articles/archive/2008/12/02/what-you-need-to-know-about-farmed-fish.aspx
- What Makes a Chicken Free-Range? Caged vs. Free-Range Eggs. (n.d.). Retrieved February 23, 2017, from http://articles.mercola.com/sites/articles/archive/2012/03/19/caged-vs-free-range-chicken-eggs.aspx
- Schuna, C. (2015, April 17). Pea Protein vs. Whey Protein. Retrieved August 26, 2016, from http://www.livestrong.com/article/281176-pea-protein-vs-whey-protein/

Chapter 8: Food Labels and Additives—Do You Know What You Are Eating?

In-text citations:

1. Are bagels and breakfast cereal as bad as cigarettes? Report shows they can raise risk of lung cancer by 49%! (n.d.). Retrieved September 09, 2017, from http://articles.mercola.com/sites/articles/archive/2016/03/23/ultra-processed-foods.aspx
2. WHO guideline : sugar consumption recommendation. (n.d.). Retrieved September 09, 2017, from http://www.who.int/mediacentre/news/releases/2015/sugar-guideline/en/

General References:

- Juntti, M. (2014, February 03). The Most Misleading Health Food Claims. Retrieved February 26, 2017, from http://www.mensjournal.com/expert-advice/the-most-misleading-health-food-claims-20140203/made-with-real-fruit
- Decoding the Nutrition Label. (n.d.). Retrieved August 5, 2016, from https://www.eatrightontario.ca/en/Articles/Nutrition-Labelling/Decoding-the-Nutrition-Label.aspx
- How to Read Food Labels Without Being Tricked. (2016, July 27). Retrieved August 5, 2016, from https://authoritynutrition.com/how-to-read-food-labels/
- Your Complete Guide to Reading Food Labels. (2015, May 25). Retrieved August 5, 2016, from http://www.besthealthmag.ca/best-eats/nutrition/your-complete-guide-to-reading-food-labels/
- Processed Foods: What's OK, What to Avoid. (n.d.). Retrieved February 5, 2016, from http://www.eatright.org/resource/food/nutrition/nutrition-facts-and-food-labels/avoiding-processed-foods

- The Shocking Truth About How Much Sugar You're Eating. (2016, June 17). Retrieved April 21, 2017, from http://www.rodalesorganiclife.com/wellbeing/the-shocking-truth-about-how-much-sugar-youre-eating

Chapter 9: Organic—Yes, It's Worth It!

In-text citations:

1. Analysis: Organic Food Really Is Healthier. (n.d.). Retrieved October 16, 2016, from http://articles.mercola.com/sites/articles/archive/2014/07/29/organic-food-healthier.aspx
2. Government of Canada,Canadian Food Inspection Agency,Food Labelling and Claims Directorate. (2016, July 04). Organic Products. Retrieved October 16, 2016, from http://www.inspection.gc.ca/food/organic-products/eng/1300139461200/1300140373901
3. Worthington, V. (2001). Nutritional Quality of Organic Versus Conventional Fruits, Vegetables, and Grains. *The Journal of Alternative and Complementary Medicine, 7*(2), 161-173. doi:10.1089/107555301750164244
4. The Haughley Experiment. (1957). *Nature, 179*(4558), 514-514. doi:10.1038/179514d0
5. Grainfed versus Grass Fed Beef, and why it matters! (n.d.). Retrieved June 27, 2016, from http://www.grass-fed-solutions.com/grassfed-beef.html
6. Hormones and antibiotics in food production. (n.d.). Retrieved February 27, 2017, from https://www.eatrightontario.ca/en/Articles/Farming-Food-production/Hormones-and-antibiotics-in-food-production.aspx
7. Farm, C. C. (n.d.). Retrieved September 09, 2017, from http://www.ccmof.com/ccmof_website_008.htm
8. Chance, G. W. (2001). Environmental contaminants and childrens health: Cause for concern, time for action. *Paediatrics & Child Health, 6*(10), 731-743. doi:10.1093/pch/6.10.731
9. Warning labels for safe stuff. (2013, November 02). Retrieved September 09, 2017, from https://www.economist.com/news/united-states/21588898-one-way-or-another-labelling-gm-food-may-be-coming-america-warning-labels-safe
10. Maternal and fetal exposure to pesticides associated to genetically modified foods in Eastern Townships of Quebec, Canada. (n.d.). Retrieved June 27, 2016, from https://www.ncbi.nlm.nih.gov/pubmed/2133867
11. E. (n.d.). EWG's Shopper's Guide to Pesticides in Produce. Retrieved October 17, 2016, from https://www.ewg.org/foodnews/dirty_dozen_list.php
12. Seafood Guide. (2017, January 18). Retrieved February 27, 2017, from http://www.foodandwaterwatch.org/live-healthy/seafood-guide

General References:

- Samsel, A., & Seneff, S. (2013). Glyphosate, pathways to modern diseases II: Celiac sprue and gluten intolerance. *Interdisciplinary Toxicology, 6*(4). doi:10.2478/intox-2013-0026
- Alavanja, M. C. (2009). Introduction: Pesticides Use and Exposure, Extensive Worldwide. *Reviews on Environmental Health, 24*(4). doi:10.1515/reveh.2009.24.4.303
- Martin, A. (2006, November 27). Free or Farmed, When Is a Fish Really Organic? Retrieved September 09, 2017, from http://www.nytimes.com/2006/11/28/business/28fish.html
- Stephanie Seneff. (n.d.). Retrieved February 27, 2017, from https://people.csail.mit.edu/seneff/
- Samsel, A., & Seneff, S. (2013). Glyphosate's Suppression of Cytochrome P450 Enzymes and Amino Acid Biosynthesis by the Gut Microbiome: Pathways to Modern Diseases. *Entropy, 15*(4), 1416-1463. doi:10.3390/e15041416
- How to Bring Minerals Back Into the Soil and Food Supply. (2016, June 17). Retrieved October 10, 2016, from http://www.wakingtimes.com/2014/05/26/bring-minerals-back-soil-food-supply/
- Vauzour, D., Kerr, J., & Czank, C. (2014). Plant Polyphenols as Dietary Modulators of Brain Functions. *Polyphenols in Human Health and Disease, 357-370*. doi:10.1016/b978-0-12-398456-2.00027-x
- Meyer, S. (1999). The use of drugs in food animals : benefits and risks, compiled by the Committee on Drug Use in Food Animals, National Research Council and Institute of Medicine, USA : book review. *Journal of the South African Veterinary Association, 70*(3). doi:10.4102/jsava.v70i3.779
- The Organic Debate - fruits and vegetables you should eat organic. (2010, October 31). Retrieved October 16, 2016, from https://drnathaliebeauchamp.com/nutrition/the-organic-debate-fruits-and-vegetables-you-should-eat-organic/
- Sen. Donna Nesselbush: three quarters of processed foods have genetically modified organisms. (n.d.). Retrieved February 27, 2017, from http://www.politifact.com/rhode-island/statements/2015/mar/22/donna-nesselbush/sen-donna-nesselbush-three-quarters-processed-food/

Chapter 10: Phytonutrients and Antioxidants—Are You Eating by Color?

In-text citations:

1. These Foods, Herb, Spices & Oils are Absolutely Bursting with Antioxidants. (2017, January 24). Retrieved February 27, 2017, from https://draxe.com/top-10-high-antioxidant-foods
2. Institute of Functional Medicine. (2015). *The Phytonutrient Spectrum* [Brochure].

General References:

- Holford, P. (2012). *The optimum nutrition bible*. London: Piatkus.
- Lobo, V., Patil, A., Phatak, A., & Chandra, N. (2010). Free radicals, antioxidants and functional foods: Impact on human health. *Pharmacognosy Reviews, 4*(8), 118. doi:10.4103/0973-7847.70902
- ORAC: Scoring Antioxidants? - Dr. Weil. (2016, August 05). Retrieved December 27, 2016, from https://www.drweil.com/vitamins-supplements-herbs/vitamins/orac-scoring-antioxidants/
- Carlsen, M. H., Halvorsen, B. L., Holte, K., Bøhn, S. K., Dragland, S., Sampson, L., . . . Blomhoff, R. (2010). The total antioxidant content of more than 3100 foods, beverages, spices, herbs and supplements used worldwide. *Nutrition Journal, 9*(1). doi:10.1186/1475-2891-9-3
- Pounis, G., Costanzo, S., Giuseppe, R. D., Lucia, F. D., Santimone, I., Sciarretta, A., . . . Iacoviello, L. (2012). Consumption of healthy foods at different content of antioxidant vitamins and phytochemicals and metabolic risk factors for cardiovascular disease in men and women of the Moli-sani study. *European Journal of Clinical Nutrition, 67*(2), 207-213. doi:10.1038/ejcn.2012.201
- Mirmiran, P., Bahadoran, Z., Moslehi, N., Bastan, S., & Azizi, F. (2015). Colors of fruits and vegetables and 3-year changes of cardiometabolic risk factors in adults: Tehran lipid and glucose study. *European Journal of Clinical Nutrition, 69*(11), 1215-1219. doi:10.1038/ejcn.2015.49

SECTION 3: GET FUELED WITH THE RIGHT FOODS AND FIGURE OUT THE DIET THAT WORKS FOR YOU

Chapter 11: Nutrition—Who Should You Believe?

In-text citations:

1. Mortillaro, N. (2016, October 24). Canada's Food Guide: What the government is changing to help Canadians eat better. Retrieved September 09, 2017, from http://globalnews.ca/news/3021864/canadas-food-guide-what-the-government-is-changing-to-help-canadians-eat-better/

2. The china study. (n.d.). Retrieved September 09, 2017, from https://issuu.com/augustinechalissery/docs/the_china_study

3. How Our Government Made Us Fat and Sick! (2016, March 07). Retrieved August 6, 2016, from http://drhyman.com/blog/2016/02/26/how-our-government-made-us-fat-and-sick/

4. Jones, D. D. (2014, October 28). Milk or Green Leafy Vegetables: Which is Better for Calcium Absorption? Retrieved February 27, 2017, from http://www.empowher.com/bones-amp-joints/content/milk-or-green-leafy-vegetables-which-better-calcium-absorption

General References:

- Revolvy, L. (n.d.). "Dietary Goals for the United States" on Revolvy.com. Retrieved September 09, 2017, from https://topics.revolvy.com/topic/Dietary%20Goals%20for%20the%20United%20States&item_type=topic
- The Effect Of Dietary Vegetable Fat On The Serum Lipids. (2009). *Nutrition Reviews,13*(1), 8-9. doi:10.1111/j.1753-4887.1955.tb03332.x

Chapter 12: Diets 101—Which One is Right for You?

General References:

1. Christianson, A. (2015). *The adrenal reset diet: strategically cycle carbs and proteins to lose weight, balance hormones, and move from stressed to thriving.* New York: Harmony.

2. Childs, V. (2015). *Hormone reset diet: balance hormones, recharge health and lose weight effortlessly!: hormone reset diet recipes included!* United States: Great Reads Publishing, LLC.

3. Bubbs, M. (2015). *The Paleo Project: the 21st century guide to looking leaner, getting stronger and living longer.* Victoria, BC: Friesen Press.

4. Davis, W. (2015). *Wheat belly: lose the wheat, lose the weight and find your path back to health.* London: Harper Thorsons.

5. Moore, J., & Westman, E. C. (2014). *Keto clarity: your definitive guide to the benefits of a low-carb, high-fat diet.* Las Vegas: Victory Belt Publishing, Inc.

6. Why I am a Pegan – or Paleo-Vegan – and Why You Should Be Too! (2016, April 06). Retrieved February 27, 2017, from http://drhyman.com/blog/2014/11/07/pegan-paleo-vegan/

Chapter 13: Intermittent Fasting—Could You Benefit from It?

In-text citations:

1. The Intermittent Fasting Dilemma. (n.d.). Retrieved September 09, 2017, from http://fitness.mercola.com/sites/fitness/archive/2012/09/14/intermittent-fasting-benefits.aspx

2. Ho, K. Y., Veldhuis, J. D., Johnson, M. L., Furlanetto, R., Evans, W. S., Alberti, K. G., & Thorner, M. O. (1988). Fasting enhances growth hormone secretion and amplifies the complex rhythms of growth hormone secretion in man. *Journal of Clinical Investigation,81*(4), 968-975. doi:10.1172/jci113450

3. The Future of Fat-Burning. (2016, November 11). Retrieved September 09, 2017, from https://philmaffetone.com/future-fat-burning/

4. The Gravity of Weight - A Clinical Guide to Weight Loss and Management. (n.d.). Retrieved September 09, 2017, from https://www.scribd.com/doc/37565304/The-Gravity-of-Weight-A-Clinical-Guide-to-Weight-Loss-and-Management

5. Marinac, C. R., Nelson, S. H., Breen, C. I., Hartman, S. J., Natarajan, L., Pierce, J. P., . . . Patterson, R. E. (2016). Prolonged Nightly Fasting and Breast Cancer Prognosis. *JAMA Oncology,2*(8), 1049. doi:10.1001/jamaoncol.2016.0164

6. Röjdmark, S. (1987). Influence of Short-Term Fasting on the Pituitary-Testicular Axis in Normal Men. *Hormone Research,25*(3), 140-146. doi:10.1159/000180645

7. Kim, I., & Lemasters, J. J. (2010). Mitochondrial degradation by autophagy (mitophagy) in GFP-LC3 transgenic hepatocytes during nutrient deprivation. *AJP: Cell Physiology,300*(2). doi:10.1152/ajpcell.00056.2010

8. Seyfried, T., Mantis, J., Todorova, M., & Greene, A. (2009). KETOGENIC DIET | Dietary Management of Epilepsy: Role of Glucose and Ketone Bodies. *Encyclopedia of Basic Epilepsy Research,687-693.* doi:10.1016/b978-012373961-2.00174-0

General References:

- Weigle, D. S. (1997). Effect of Fasting, Refeeding, and Dietary Fat Restriction on Plasma Leptin Levels. *Journal of Clinical Endocrinology & Metabolism,82*(2), 561-565. doi:10.1210/jc.82.2.561
- Varady, K. A. (2012). Alternate Day Fasting: Effects on Body Weight and Chronic Disease Risk in Humans and Animals. *Comparative Physiology of Fasting, Starvation, and Food Limitation,395-408.* doi:10.1007/978-3-642-29056-5_23
- Kraemer, F. B. (2002). Hormone-sensitive lipase: control of intracellular tri-(di-)acylglycerol and cholesteryl ester hydrolysis. *The Journal of Lipid Research,43*(10), 1585-1594. doi:10.1194/jlr.r200009-jlr200
- Varady, K. A., Bhutani, S., Church, E. C., & Klempel, M. C. (2009). Short-term modified alternate-day fasting: a novel dietary strategy for weight loss and cardioprotection in obese adults. *American Journal of Clinical Nutrition,90*(5), 1138-1143. doi:10.3945/ajcn.2009.28380
- Halberg, N. (2005). Effect of intermittent fasting and refeeding on insulin action in healthy men. *Journal of Applied Physiology,99*(6), 2128-2136. doi:10.1152/japplphysiol.00683.2005
- Tikoo, K., Tripathi, D. N., Kabra, D. G., Sharma, V., & Gaikwad, A. B. (2007). Intermittent fasting prevents the progression of type I diabetic nephropathy in rats and changes the expression of Sir2 and p53. *FEBS Letters,581*(5), 1071-1078. doi:10.1016/j.febslet.2007.02.006
- Varady, K. A. (2011). Intermittent versus daily calorie restriction: which diet regimen is more effective for weight loss? *Obesity Reviews,12*(7). doi:10.1111/j.1467-789x.2011.00873.x
- Seyfried. (2012). Mitochondrial Respiratory Dysfunction and the Extrachromosomal Origin of Cancer. *Cancer as a Metabolic Disease,253-259.* doi:10.1002/9781118310311.ch14
- Stewart, W. K., & Fleming, L. W. (1973). Features of a successful therapeutic fast of 382 days' duration. *Postgraduate Medical Journal,49*(569), 203-209. doi:10.1136/pgmj.49.569.203
- Taylor, M. A., & Garrow, J. S. (2001). Compared with nibbling, neither gorging nor a morning fast affect short-term energy balance in obese patients in a chamber calorimeter. *International Journal of Obesity,25*(4), 519-528. doi:10.1038/sj.ijo.0801572
- Gelino, S., Chang, J. T., Kumsta, C., She, X., Davis, A., Nguyen, C., . . . Hansen, M. (2016). Intestinal Autophagy Improves Healthspan and Longevity in C. elegans during Dietary Restriction. *PLOS Genetics,12*(7). doi:10.1371/journal.pgen.1006135
- Good, R. A., Lorenz, E., Engelman, R. W., & Day, N. K. (1991). Chronic Energy Intake Restriction: Influence on Longevity, Autoimmunity, Immunodeficiency, and Cancer in Autoimmune-Prone Mice. *Biological Effects of Dietary Restriction,147-156.* doi:10.1007/978-3-642-58181-6_14
- Diet, hormones and cancer. (1996). *European Journal of Cancer Prevention,5*(5), 413-416. doi:10.1097/00008469-199610000-00013

- Choi, I., Piccio, L., Childress, P., Bollman, B., Ghosh, A., Brandhorst, S., . . . Longo, V. (2016). A Diet Mimicking Fasting Promotes Regeneration and Reduces Autoimmunity and Multiple Sclerosis Symptoms. *Cell Reports,15*(10), 2136-2146. doi:10.1016/j.celrep.2016.05.009
- Mattson, M. P., Allison, D. B., Fontana, L., Harvie, M., Longo, V. D., Malaisse, W. J., . . . Panda, S. (2014). Meal frequency and timing in health and disease. *Proceedings of the National Academy of Sciences, 111*(47), 16647-16653. doi:10.1073/pnas.1413965111
- Mattson, M. P., Duan, W., Wan, R., & Guo, Z. (2004). Prophylactic activation of neuroprotective stress response pathways by dietary and behavioral manipulations. *Neurotherapeutics, 1*(1), 111-116. doi:10.1007/bf03206571

Chapter 14: The Ketogenic Diet—A Way to Stay Lean & Prevent Disease

In-text citations:

1. Good, R. A., Lorenz, E., Engelman, R. W., & Day, N. K. (1991). Chronic Energy Intake Restriction: Influence on Longevity, Autoimmunity, Immunodeficiency, and Cancer in Autoimmune-Prone Mice. *Biological Effects of Dietary Restriction,*147-156. doi:10.1007/978-3-642-58181-6_14

General References:

- Moore, J., & Westman, E. C. (2014). *Keto clarity: your definitive guide to the benefits of a low-carb, high-fat diet.* Las Vegas: Victory Belt Publishing, Inc.
- Verdy, M. (1966). BSP retention during total fasting. *Metabolism,15*(9), 769-772. doi:10.1016/0026-0495(66)90168-5
- Szot, P. (2004). The Role of Norepinephrine in the Anticonvulsant Mechanism of Action of the Ketogenic Diet. *Epilepsy and the Ketogenic Diet,*265-278. doi:10.1007/978-1-59259-808-3_20
- Bough, K. (2008). Energy metabolism as part of the anticonvulsant mechanism of the ketogenic diet. *Epilepsia,*49, 91-93. doi:10.1111/j.1528-1167.2008.01846.x
- Youm, Y., Nguyen, K. Y., Grant, R. W., Goldberg, E. L., Bodogai, M., Kim, D., . . . Dixit, V. D. (2015). The ketone metabolite beta-hydroxybutyrate blocks NLRP3 inflammasome–mediated inflammatory disease. *Nature Medicine.* doi:10.1038/nm.3804
- Egan, B., & D'Agostino, D. (2016). Fueling Performance: Ketones Enter the Mix. *Cell Metabolism,*24(3), 373-375. doi:10.1016/j.cmet.2016.08.021
- Egan, B. (n.d.). Faculty of 1000 evaluation for Nutritional Ketosis Alters Fuel Preference and Thereby Endurance Performance in Athletes. F1000 - *Post-publication peer review of the biomedical literature.* doi:10.3410/f.726590927.793524634
- Veech, R. L. (2004). The therapeutic implications of ketone bodies: the effects of ketone bodies in pathological conditions: ketosis, ketogenic diet, redox states, insulin resistance, and mitochondrial metabolism. *Prostaglandins, Leukotrienes and Essential Fatty Acids,70(3),* 309-319. doi:10.1016/j.plefa.2003.09.007
- Jarrett, S. G., Milder, J. B., Liang, L., & Patel, M. (2008). The ketogenic diet increases mitochondrial glutathione levels. *Journal of Neurochemistry,106*(3), 1044-1051. doi:10.1111/j.1471-4159.2008.05460.x
- Insulin Signaling/Insulin Action. (2011). *Diabetes,60*(Supplement_1). doi:10.2337/db11-2552-2584
- Bruce Keller, A. J., Umberger, G., Mcfall, R., & Mattson, M. P. (1999). Food restriction reduces brain damage and improves behavioral outcome following excitotoxic and metabolic insults. *Annals of Neurology,45*(1), 8-15. doi:10.1002/1531-8249(199901)45:1<8::aid-art4>3.3.co;2-m
- Gerschcovich, E. R., & Tseng, K. Y. (2008). *Cognitive Deficits in Parkinson's Disease. Cortico-Subcortical Dynamics in Parkinson's Disease,*1-15. doi:10.1007/978-1-60327-252-0_19
- Volek, J. S., & Phinney, S. D. (2012). *The art and science of low carbohydrate performance.* Berlín: Beyond Obesity LLC.
- Hyman, M. (2016). *Eat fat, get thin: why the fat we eat is the key to sustained weight loss and vibrant health.* New York: Little, Brown and Company.
- *ATKINS' diet.* (1999).ILC Prime Limited.
- Perform, E. T. (2016, July 10). "Are Carbs the Body's Preferred Fuel Source?" by James Barnum. Retrieved February 27, 2017, from http://www.eattoperform.com/2014/03/26/are-carbs-the-bodys-preferred-fuel-source/

Chapter 15: pH Balance—Don't Be So Acidic!

General References:

- Alkaline diet. (n.d.). Retrieved February 27, 2017, from http://growyouthful.com/remedy/diet-alkaline.php
- Aloisio, T. (2004). *Blood never lies: a practical guide to health and nutrition.* Coral Springs: Llumina Press.
- Body pH and Alkaline Diet Explained by Holistic Medical Doctor. (n.d.). Retrieved February 27, 2017, from http://www.drfostersessentials.com/store/ph_bal.php#sthash.rLgTkFDg.dpbs
- Canadian Consumer Raw Milk Advocacy Group. (n.d.). Retrieved February 27, 2017, from http://rawmilkconsumer.ca/information/raw-milk-laws/
- The Acid & Alkaline Foods List. (2016, November 11). Retrieved February 27, 2017, from http://asanafoods.com/blog/the-acid-alkaline-foods-list/
- Food pH List - Balancing Acid/Alkaline Foods. (n.d.). Retrieved February 27, 2017, from https://trans4mind.com/nutrition/pH.html
- Young, R. O., & Young, S. R. (2010). *The pH miracle: balance your diet, reclaim your health.* New York, NY: Wellness Central.

SECTION 4: GET RID OF TOXINS—THE KEY TO REAL CELLULAR DETOX FOR OPTIMAL HEALTH

Chapter 16: Toxins—What Are You Exposed To?

In-text citations:

1. Scialla, M. (n.d.). It could take centuries for EPA to test all the unregulated chemicals under a new landmark bill. Retrieved August 14, 2017, from http://www.pbs.org/newshour/updates/it-could-take-centuries-for-epa-to-test-all-the-unregulated-chemicals-under-a-new-landmark-bill/
2. Chemicals under the Toxic Substances Control Act (TSCA). (2017, January 24). Retrieved January 28, 2017, from https://www.epa.gov/chemicals-under-tsca
3. Mittelstaedt, M. (2009, March 17). Risk of 4,000 everyday chemicals to be studied. Retrieved August 14, 2017, from https://www.theglobeandmail.com/life/risk-of-4000-everyday-chemicals-to-be-studied/article4110626/
4. Wingspread Conference on the Precautionary Principle. (2016, February 08). Retrieved January 28, 2017, from http://www.sehn.org/wing.html
5. Body Burden: The Pollution in Newborns. (n.d.). Retrieved January 28, 2017, from http://www.ewg.org/research/body-burden-pollution-newborns
6. Reducing "High-Priority" Toxic Exposures. (2016, April 07). Retrieved January 28, 2017, from https://trmorrisnd.com/2016/02/25/reducing-high-priority-toxic-exposures/

General References:

- Janjua, N. R., Frederiksen, H., Skakkebæk, N. E., Wulf, H. C., & Andersson, A. (2008). Urinary excretion of phthalates and paraben after repeated whole-body topical application in humans. *International Journal of Andrology,31*(2), 118-130. doi:10.1111/j.1365-2605.2007.00841.x

- Harvey, P. W., & Everett, D. J. (2012). Parabens detection in different zones of the human breast: consideration of source and implications of findings. *Journal of Applied Toxicology,*32(5), 305-309. doi:10.1002/jat.2743

- State of the science of Endocrine Disturbing Chemicals (2012). World Health Organization

- Summary of the Toxic Substances Control Act. (2016, December 14). Retrieved January 28, 2017, from https://www.epa.gov/laws-regulations/summary-toxic-substances-control-act

- (2017, January 31). Retrieved February 28, 2017, from http://www.cdc.gov/exposurereport/

- Adams, M. (2016). *Food forensics: the hidden toxins lurking in your food and how you can avoid them for lifelong health.* Dallas, TX: BenBella Books, Inc.

- Lourie, B., & Smith, R. (2015). *Toxin toxout: getting harmful chemicals out of our bodies and our world.* Strawberry Hills, N.S.W.: ReadHowYouWant.

- Westervelt, A. (2015, February 10). Chemical enemy number one: how bad are phthalates really? Retrieved February 28, 2017, from https://www.theguardian.com/lifeandstyle/2015/feb/10/phthalates-plastics-chemicals-research-analysis

- Thornton, J. W. (2002). Biomonitoring of Industrial Pollutants: Health and Policy Implications of the Chemical Body Burden. *Public Health Reports,117*(4), 315-323. doi:10.1093/phr/117.4.315

- Fish Women Should Avoid. (n.d.). Retrieved February 28, 2017, from http://www.ewg.org/safefishlist

- EWG's Consumer Guide to Seafood. (n.d.). Retrieved February 28, 2017, from http://www.ewg.org/tunacalculator

- Pumarega, J., Gasull, M., Lee, D., López, T., & Porta, M. (2016). Number of Persistent Organic Pollutants Detected at High Concentrations in Blood Samples of the United States Population. Plos One, 11(8). doi:10.1371/journal.pone.0160432

- Banerjee, B. (1999). The influence of various factors on immune toxicity assessment of pesticide chemicals. *Toxicology Letters, 107*(1-3), 21-31. doi:10.1016/s0378-4274(99)00028-4

- Aydin, N., Karaoglanoglu, S., Yigit, A., Keles, M. S., Kirpinar, I., & Seven, N. (2003). Neuropsychological effects of low mercury exposure in dental staff in Erzurum, Turkey. *International Dental Journal, 53*(2), 85-91. doi:10.1111/j.1875-595x.2003.tb00664.x

- Bouchard, M. F., Bellinger, D. C., Wright, R. O., & Weisskopf, M. G. (2010). Attention-Deficit/Hyperactivity Disorder and Urinary Metabolites of Organophosphate Pesticides. *Pediatrics, 125*(6). doi:10.1542/peds.2009-3058

- Rudel, R. A., Gray, J. M., Engel, C. L., Rawsthorne, T. W., Dodson, R. E., Ackerman, J. M., . . . Brody, J. G. (2011). Food Packaging and Bisphenol A and Bis(2-Ethyhexyl) Phthalate Exposure: Findings from a Dietary Intervention. *Environmental Health Perspectives, 119*(7), 914-920. doi:10.1289/ehp.1003170

- Bae, S., & Hong, Y. (2014). Exposure to Bisphenol A From Drinking Canned Beverages Increases Blood Pressure: Randomized Crossover Trial. *Hypertension,65*(2), 313-319. doi:10.1161/hypertensionaha.114.04261

- Belyaeva, E. A., Sokolova, T. V., Emelyanova, L. V., & Zakharova, I. O. (2012). Mitochondrial Electron Transport Chain in Heavy Metal-Induced Neurotoxicity: Effects of Cadmium, Mercury, and Copper. *The Scientific World Journal, 2012*, 1-14. doi:10.1100/2012/136063

- Xu, Y., Wang, Y., Zheng, Q., Li, B., Li, X., Jin, Y., . . . Sun, G. (2008). Clinical Manifestations and Arsenic Methylation after a Rare Subacute Arsenic Poisoning Accident. *Toxicological Sciences, 103*(2), 278-284. doi:10.1093/toxsci/kfn041

- Lim, S., Cho, Y. M., Park, K. S., & Lee, H. K. (2010). Persistent organic pollutants, mitochondrial dysfunction, and metabolic syndrome. *Annals of the New York Academy of Sciences, 1201*(1), 166-176. doi:10.1111/j.1749-6632.2010.05622.x

- Lee, J., & Kim, Y. (2012). Association between bone mineral density and blood lead level in menopausal women: Analysis of 2008–2009 Korean national health and nutrition examination survey data. *Environmental Research, 115*, 59-65. doi:10.1016/j.envres.2012.03.010

- Baillie-Hamilton, P. F. (2002). Chemical Toxins: A Hypothesis to Explain the Global Obesity Epidemic. *The Journal of Alternative and Complementary Medicine, 8*(2), 185-192. doi:10.1089/107555302317371479

- Clayton, E. M., Todd, M., Dowd, J. B., & Aiello, A. E. (2010). The Impact of Bisphenol A and Triclosan on Immune Parameters in the U.S. Population, NHANES 2003–2006. *Environmental Health Perspectives, 119*(3), 390-396. doi:10.1289/ehp.1002883

- Dodson, R. E., Nishioka, M., Standley, L. J., Perovich, L. J., Brody, J. G., & Rudel, R. A. (2012). Endocrine Disruptors and Asthma-Associated Chemicals in Consumer Products. *Environmental Health Perspectives, 120*(7), 935-943. doi:10.1289/ehp.1104052

- Savage, J. H., Matsui, E. C., Wood, R. A., & Keet, C. A. (2012). Urinary levels of triclosan and parabens are associated with aeroallergen and food sensitization. *Journal of Allergy and Clinical Immunology, 130*(2). doi:10.1016/j.jaci.2012.05.006

- Sharma, R., Kotyk, M. W., & Wiltshire, W. A. (2016). An investigation into bisphenol A leaching from materials used intraorally. *The Journal of the American Dental Association, 147*(7), 545-550. doi:10.1016/j.adaj.2016.01.013

Chapter 17: Detoxification—Is Your Body Flushing Out Toxins Efficiently?

In-text citations:

1. Why Measure Lead in Bone? (n.d.). Retrieved February 28, 2017, from http://research.mssm.edu/xrf/why.html

2. II. Lourie, B., & Smith, R. (2015). *Toxin toxout: getting harmful chemicals out of our bodies and our world.* Strawberry Hills, N.S.W.: ReadHowYouWant.

3. True Cellular Detox™. (n.d.). Retrieved February 28, 2017, from https://cytodetox.com/about-cytodetox/

4. Lipton, B. H. (2003). *The biology of belief.* Memphis, TN: Spirit 2000, Inc.

General References:

- Rosa, C. T., Hicks, H. E., Ashizawa, A. E., Pohl, H. R., & Mumtaz, M. M. (2006). A Regional Approach to Assess the Impact of Living in a Chemical World. *Annals of the New York Academy of Sciences,1076*(1), 829-838. doi:10.1196/annals.1371.028

- E. (n.d.). How American Industry Skips Some Chemical Safety Checks. Retrieved January 28, 2017, from http://www.ewg.org/enviroblog/2015/04/how-american-industry-skips-some-chemical-safety-checks

- Purohit, V., Bode, J. C., Bode, C., Brenner, D. A., Choudhry, M. A., Hamilton, F., . . . Turner, J. R. (2008). Alcohol, intestinal bacterial growth, intestinal permeability to endotoxin, and medical consequences: Summary of a symposium. *Alcohol,42*(5), 349-361. doi:10.1016/j.alcohol.2008.03.131

- Health and Environmental Impacts of Monsanto's Roundup Pesticide. (n.d.). Retrieved February 28, 2017, from https://www.organicconsumers.org/old_articles/monsanto/roundup.cfm

- Methylation Problems Lead to 100s of Diseases. (2016, April 22). Retrieved January 28, 2017, from http://suzycohen.com/articles/methylation-problems/

- Writer, S. V. (2015, January 08). Best herbs to improve kidney function. Retrieved February 28, 2017, from http://www.naturalhealth365.com/chronic-kidney-disease-conventional-medicine-1274.html

- Hevesy, G., & Hofer, E. (1934). Elimination of Water from the Human Body. *Nature,134*(3397), 879-879. doi:10.1038/134879a0

- Jeong, H. G., Kang, M. J., Kim, H. G., Oh, D. G., Kim, J. S., Lee, S. K., & Jeong, T. C. (2012). Role of intestinal microflora in xenobiotic-induced toxicity. *Molecular Nutrition & Food Research,57*(1), 84-99. doi:10.1002/mnfr.201200461

- Sunscreens, E. 2. (n.d.). EWG's 10th Annual Guide to Safer Sunscreens. Retrieved February 28, 2017, from http://www.ewg.org/sunscreen/report/skin-cancer-on-the-rise/

- Vitamin D May Help Prevent Your Risk of Cancer By 77 Percent. (n.d.). Retrieved February 28, 2017, from http://articles.mercola.com/sites/articles/archive/2013/05/12/vitamin-d-may-prevent-breast-cancer.aspx
- Uncovering the Truth: Sun Exposure, Sunscreen and Skin Cancer. (n.d.). Retrieved February 28, 2017, from http://pathwaystofamilywellness.org/Holistic-Healthcare/uncovering-the-truth-sun-exposure-sunscreen-and-skin-cancer.html
- Jeong, H. G., Kang, M. J., Kim, H. G., Oh, D. G., Kim, J. S., Lee, S. K., & Jeong, T. C. (2012). Role of intestinal microflora in xenobiotic-induced toxicity. *Molecular Nutrition & Food Research, 57*(1), 84-99. doi:10.1002/mnfr.201200461
- Hodges, R. E., & Minich, D. M. (2015). Modulation of Metabolic Detoxification Pathways Using Foods and Food-Derived Components: A Scientific Review with Clinical Application. *Journal of Nutrition and Metabolism, 2015*, 1-23. doi:10.1155/2015/760689
- Liu, R. H. (2013). Health-Promoting Components of Fruits and Vegetables in the Diet. *Advances in Nutrition: An International Review Journal, 4*(3). doi:10.3945/an.112.003517
- Agarwal, R., Goel, S. K., & Behari, J. R. (2010). Detoxification and antioxidant effects of curcumin in rats experimentally exposed to mercury. *Journal of Applied Toxicology.* doi:10.1002/jat.1517
- Ryan, P. B., Burke, T. A., Hubal, E. A., Cura, J. J., & Mckone, T. E. (2007). Using Biomarkers to Inform Cumulative Risk Assessment. *Environmental Health Perspectives, 115*(5), 833-840. doi:10.1289/ehp.9334
- Eliaz, I., Hotchkiss, A. T., Fishman, M. L., & Rode, D. (2006). The effect of modified citrus pectin on urinary excretion of toxic elements. *Phytotherapy Research,20*(10), 859-864. doi:10.1002/ptr.1953
- Geier, D., Kern, J., King, P., Sykes, L., & Geier, M. (2012). Hair Toxic Metal Concentrations and Autism Spectrum Disorder Severity in Young Children. *International Journal of Environmental Research and Public Health, 9*(12), 4486-4497. doi:10.3390/ijerph9124486
- Xie, L., Kang, H., Xu, Q., Chen, M. J., Liao, Y., Thiyagarajan, M., . . . Nedergaard, M. (2013). Sleep Drives Metabolite Clearance from the Adult Brain. *Science,342*(6156), 373-377. doi:10.1126/science.1241224
- Zmrzljak, U. P., & Rozman, D. (2012). Circadian Regulation of the Hepatic Endobiotic and Xenobitoic Detoxification Pathways: The Time Matters. *Chemical Research in Toxicology, 25*(4), 811-824. doi:10.1021/tx200538r
- Chung, R. T. (2015). Detoxification effects of phytonutrients against environmental toxicants and sharing of clinical experience on practical applications. *Environmental Science and Pollution Research.* doi:10.1007/s11356-015-5263-3
- Samsel, A., & Seneff, S. (2013). Glyphosate's Suppression of Cytochrome P450 Enzymes and Amino Acid Biosynthesis by the Gut Microbiome: Pathways to Modern Diseases. *Entropy, 15*(4), 1416-1463. doi:10.3390/e15041416
- Reinholds, I., Pugajeva, I., Bavrins, K., Kuckovska, G., & Bartkevics, V. (2016). Mycotoxins, pesticides and toxic metals in commercial spices and herbs. *Food Additives & Contaminants: Part B, 10*(1), 5-14. doi:10.1080/19393210.2016.1210244

Chapter 18: Your Skin—What Are You Soaking Up?

In-text citations:

1. I. If You Wear Make-Up, Your Body Could be Absorbing Up to 5 Lbs of Chemicals Per Year. *Organic Consumers Association,* www.organicconsumers.org/news/if-you-wear-make-your-body-could-be-absorbing-5-lbs-chemicals-year. Accessed 14 Aug. 2017.
2. II. Mean 15. (n.d.). Retrieved January 28, 2017, from http://adriavasil.com/mean15
3. Sunscreens, E. 2. (n.d.). EWG's 2017 Guide to Safer Sunscreens. Retrieved January 09, 2018, from https://www.ewg.org/sunscreen/report/imperfect-protection/#.WlUEOCOZOCQ
4. What You Need to Know About Sunscreen Protection. (n.d.). Retrieved December 20, 2017, from https://articles.mercola.com/sites/articles/archive/2016/06/08/the-truth-about-sunscreen-protection.aspx
5. Vitamin D Resource Page | Resources for More Information on Vitamin D. (n.d.). Retrieved December 20, 2017, from http://www.mercola.com/article/vitamin-d-resources.htm

General References:

- Vasil, A., & Glatt, A. (2013). *Ecoholic body: your ultimate earth-friendly guide to living healthy and looking good.* Toronto: CNIB.
- Deacon, G. (2011). *There's lead in your lipstick: toxins in our everyday body care and how to avoid them.* Toronto: Penguin Canada.
- Skin Deep° Cosmetics Database | EWG. (n.d.). Retrieved February 28, 2017, from http://www.ewg.org/skindeep/
- Ingredients. (n.d.). Retrieved February 28, 2017, from http://www.cir-safety.org/ingredients
- Campaign for Safe Cosmetics-working for safer cosmetics. (n.d.). Retrieved February 28, 2017, from http://www.safecosmetics.org/
- Dirty Dozen Endocrine Disruptors. (n.d.). Retrieved February 28, 2017, from http://www.ewg.org/research/dirty-dozen-list-endocrine-disruptors
- Miessence - Miessence: home to probiotic, antioxidant and green alkalising certified organic superfood nutrition. (n.d.). Retrieved February 28, 2017, from http://www.miessence.com/shop/en/
- How Dangerous Are Your Cosmetics? 7/17/04. (n.d.). Retrieved January 28, 2017, from http://articles.mercola.com/sites/articles/archive/2004/07/17/dangerous-cosmetics.aspx
- Kounang, N. (2015, November 13). What's in your pad or tampon? Retrieved August 14, 2017, from http://www.cnn.com/2015/11/13/health/whats-in-your-pad-or-tampon/index.html
- U.S. Sunscreens Get Flunking Grade for UVA Protection 9/28/10. (n.d.). Retrieved January 28, 2017, from http://www.ewg.org/release/Sunscreens-Get-Flunking-Grade-for-UVA-Protection
- Uncovering the Truth: Sun Exposure, Sunscreen and Skin Cancer. (n.d.). Retrieved January 28, 2017, from http://pathwaystofamilywellness.org/Holistic-Healthcare/uncovering-the-truth-sun-exposure-sunscreen-and-skin-cancer.html
- New Study Shows Many Sunscreens are Accelerating not Preventing Cancer. (n.d.). Retrieved December 20, 2017, from https://articles.mercola.com/sites/articles/archive/2011/04/22/new-study-shows-many-sunscreens-are-accelerating-not-preventing-cancer.aspx

Chapter 19: Cookware—Is Yours Safe or Toxic?

In-text citations:

1. The Real Facts About Alzheimer's and Aluminum - from EHSO. (n.d.). Retrieved February 28, 2017, from http://www.ehso.com/ehshome/alzheimers.htm
2. Summer Grilling Could Be Dangerous to Your Health. (n.d.). Retrieved August 14, 2017, from http://articles.mercola.com/sites/articles/archive/2009/05/16/Summer-Grilling-Could-Be-Dangerous-to-Your-Health.aspx

General References:

- Ceramic Cookware | Safe & Healthy Cookware Set. (n.d.). Retrieved February 28, 2017, from http://cookware.mercola.com/ceramic-cookware.aspx
- Wood, R. (2016, February 11). Healthy Cookware. Retrieved February 28, 2017, from http://www.rwood.com/Articles/Healthy_Cookware.htm

- The Real Facts About Alzheimer's and Aluminum - from EHSO. (n.d.). Retrieved February 28, 2017, from http://www.ehso.com/ehshome/alzheimers.htm
- Walling, E. (2016, November 29). How to Find the Healthiest Cooking Pans Safe Cookware. Retrieved February 28, 2017, from http://www.livingthenourishedlife.com/cookware-what-is-safe-and-what-is-toxic/

Chapter 20: Air Quality—What Are You Breathing?

In-text citations:

1. The Inside Story: A Guide to Indoor Air Quality. (2016, May 31). Retrieved February 28, 2017, from https://www.epa.gov/indoor-air-quality-iaq/inside-story-guide-indoor-air-quality

2. Your Indoor Air Quality Could Be Worse than Outdoor Air. (n.d.). Retrieved August 14, 2017, from http://articles.mercola.com/sites/articles/archive/2011/07/25/poor-indoor-air-quality-could-be-jeopardizing-your-health.aspxThe dirt on toxic chemicals in household cleaning products. (n.d.). Retrieved January 28, 2017, from http://www.davidsuzuki.org/issues/health/science/toxics/the-dirt-on-toxic-chemicals-in-household-cleaning-products/

3. Lloyd-Smith, M., & Sheffield-Brotherton, B. (2008, October). Children's environmental health: intergenerational equity in action--a civil society perspective. Retrieved August 14, 2017, from https://www.ncbi.nlm.nih.gov/pubmed/18991917

4. Not so spotless. (n.d.). Retrieved December 20, 2017, from http://www.spotlessliving.info/about/not-so-spotless/

5. (n.d.). Retrieved January 09, 2018, from http://rense.com/general19/chemical.htm

6. Watch List: Synthetic Fragrance Exposes You to Hundreds of Chemicals. (2017, October 12). Retrieved December 20, 2017, from https://www.annmariegianni.com/ingredient-watch-list-synthetic-fragrance-exposes-you-to-hundreds-of-chemicals/

7. Environmental Working Group || BodyBurden. (n.d.). Retrieved August 14, 2017, from http://www.ewg.org/sites/bodyburden1/findings.php

8. 8 Sickening Facts About Flame Retardants. (n.d.). Retrieved February 28, 2017, from http://articles.mercola.com/sites/articles/archive/2013/12/11/8-flame-retardant-facts.aspx

9. (n.d.). Retrieved December 20, 2017, from https://aircleaners.com/comparisons/

10. Advantages of Aroma Diffusers. (2017, January 11). Retrieved February 28, 2017, from http://2brighteyes.com/en/articles/7-advantages-of-aroma-diffusers/

General References:

- Indoor Air Quality (IAQ). (2017, February 02). Retrieved February 28, 2017, from http://www.epa.gov/iaq/pubs/ozonegen.html
- Ingredient Cosmetics chemicals of concern. (n.d.). Retrieved December 20, 2017, from https://www.ewg.org/research/teen-girls-body-burden-hormone-altering-cosmetics-chemicals/cosmetics-chemicals-concern#.Wjp0s9-nG70
- Kitchen Appliances | Home Appliances. (n.d.). Retrieved February 28, 2017, from http://www.consumerreports.org/cro/appliances/air-cleaners-1005/overview/index.htm
- News Release: 2005-01-20 ARB Warns - Danger from Popular "Air Purifying" Machines. (n.d.). Retrieved February 28, 2017, from http://www.arb.ca.gov/newsrel/nr012005.htm
- Harrington, M. (2011). Air pollution linked to obesity, inflammation. *Lab Animal,40*(1), 3-3. doi:10.1038/laban0111-3a
- Government of Canada, Health Canada, Public Affairs, Consultation and Communications Branch. (2017, February 21). Health Canada - Home Page. Retrieved February 28, 2017, from http://www.hc-sc.gc.ca/english/protection/warnings/1999/99_62e.html
- Board, C. A. (n.d.). Hazardous Ozone-Generating "Air Purifiers." Retrieved January 26, 2017, from http://www.arb.ca.gov/research/indoor/ozone.htm
- 12, 2. J., 29, 2. N., & 14, 2. O. (n.d.). Welcome to NAFA. Retrieved February 28, 2017, from http://www.nafahq.org/
- Care, A. S. (2016, October 20). Ingredient Watch List: Synthetic Fragrance Exposes You to Hundreds of Chemicals. Retrieved February 28, 2017, from https://www.annmariegianni.com/ingredient-watch-list-synthetic-fragrance-exposes-you-to-hundreds-of-chemicals/
- The Pitfalls of the New "Ozone Initiative." (n.d.). Retrieved February 28, 2017, from http://articles.mercola.com/sites/articles/archive/2012/04/25/controversial-ozone-initiative-that-could-cost-you-your-job.aspx

Chapter 21: Molds—Are They Making You Sick?

In-text citations:

1. Shoemaker, R. C. (2010). *Surviving mold: life in the era of dangerous buildings.* Baltimore, MD: Otter Bay Books, LLC.

2. Amen, D. G. (2015). *Change your brain, change your life: the breakthrough program for conquering anxiety, depression, obsessiveness, lack of focus, anger, and memory problems.* New York: Harmony Books.

3. ERMI Testing - Environmental Relative Moldiness Index. (n.d.). Retrieved February 28, 2017, from http://www.survivingmold.com/diagnosis/ermi-testing

General References:

- Myers, A. (2016). *Autoimmune solution: prevent and reverse the full spectrum of inflammatory symptoms and diseases.* Place of publication not identified: Harperone.
- Black Mold Mental Symptoms And Mental Illness. (2017, January 05). Retrieved February 28, 2017, from http://www.amenclinics.com/blog/mental-illness-mold-toxicity/

Chapter 22: Water—What Should You Be Concerned About?

In-text citations:

1. (n.d.). Retrieved February 28, 2017, from http://fluoridealert.org/

2. What Happens to Your Body When You Drink Fluoride? (n.d.). Retrieved December 20, 2017, from https://articles.mercola.com/sites/articles/archive/2014/12/13/fluoride-deception.aspx

3. Group, E. W. (n.d.). EWG's Tap Water Database: What's in Your Drinking Water? Retrieved August 14, 2017, from https://www.ewg.org/tapwater/#.WZH563eGPL8

4. Public Works & Environmental Services Dept. (2017, March 17). What's in your water? Retrieved December 20, 2017, from https://ottawa.ca/en/residents/water-and-environment/drinking-water/drinking-water-quality/whats-your-water

5. Plastic. (n.d.). Retrieved February 28, 2017, from http://www.thegreenguide.com/doc/101/plastic

General References:

- Public Works & Environmental Services Dept. (2017, February 14). What's in your water? Retrieved February 28, 2017, from http://ottawa.ca/en/residents/water-and-environment/drinking-water/drinking-water-quality/whats-your-water
- Pure & Clear Drinking Water Filter System. (n.d.). Retrieved February 28, 2017, from http://waterfilters.mercola.com/drinking-water-filter.aspx

- Product Technologies. (n.d.). Retrieved February 28, 2017, from http://www.nikken.com/product/technology?hash=pimag#pimag
- Travel Berkey Water Filter. (n.d.). Retrieved February 28, 2017, from http://www.bigberkeywaterfilters.com/
- Your Guide to Plastic Recycling Symbols: The Numbers on Plastic. (2014, May 21). Retrieved February 28, 2017, from http://naturalsociety.com/recycling-symbols-numbers-plastic-bottles-meaning/
- A Natural Health & Wellness Magazine. (n.d.). Retrieved February 28, 2017, from http://www.alive.com/
- "You're not sick; you're thirsty. Don't treat thirst with medication." Dr. F. Batmanghelidj. (n.d.). Retrieved February 28, 2017, from http://www.watercure.com/
- Batmanghelidj, F. (2004). *Your body's many cries for water.* Tagman Press.
- Your Drinking Water and the Whole House Water Filtration. (n.d.). Retrieved February 28, 2017, from http://articles.mercola.com/sites/articles/archive/2011/01/26/whole-house-water-filtration.aspx
- Makino, S. (1999). *The miracle of Pi-water: a gift from the cosmos: the revolutionary technology of water that will save our planet and its people.* Nagoya, Japan: IBE Company.
- PlasticFreeBottles.com. (n.d.). Retrieved February 28, 2017, from http://www.plasticfreebottles.com/
- Xenoestrogens Cause Fibrocystic Breast Disease. (n.d.). Retrieved February 28, 2017, from http://www.fibrocystic.com/xeno.htm
- Home. (2015, March 26). Retrieved February 28, 2017, from http://www.alkalife.com/

SECTION 5: GET THE RIGHT VITAMINS TO HELP YOUR BODY PERFORM AT ITS BEST

Chapter 23: Low-Down on Vitamins—Do We Need Them, and Are They All Created Equal?

In-text citations:

1. 2015 CRN CONSUMER SURVEY ON DIETARY SUPPLEMENTS. (n.d.). Retrieved October 23, 2017, from http://www.crnusa.org/CRNconsumersurvey/2015/
2. Vitamins and Minerals. (2017, September 24). Retrieved October 23, 2017, from https://nccih.nih.gov/health/vitamins
3. No Deaths from Vitamins and Millions From Prescription Drugs. (2012, November 17). Retrieved October 23, 2017, from http://naturalsociety.com/27-years-no-deaths-from-vitamins-3-million-prescription-drug-deaths/
4. How Organic Farming Prevents the Use of Fertilizers. (n.d.). Retrieved October 23, 2017, from https://articles.mercola.com/sites/articles/archive/2013/07/02/fertilizer.aspx
5. Adults Meeting Fruit and Vegetable Intake Recommendations—United States, 2013. (2015, July 10). Retrieved October 23, 2017, from https://www.cdc.gov/mmwr/preview/mmwrhtml/mm6426a1.htm
6. W. (n.d.). NutrEval® FMV. Retrieved October 23, 2017, from https://www.gdx.net/product/nutreval-fmv-nutritional-test-blood-urine
7. Product Rating Criteria. (n.d.). Retrieved October 23, 2017, from https://www.nutrisearch.ca/criteria.html
8. What Is NSF Certification? (n.d.). Retrieved October 23, 2017, from http://www.nsf.org/consumer-resources/what-is-nsf-certification
9. International, I. A. (n.d.). NPA GMP Certification Program Overview. Retrieved October 23, 2017, from http://www.npainfo.org/NPA/EducationandCertification/GMPCertification/ProgramOverview/NPA/EducationCertification/NPAGMPCertificationProgramOverview.aspx?hkey=8ebad406-b72e-4a98-92b0-31e30176ab2e

General References:

- King, D. E., Mainous, A. G., Geesey, M. E., & Woolson, R. F. (2005). Dietary Magnesium and C-reactive Protein Levels. *Journal of the American College of Nutrition, 24*(3), 166-171. doi:10.1080/07315724.2005.10719461
- Jagadamma, S., Lal, R., & Rimal, B. (2009). Effects of topsoil depth and soil amendments on corn yield and properties of two Alfisols in central Ohio. *Journal of Soil and Water Conservation, 64*(1), 70-80. doi:10.2489/jswc.64.1.70
- Government of Canada, Health Canada, Health Products and Food Branch, Natural Health Products Directorate. (2016, August 11). About Natural Health Product Regulations in Canada - Health Canada. Retrieved September 01, 2016, from http://www.hc-sc.gc.ca/dhp-mps/prodnatur/about-apropos/index-eng.php
- Publications, H. H. (n.d.). Listing of vitamins. Retrieved October 24, 2016, from http://www.health.harvard.edu/staying-healthy/listing_of_vitamins
- Critics: To Take Vitamin Supplements or Not? (n.d.). Retrieved March 01, 2017, from http://articles.mercola.com/sites/articles/archive/2014/01/20/food-nutrients-vitamin-supplements.aspx
- MacWilliam, L. D., & MacWilliam, L. D. (2008). *NutriSearch comparative guide to nutritional supplements.* Vernon, B.C.: Northern Dimensions Pub.
- Aloisio, T. (2004). *Blood never lies: a practical guide to health and nutrition.* Coral Springs: Llumina Press.
- 18. Holford, P. (2012). *The optimum nutrition bible.* London: Piatkus.
- FDA. (n.d.). Retrieved March 01, 2017, from http://articles.mercola.com/sites/articles/archive/2012/04/23/defend-your-right-to-access-safe-dietary-supplements.aspx

Chapter 24: Vitamins and Minerals—Understanding Their Specific Roles

In-text citations:

1. Vitamin A and Bone Health. (n.d.). Retrieved October 23, 2017, from https://www.bones.nih.gov/health-info/bone/bone-health/nutrition/vitamin-and-bone-health
2. Vitamin A (retinol) Safety. (2013, November 01). Retrieved October 23, 2017, from https://www.mayoclinic.org/drugs-supplements/vitamin-a/safety/hrb-20060201
3. Tidy, D. C. (2015, July 09). Vitamin A Deficiency | Health. Retrieved October 23, 2017, from https://patient.info/health/vitamin-a-deficiency-leaflet
4. Vitamin D Deficiency. (n.d.). Retrieved October 23, 2017, from https://www.webmd.com/diet/guide/vitamin-d-deficiency#1
5. Vitamin E. (n.d.). Retrieved October 23, 2017, from http://www.nytimes.com/health/guides/nutrition/vitamin-e/overview.html
6. Vitamin E - Nutritional Disorders. (n.d.). Retrieved October 23, 2017, from http://www.msdmanuals.com/professional/nutritional-disorders/vitamin-deficiency,-dependency,-and-toxicity/vitamin-e
7. Eat Foods Rich In This Vitamin to Help Prevent Vision Problems, Kidney Failure, and Blindness. (n.d.). Retrieved October 23, 2017, from https://articles.mercola.com/sites/articles/archive/2016/08/08/vitamin-e-deficiency.aspx
8. Vitamin K. (n.d.). Retrieved October 23, 2017, from http://www.umm.edu/health/medical/altmed/supplement/vitamin-k

9. Babcock, J. (2017, June 21). Vitamin K Deficiency, Foods & Health Benefits! Retrieved October 23, 2017, from https://draxe.com/vitamin-k-deficiency/

10. Vitamin B1 (Thiamine). (n.d.). Retrieved October 23, 2017, from http://www.umm.edu/health/medical/altmed/supplement/vitamin-b1-thiamine

11. Vitamin B2. (n.d.). Retrieved October 23, 2017, from http://www.nutri-facts.org/en_US/nutrients/vitamins/b2.html

12. Niacin Deficiency. (n.d.). Retrieved October 23, 2017, from https://www.webmd.com/diet/niacin-deficiency-symptoms-and-treatments#1

13. A. (n.d.). Vitamin B5 Functions, Sources, Deficiency Symptoms, Dose. Retrieved October 23, 2017, from http://www.medasq.com/article/28/vitamin-b5/

14. Babcock, J. (2017, June 21). Prime Your Brain to Create More 'Happy Hormones' with These Foods. Retrieved October 23, 2017, from https://draxe.com/vitamin-b6-benefits/

15. Vitamin B7, Biotin | What is Biotin? | Andrew Weil, M.D. (2017, September 21). Retrieved October 23, 2017, from https://www.drweil.com/vitamins-supplements-herbs/vitamins/vitamin-b7-for-metabolism/

16. Vitamin B9 | Folic Acid | Folate | Andrew Weil, M.D. (2017, September 21). Retrieved October 23, 2017, from https://www.drweil.com/vitamins-supplements-herbs/vitamins/vitamin-b9-folate/

17. Office of Dietary Supplements - Dietary Supplement Fact Sheet: Vitamin B12. (n.d.). Retrieved October 23, 2017, from https://ods.od.nih.gov/factsheets/VitaminB12-HealthProfessional/

18. Vitamin C (Ascorbic acid). (n.d.). Retrieved October 23, 2017, from http://www.umm.edu/health/medical/altmed/supplement/vitamin-c-ascorbic-acid

19. Office of Dietary Supplements - Calcium. (n.d.). Retrieved October 23, 2017, from https://ods.od.nih.gov/factsheets/Calcium-HealthProfessional/

20. Office of Dietary Supplements - Magnesium. (n.d.). Retrieved October 23, 2017, from https://ods.od.nih.gov/factsheets/Magnesium-HealthProfessional/

21. Canada, H. (2012, March 15). Do Canadian Adults Meet Their Nutrient Requirements Through Food Intake Alone? Retrieved October 23, 2017, from https://www.canada.ca/en/health-canada/services/food-nutrition/food-nutrition-surveillance/health-nutrition-surveys/canadian-community-health-survey-cchs/canadian-adults-meet-their-nutrient-requirements-through-food-intake-alone-health-canada-2012.html

22. Babcock, J. (2017, September 12). Phosphorus Helps Your Body Detox & Strengthen. Retrieved October 23, 2017, from https://draxe.com/foods-high-in-phosphorus/

23. Himalayan Salt | Pure Cooking Salt. (n.d.). Retrieved December 20, 2017, from http://products.mercola.com/himalayan-salt/

24. What Are the Roles of Sodium? (n.d.). Retrieved October 23, 2017, from http://healthyeating.sfgate.com/roles-sodium-2999.html

25. Potassium. (n.d.). Retrieved October 23, 2017, from http://www.umm.edu/health/medical/altmed/supplement/potassium

26. GUARNERI, N. E. (2017). SUGAROCRACY. S.l.: LULU COM.

27. Zinc In diet . (n.d.). Retrieved October 23, 2017, from http://www.nytimes.com/health/guides/nutrition/zinc-in-diet/overview.html

28. IODINE: Uses, Side Effects, Interactions and Warnings. (n.d.). Retrieved October 23, 2017, from https://www.webmd.com/vitamins-supplements/ingredientmono-35-iodine.aspx?activeingredientid=35

29. Selenium in Diet . (n.d.). Retrieved October 23, 2017, from http://www.nytimes.com/health/guides/nutrition/selenium-in-diet/overview.html

30. Babcock, J. (2017, June 21). What Is Chromium? Chromium Controls Blood Sugar. Retrieved October 23, 2017, from https://draxe.com/what-is-chromium/

General References:

- Critics: To Take Vitamin Supplements or Not? (n.d.). Retrieved March 01, 2017, from http://articles.mercola.com/sites/articles/archive/2014/01/20/food-nutrients-vitamin-supplements.aspx

- Holford, P. (2012). *The optimum nutrition bible*. London: Piatkus.

- Liska, D., & Bland, J. (2004). *Clinical nutrition: a functional approach*. Gig Harbor, WA: Institute for Functional Medicine.

- CRN 2015 Consumer Survey on Dietary Supplements. (n.d.). Retrieved March 01, 2017, from http://www.crnusa.org/CRNconsumersurvey/2015/

- National Library of Medicine - National Institutes of Health. (n.d.). Retrieved March 01, 2017, from https://www.nlm.nih.gov/

- Himalayan Salt | Pure Cooking Salt. (n.d.). Retrieved March 01, 2017, from http://products.mercola.com/himalayan-salt/

- CRN 2015 Consumer Survey on Dietary Supplements. (n.d.). Retrieved March 01, 2017, from http://www.crnusa.org/CRNconsumersurvey/2015/

Chapter 25: Vitamin D—Are You Operating on Low?

In-text citations:

1. LD, M. W. (2017, October 01). Vitamin D: Health benefits, facts, and research. Retrieved October 24, 2017, from https://www.medicalnewstoday.com/articles/161618.php

2. Grant, W. B. (2006). Epidemiology of disease risks in relation to vitamin D insufficiency. *Progress in Biophysics and Molecular Biology,92*(1), 65-79. doi:10.1016/j.pbiomolbio.2006.02.013

3. Hoel, D. G., Berwick, M., Gruijl, F. R., & Holick, M. F. (2016). The risks and benefits of sun exposure 2016. Retrieved October 24, 2017, from https://www.ncbi.nlm.nih.gov/pmc/articles/PMC5129901/

4. Grant, W. B. (2002). An estimate of premature cancer mortality in the U.S. due to inadequate doses of solar ultraviolet-B radiation. *Cancer,94*(6), 1867-1875. doi:10.1002/cncr.10427

5. Which Vitamin K2 Supplement is Best - MK-4 or MK-7? (2017, July 08). Retrieved October 24, 2017, from https://www.thehealthyhomeeconomist.com/which-vitamin-k2-supplement-is-best-mk-4-or-mk-7/

6. *Vitamin D Functional Ranges* . (n.d.).

General References:

- Borissova, A. M., Djambazova, A., Todorov, K., Dakovska, L., Tankova, T., & Kirilov, G. (1993). Effect of erythropoietin on the metabolic state and peripheral insulin sensitivity in diabetic patients on haemodialysis. *Nephrology Dialysis Transplantation,8*(1), 93-93. doi:10.1093/oxfordjournals.ndt.a092282

- Chakraborti, C. (2011). Vitamin D as a promising anticancer agent. *Indian Journal of Pharmacology, 43*(2), 113. doi:10.4103/0253-7613.77335

- Holick, M. F., Binkley, N. C., Bischoff-Ferrari, H. A., Gordon, C. M., Hanley, D. A., Heaney, R. P., . . . Weaver, C. M. (2011). Evaluation, Treatment, and Prevention of Vitamin D Deficiency: an Endocrine Society Clinical Practice Guideline. *The Journal of Clinical Endocrinology & Metabolism, 96*(7), 1911-1930. doi:10.1210/jc.2011-0385

- Holford, P. (2012). *The optimum nutrition bible*. London: Piatkus.

- Giovannucci, E., Liu, Y., Rimm, E. B., Hollis, B. W., Fuchs, C. S., Stampfer, M. J., & Willett, W. C. (2006). Prospective Study of Predictors of Vitamin D Status and Cancer Incidence and Mortality in Men. *JNCI Journal of the National Cancer Institute, 98*(7), 451-459. doi:10.1093/jnci/djj101

- Vitamin D: The Simplest Solution to Most Health Problems. (n.d.). Retrieved March 01, 2017, from http://articles.mercola.com/sites/articles/archive/2013/12/22/dr-holick-vitamin-d-benefits.aspx

- Vitamin D 101 - A Detailed Beginner's Guide. (2016, August 18). Retrieved March 01, 2017, from https://authoritynutrition.com/vitamin-d-101/

- D-Spot. (2017, February 01). Retrieved March 01, 2017, from http://rmalab.com/d-spot

- Vitamin D: Vital Role in Your Health. (n.d.). Retrieved March 01, 2017, from http://www.webmd.com/food-recipes/features/vitamin-d-vital-role-in-your-health

- Agar, N. S., Halliday, G. M., Barnetson, R. S., Ananthaswamy, H. N., Wheeler, M., & Jones, A. M. (2004). The basal layer in human squamous tumors harbors more UVA than UVB fingerprint mutations: A role for UVA in human skin carcinogenesis. *Proceedings of the National Academy of Sciences, 101*(14), 4954-4959. doi:10.1073/pnas.0401141101

- Bestak, R., Barnetson, R. C., Nearn, M. R., & Halliday, G. M. (1995). Sunscreen Protection of Contact Hypersensitivity Responses from Chronic Solar-Simulated Ultraviolet Irradiation Correlates with the Absorption Spectrum of the Sunscreen. *Journal of Investigative Dermatology, 105*(3), 345-351. doi:10.1111/1523-1747.ep12320580

- Reduce Your Risk of Cancer With Sunlight Exposure 3/31/04. (n.d.). Retrieved March 01, 2017, from http://articles.mercola.com/sites/articles/archive/2004/03/31/cancer-sunlight.aspx

- Trash Your Sunscreen and Other Summer Sun Tips 5/26/04. (n.d.). Retrieved March 01, 2017, from http://articles.mercola.com/sites/articles/archive/2004/05/26/summer-sun.aspx

- Ask the Doc: Worrying About Sunblock Ingredients. (n.d.). Retrieved March 01, 2017, from http://beauty-grooming.healthguru.com/video/ask-the-doc-worrying-about-sunblock-ingredients

- The Dark Side of Sunscreens - Organic Consumers Association. (n.d.). Retrieved March 1, 2017.

- Zittermann, A. (2006). Vitamin D and disease prevention with special reference to cardiovascular disease. *Progress in Biophysics and Molecular Biology, 92*(1), 39-48. doi:10.1016/j.pbiomolbio.2006.02.001

Chapter 26: Essential Fatty Acids—Their Roles In Your Overall Health

In-text citations:

1. Asia Pac J Clin Nutr 2008;17 (S1):131-134

2. https://www.ncbi.nlm.nih.gov/pubmed/12442909

3. Am J Clin Nutr. 2003:78 (suppl):640S-646S

4. Kharrazian, D. (2017). *Why Isn't My Brain Working? A Revolutionary Understanding of Brain Decline and Effective Strategies to Recover Your Brain Health.* Elephant Press.

General References:

- Exp Biol Med 233:674-688, 20018 Biomed Pharmacother, 2001 Oct;56(8):365-379.

- Chestnut, J. L. (2017). *Live Right For Your Species Type: The Biological Wellness and Prevention Solution.* TWP Press.

- Malavolta, M., & Mocchegiani, E. (2016). *Molecular basis of nutrition and aging: A volume in the molecular nutrition series.* Amsterdam: Elsevier, AP. 155-176

- Recent. (n.d.). Retrieved from https://articles.mercola.com/sites/articles/archive/2012/01/12/aha-position-on-omega-6-fats.aspx

- Simopoulos, A. P. (2008). The Importance of the Omega-6/Omega-3 Fatty Acid Ratio in Cardiovascular Disease and Other Chronic Diseases. *Experimental Biology and Medicine, 233*(6), 674-688.

- Recent. (n.d.). Retrieved from http://www.drmirkin.com/heart/fish-oil-pills-have-not-been-shown-to-prevent-heart-attacks.html

- Citation (APA): Peskin, B. S., & Rowen, M.D. R. J. (2015). *PEO Solution - Conquering Cancer, Diabetes and Heart Disease with Parent Essential Oils* [Kindle iOS version]. Retrieved from Amazon.com

- FACLM, M. G. (n.d.). Is Fish Oil Just Snake Oil? Retrieved from https://nutritionfacts.org/video/is-fish-oil-just-snake-oil/

- Oxidation levels of North American over-the-counter n-3 (omega-3) supplements and the influence of supplement formulation and delivery form on evaluating oxidative safety. *Journal of Nutritional Science, 4*. doi:10.1017/jns.2015.21

- Omega-3 fatty acid supplementation and weekly consumption of fish may prevent Alzheimer's disease,. *Inpharma Weekly, &NA;*(1400), 15. doi:10.2165/00128413-200314000-00038

- Jackowski, S. A., Alvi, A. Z., Mirajkar, A., Imani, Z., Gamalevych, Y., Shaikh, N. A., & Jackowski, G. (2015). Oxidation levels of North American over-the-counter n-3 (omega-3) supplements and the influence of supplement formulation and delivery form on evaluating oxidative safety. *Journal of Nutritional Science, 4*. doi:10.1017/jns.2015.21

- Learn your Lipids: A Quick Guide to Bulletproof Fats. (2018, February 23). Retrieved from https://blog.bulletproof.com/omega-3-vs-omega-6-fat-supplements/

- Mozaffarian, D., Aro, A., & Willett, W. C. (2009). Health effects of trans-fatty acids: experimental and observational evidence. *European Journal of Clinical Nutrition, 63*. doi:10.1038/sj.ejcn.1602973

- Fascinating Facts You Never Knew About the Human Brain. (n.d.). Retrieved March 01, 2017, from http://articles.mercola.com/sites/articles/archive/2009/01/22/fascinating-facts-you-never-knew-about-the-human-brain.aspx

Chapter 27: Probiotics—Keep Your Bugs Happy!

In-text citations:

1. Guinane, C. M., & Cotter, P. D. (2013, July). Role of the gut microbiota in health and chronic gastrointestinal disease: understanding a hidden metabolic organ. Retrieved October 24, 2017, from https://www.ncbi.nlm.nih.gov/pmc/articles/PMC3667473/

2. Vighi, G., Marcucci, F., Sensi, L., Cara, G. D., & Frati, F. (2008, September). Allergy and the gastrointestinal system. Retrieved October 24, 2017, from https://www.ncbi.nlm.nih.gov/pmc/articles/PMC2515351/

3. Plummer, D. (n.d.). *The Human Microbiome: A Key Driver in Lifelong Health & Disease.*

4. Bray, K. (2016, December 08). The health benefits of fermented foods - Nutrition. Retrieved October 24, 2017, from https://www.choice.com.au/food-and-drink/nutrition/superfoods/articles/fermented-foods

5. Antibiotic / Antimicrobial Resistance. (2017, September 19). Retrieved October 24, 2017, from https://www.cdc.gov/drugresistance/about.html

6. RP Siegel on Friday, Dec 17th, 2010. (2015, February 07). FDA Reports Alarmingly High Levels of Antibiotics in Farm Animals. Retrieved October 24, 2017, from http://www.triplepundit.com/2010/12/fda-reports-alarmingly-high-levels-antibiotics-farm-animals/

7. Phillips, M. L. (2009, May). Gut Reaction: Environmental Effects on the Human Microbiota. Retrieved October 24, 2017, from https://www.ncbi.nlm.nih.gov/pmc/articles/PMC2685866/

8. Zhang, Y., Li, S., Gan, R., Zhou, T., Xu, D., & Li, H. (2015, April). Impacts of Gut Bacteria on Human Health and Diseases. Retrieved October 24, 2017, from https://www.ncbi.nlm.nih.gov/pmc/articles/PMC4425030/

General References:

- Antibiotics Kill Your Body's Good Bacteria, Too, Leading to Serious Health Risks 6/14/03. (n.d.). Retrieved March 01, 2017, from http://articles.mercola.com/sites/articles/archive/2003/06/18/antibiotics-bacteria.aspx
- Firmicutes Versus Bacteroides. (n.d.). Retrieved March 01, 2017, from http://www.drperlmutter.com/?s=Firmicutes%2Bversus%2Bbacteroidetes
- Probiotics are Essential to a Healthy Gut Flora. (n.d.). Retrieved March 01, 2017, from http://articles.mercola.com/sites/articles/archive/2011/09/24/one-of-the-most-important-steps-you-can-take-to-improve-your-health.aspx
- About Antimicrobial Resistance. (2015, September 08). Retrieved March 01, 2017, from https://www.cdc.gov/drugresistance/about.html
- Mercola, J. (2016). *Effortless healing: 9 simple ways to sidestep illness, shed excess weight, and help your body fix itself.* New York: Harmony Book.
- Probiotics Benefits, Foods and Supplements. (2016, December 22). Retrieved March 01, 2017, from https://draxe.com/probiotics-benefits-foods-supplements/
- 8 Health Benefits of Probiotics. (2016, October 12). Retrieved March 01, 2017, from https://authoritynutrition.com/8-health-benefits-of-probiotics/
- How Your Gut Flora Influences Your Health. (n.d.). Retrieved March 01, 2017, from http://articles.mercola.com/sites/articles/archive/2012/06/27/probiotics-gut-health-impact.aspx
- See How Bacteria Plays a Role in Depression, Obesity, Spinal Cord Recover More Conditions. (2016, October 22). Retrieved March 01, 2017, from https://draxe.com/gut-bacteria-benefits/
- How to Choose the Best Probiotic Supplement | Dr. Williams. (n.d.). Retrieved March 01, 2017, from https://www.drdavidwilliams.com/how-to-choose-the-best-probiotic-supplement/
- Gibson, G. R., Beatty, E. R., Wang, X., & Cummings, J. H. (1995). Selective stimulation of bifidobacteria in the human colon by oligofructose and inulin. Gastroenterology, 108(4), 975-982. doi:10.1016/0016-5085(95)90192-2
- Giudice, M. M., Rocco, A., & Capristo, C. (2006). Probiotics in the atopic march: highlights and new insights. Digestive and Liver Disease, 38. doi:10.1016/s1590-8658(07)60012-7

SECTION 6: GET FIT AND STRONG IN LESS TIME

Chapter 28: Goal of Fitness—Use it or Lose It

In-text citations:

1. Constitution of WHO: principles. (n.d.). Retrieved October 24, 2017, from http://www.who.int/about/mission/en/

General References:

- Schober, T., LeClair, E., Calorie, C., Hartley, J., M., Blakrishnan, P., . . . R. (n.d.). 50 Amazing Health Benefits of Exercise and Physical Activity. Retrieved March 01, 2017, from http://www.coachcalorie.com/health-benefits-of-exercise-and-physical-activity/
- Kyu, H. H., Bachman, V. F., Alexander, L. T., Mumford, J. E., Afshin, A., Estep, K., . . . Forouzanfar, M. H. (2016). Physical activity and risk of breast cancer, colon cancer, diabetes, ischemic heart disease, and ischemic stroke events: systematic review and dose-response meta-analysis for the Global Burden of Disease Study 2013. *Bmj,* I3857. doi:10.1136/bmj.i3857
- Tsai, S., Chan, Y., Liang, F., Hsu, C., & Lee, I. (2015). Brain-derived neurotrophic factor correlated with muscle strength in subjects undergoing stationary bicycle exercise training. *Journal of Diabetes and its Complications, 29*(3), 367-371. doi:10.1016/j.jdiacomp.2015.01.014
- Håkansson, K., Ledreux, A., Daffner, K., Terjestam, Y., Bergman, P., Carlsson, R., . . . Mohammed, A. K. (2016). BDNF Responses in Healthy Older Persons to 35 Minutes of Physical Exercise, Cognitive Training, and Mindfulness: Associations with Working Memory Function. *Journal of Alzheimer's Disease, 55*(2), 645-657. doi:10.3233/jad-160593
- Powers, M. B., Medina, J. L., Burns, S., Kauffman, B. Y., Monfils, M., Asmundson, G. J., . . . Smits, J. A. (2015). Exercise Augmentation of Exposure Therapy for PTSD: Rationale and Pilot Efficacy Data. *Cognitive Behaviour Therapy, 44*(4), 314-327. doi:10.1080/16506073.2015.1012740
- Ruscheweyh, R., Willemer, C., Krüger, K., Duning, T., Warnecke, T., Sommer, J., . . . Flöel, A. (2011). Physical activity and memory functions: An interventional study. *Neurobiology of Aging, 32*(7), 1304-1319. doi:10.1016/j.neurobiolaging.2009.08.001

Chapter 29: Beyond Being Fit—Be Functional

In-text citations:

1. What can functional fitness training do for you? (2016, October 29). Retrieved October 24, 2017, from https://www.mayoclinic.org/healthy-lifestyle/fitness/in-depth/functional-fitness/art-20047680
2. What is FMS? (n.d.). Retrieved March 01, 2017, from http://functionalmovement.com/fms

General References:

- What Are Functional Patterns. (n.d.). Retrieved March 01, 2017, from http://www.functionalpatterns.com/about-us/what-is-functional-patterns/
- The Importance of Functional Training for Women. (2015, May 08). Retrieved March 01, 2017, from http://www.top.me/fitness/the-importance-of-functional-fitness-for-women-454.html

Chapter 30: High-Intensity Interval Training (HIIT)—Keep It Short and Efficient

In-text citations:

1. Tabata, I., Nishimura, K., Kouzaki, M., Hirai, Y., Ogita, F., Miyachi, M., & Yamamoto, K. (1996). Effects of moderate-intensity endurance and high-intensity intermittent training on anaerobic capacity and VO2max. *Medicine & Science in Sports & Exercise,28*(10), 1327-1330. doi:10.1097/00005768-199610000-00018
2. Effects of Moderate- and High-Intensity Intermittent Training. (n.d.). Retrieved October 24, 2017, from https://www.bodyrecomposition.com/research-review/effects-of-moderate-intensity-endurance-and-high-intensity-intermittent-training-on-anaerobic-capacity-and-vo2-max.html/
3. Gibala, M. J., & Mcgee, S. L. (2008). Metabolic Adaptations to Short-term High-Intensity Interval Training. *Exercise and Sport Sciences Reviews, 36*(2), 58-63. doi:10.1097/jes.0b013e318168ec1f
4. Madsen, S. M., Thorup, A. C., Overgaard, K., & Jeppesen, P. B. (2015). High Intensity Interval Training Improves Glycaemic Control and Pancreatic Beta Cell Function of Type 2 Diabetes Patients. *Plos One, 10*(8). doi:10.1371/journal.pone.0133286
5. Wu, L., Chang, S., Fu, T., Huang, C., & Wang, J. (2017). High-intensity Interval Training Improves Mitochondrial Function and Suppresses Thrombin Generation in Platelets undergoing Hypoxic Stress. Retrieved October 24, 2017, from https://www.ncbi.nlm.nih.gov/pmc/articles/PMC5482849/
6. Lewis-McCormick, I. (2016). *The HIIT advantage: high-intensity workouts for women.* Champaign, IL: Human Kinetics.

General References:

- High-Intensity Interval Training: Efficient, Effective, and... : ACSM's Health & Fitness Journal. (n.d.). Retrieved April 02, 2017, from http://journals.lww.com/acsm-healthfitness/Citation/2013/05000/High_Intensity_Interval_Training___Efficient,.3.aspx
- Roy, B. A. (2013). High-Intensity Interval Training. *ACSM's Health & Fitness Journal, 17*(3), 3. doi:10.1249/fit.0b013e31828cb21c
- Jelleyman, C., Yates, T., O'donovan, G., Gray, L. J., King, J. A., Khunti, K., & Davies, M. J. (2015). The effects of high-intensity interval training on glucose regulation and insulin resistance: a meta-analysis. *Obesity Reviews, 16*(11), 942-961. doi:10.1111/obr.12317
- Guiraud, T., Nigam, A., Gremeaux, V., Meyer, P., Juneau, M., & Bosquet, L. (2012). High-Intensity Interval Training in Cardiac Rehabilitation. *Sports Medicine, 42*(7), 587-605. doi:10.2165/11631910-000000000-00000
- Haykowsky, M. J., Timmons, M. P., Kruger, C., Mcneely, M., Taylor, D. A., & Clark, A. M. (2013). Meta-Analysis of Aerobic Interval Training on Exercise Capacity and Systolic Function in Patients With Heart Failure and Reduced Ejection Fractions. *The American Journal of Cardiology, 111*(10), 1466-1469. doi:10.1016/j.amjcard.2013.01.303
- Driver, J. (2012). *HIIT: high intensity interval training explained.* Lexington, KY: James Driver.
- Salassi, J. W. (2014). *The acute effects of various high-intensity interval training (HIIT) protocols on cardiopulmonary and metabolic function.*
- High-Intensity Interval Training 101 | HIIT Benefits. (n.d.). Retrieved March 01, 2017, from http://fitness.mercola.com/sites/fitness/archive/2013/06/21/interval-training.aspx
- High-Intensity Interval Training Workout Benefits. (n.d.). Retrieved March 01, 2017, from http://fitness.mercola.com/sites/fitness/archive/2016/05/13/intense-exercises.aspx
- Crandall, K. J., & Dennehy, C. A. (1999). The Effects Of Exercise Intensity On Macronutrient Composition, Caloric Intake, Body Composition, And Body Weight. *Medicine & Science in Sports & Exercise, 31*(Supplement). doi:10.1097/00005768-199905001-00171
- Gibala, M. J., Little, J. P., Essen, M. V., Wilkin, G. P., Burgomaster, K. A., Safdar, A., . . . Tarnopolsky, M. A. (2006). Short-term sprint interval versus traditional endurance training: similar initial adaptations in human skeletal muscle and exercise performance. *The Journal of Physiology, 575*(3), 901-911. doi:10.1113/jphysiol.2006.112094

Chapter 31: Strength Training—Strong Is The New Sexy

In-text citations:

1. How to Make Sure You Burn Calories for Hours after Your Workout. (n.d.). Retrieved October 24, 2017, from https://fitness.mercola.com/sites/fitness/archive/2011/05/05/how-to-make-sure-you-burn-calories-for-hours-after-your-workout.aspx
2. Schoenfeld, B. J. (2010). The Mechanisms of Muscle Hypertrophy and Their Application to Resistance Training. *Journal of Strength and Conditioning Research, 24*(10), 2857-2872. doi:10.1519/jsc.0b013e3181e840f3
3. Tumminello, N. (2014). *Strength training for fat loss.* Champaign, IL: Human Kinetics.
4. What is Muscle Imbalance. (n.d.). Retrieved October 24, 2017, from http://www.muscleimbalancesyndromes.com/what-is-muscle-imbalance/
5. The Danger of Muscle Imbalances and the Importance of Symmetry. (2014, March 27). Retrieved March 01, 2017, from http://www.marksdailyapple.com/muscle-imbalances/

General References:

- Warburton, D. E., & Nicol, C. W. (2006, March 14). Darren E.R. Warburton. Retrieved April 02, 2017, from http://www.cmaj.ca/content/174/6/801.full
- Stoever, K., Heber, A., Eichberg, S., & Brixius, K. (2016). Influences of Resistance Training on Physical Function in Older, Obese Men and Women With Sarcopenia. *Journal of Geriatric Physical Therapy*, 1. doi:10.1519/jpt.0000000000000105
- Garber, C. E., Blissmer, B., Deschenes, M. R., Franklin, B. A., Lamonte, M. J., Lee, I., . . . Swain, D. P. (2011). Quantity and Quality of Exercise for Developing and Maintaining Cardiorespiratory, Musculoskeletal, and Neuromotor Fitness in Apparently Healthy Adults. *Medicine & Science in Sports & Exercise, 43*(7), 1334-1359. doi:10.1249/mss.0b013e318213fefb
- Weight training: Free weights vs. machine weights. (n.d.). Retrieved March 01, 2017, from http://www.mayoclinic.org/healthy-lifestyle/fitness/expert-answers/weight-training/faq-20058479
- Macdonald, R. (2016). *Canfitpro: foundations of professional personal training.* Place of publication not identified: Human Kinetics.
- Nelson, M. E. (2009). Strength Training for Older Adults. *Medicine & Science in Sports & Exercise, 41*, 51. doi:10.1249/01.mss.0000353077.05953.08
- Vehrs, P. R. (2005). Strength Training in Children and Teens. *ACSM's Health & Fitness Journal, 9*(4), 8-12. doi:10.1097/00135124-200507000-00006
- Carpinelli, R. N. (2009). Challenging the American College of Sports Medicine 2009 Position Stand on Resistance Training. *Medicina Sportiva, 13*(2), 131-137. doi:10.2478/v10036-009-0020-7
- Singulani, M. P., Stringhetta-Garcia, C. T., Santos, L. F., Morais, S. R., Louzada, M. J., Oliveira, S. H., . . . Dornelles, R. C. (2017). Effects of strength training on osteogenic differentiation and bone strength in aging female Wistar rats. *Scientific Reports, 7*, 42878. doi:10.1038/srep42878
- Station, T. T. (2016, November 04). The Benefits Of Strength Training! Retrieved March 01, 2017, from http://www.bodybuilding.com/fun/trainingstation1.htm
- Strength Training 101: Where do I start? (2016, October 24). Retrieved March 01, 2017, from https://www.nerdfitness.com/blog/strength-training-101-where-do-i-start/

Chapter 32: Yoga—You Don't Have to Be a Pretzel

In-text citations:

1. Woodyard, C. (2011). Exploring the therapeutic effects of yoga and its ability to increase quality of life. Retrieved October 24, 2017, from https://www.ncbi.nlm.nih.gov/pmc/articles/PMC3193654/

General References:

- Norberg, U. (2008). *Hatha yoga.* New York, NY: Skyhorse Pub.
- 38 Health Benefits of Yoga | Yoga Benefits. (2015, April 21). Retrieved March 01, 2017, from http://www.yogajournal.com/article/health/count-yoga-38-ways-yoga-keeps-fit/
- Yu, %. (2016, July 14). Yoga for Beginners: 9 Types of Yoga to Try. Retrieved March 01, 2017, from http://dailyburn.com/life/fitness/yoga-for-beginners-kundalini-yin-bikram/
- Chu, P., Gotink, R. A., Yeh, G. Y., Goldie, S. J., & Hunink, M. M. (2016). The effectiveness of yoga in modifying risk factors for cardiovascular disease and metabolic syndrome: A systematic review and meta-analysis of randomized controlled trials. *European Journal of Preventive Cardiology, 23*(3), 291-307. doi:10.1177/2047487314562741

Chapter 33: Straighten-Up! Is Your Posture Wearing You Out?

In-text citations:

1. The Importance of Good Posture. (n.d.). Retrieved October 24, 2017, from https://www.scoi.com/importance-good-posture

2. Anterior Head Carriage. (2015, December 04). Retrieved March 01, 2017, from http://vancouverbackpain.com/anterior-head-carriage/

3. Hyman, M. (2017, March 24). Lecture presented at Institute of Functional Medicine Annual Conference .

General References:

- Good Posture...just how important is it? (n.d.). Retrieved March 01, 2017, from http://www.kansaschirofoundation.org/goodposture-article.html

- Chiropractic Care for Back Pain. (n.d.). Retrieved March 01, 2017, from http://www.webmd.com/pain-management/guide/chiropractic-pain-relief#1

- 10 Proven Benefits of Good Posture. (n.d.). Retrieved March 01, 2017, from http://www.uprightpose.com/blog-10-proven-benefits-of-good-posture/

- How to sit at a computer. (2016, June 28). Retrieved March 01, 2017, from http://www.ergonomics.com.au/how-to-sit-at-a-computer/

- Buckley, J. P., Hedge, A., Yates, T., Copeland, R. J., Loosemore, M., Hamer, M., . . . Dunstan, D. W. (2015). The sedentary office: an expert statement on the growing case for change towards better health and productivity. *British Journal of Sports Medicine, 49*(21), 1357-1362. doi:10.1136/bjsports-2015-094618

- Katzmarzyk, P. T., Church, T. S., Craig, C. L., & Bouchard, C. (2009). Sitting Time and Mortality from All Causes, Cardiovascular Disease, and Cancer. *Medicine & Science in Sports & Exercise, 41*(5), 998-1005. doi:10.1249/mss.0b013e3181930355

SECTION 7: GET TO KNOW YOUR HORMONES AND FEEL BETTER

Chapter 34: Your Adrenals—Stress is Not Overrated!

In-text citation:

1. Selye's Concept of a "General Adaptation Syndrome" | in Chapter 14: Frontiers | from Psychology: An Introduction by Russ Dewey. (n.d.). Retrieved March 02, 2017, from http://www.intropsych.com/ch14_frontiers/selyes_concept_of_a_general_adaptation_syndrome.html

General References:

- Bitenieks, M. (n.d.). Reporting with the COREscore™. Retrieved March 02, 2017, from http://www.subluxation.com/productsservices/corescore/

- Study supporting DUTCH testing – Cortisol. (n.d.). Retrieved March 02, 2017, from https://dutchtest.com/2016/06/20/more-data-supporting-dutch-testing-cortisol/

- Wahbeh, H., & Oken, B. S. (2013). Salivary Cortisol Lower in Posttraumatic Stress Disorder. *Journal of Traumatic Stress, 26*(2), 241-248. doi:10.1002/jts.21798

- Gold, P. W. (2014). The organization of the stress system and its dysregulation in depressive illness. *Molecular Psychiatry, 20*(1), 32-47. doi:10.1038/mp.2014.163

- Sarris, J., O'Neil, A., Coulson, C. E., Schweitzer, I., & Berk, M. (2014). Lifestyle medicine for depression. *BMC Psychiatry, 14,* 107. doi:10.1186/1471 244X 14 107

- Turakitwanakan, W. et al. (2013). Effects of mindfulness meditation on serum cortisol of medical students. *Journal of the Medical Association of Thailand,* 2013 Jan; 96 Suppl 1:S90 5.

- Milagros, C. et al. (2010). Stress, social support, and cortisol: inverse associations? Behavioral Medicine, 30(1):11 22. doi:10.3200/bmed.30.1.11 22

- Panossian, A. et al. (2009) Adaptogens exert a stress protective effect by modulation of molecular chaperones. *Phytomedicine,* 2009 Jun;16(6 7):617 22. doi: 10.1016/j.phymed.2008.12.003. Epub 2009 Feb 1.

- Panossian, A. et al. (2012). Adaptogens Stimulate Neuropeptide Y and Hsp72 Expression and Release in Neuroglia Cells. Frontiers in Neuroscience, 6, 6. doi:10.3389/fnins.2012.00006

- Nobre AC, Rao A, and Owen GN. L theanine, a natural constituent in tea, and its effect on mental state. *Asia Pac J Clin Nutr.* 2008;17 Suppl 1:167 8.

- Singh N, et al. *Withania somnifera* (Ashwagandha), a rejuvenating herbal drug which enhances survival during stress (an adaptogen). *Int J Crude Drug Res* 1982;20(1):29-3

- Elsas, S. et al. (2010). Passiflora incarnata L. (Passionflower) extracts elicit GABA currents in hippocampal neurons in vitro, and show anxiogenic and anticonvulsant effects in vivo, varying with extraction method. *Phytomedicine : International Journal of Phytotherapy and Phytopharmacology,* 17(12), 940–949. doi:10.1016/j.phymed.2010.03.002

- Panossian A, et al. (2012). Adaptogens stimulate neuropeptide y and hsp72 expression and release in neuroglia cells. Front Neurosci. Feb. 2012.

- Russell, E., Koren, G., Rieder, M., & Uum, S. V. (2012). Hair cortisol as a biological marker of chronic stress: Current status, future directions and unanswered questions. *Psychoneuroendocrinology,37*(5), 589-601. doi:10.1016/j.psyneuen.2011.09.009

Chapter 35: Thyroid—Slow and Sluggish = Fatigue and Weight Gain

In-text citations:

1. Thyroid. (2017, April 17). Retrieved September 10, 2017, from http://www.humannaturenaturalhealth.com/Thyroid

2. Bazayev, A. (n.d.). Thyroid. Retrieved September 10, 2017, from http://www.healthyimmunity.com/books/An-A-Z-Woman-s-Guide-to-Vibrant-Health/Thyroid.asp

3. Hoang, T. D., Olsen, C. H., Mai, V. Q., Clyde, P. W., & Shakir, M. K. (2013). Desiccated Thyroid Extract Compared With Levothyroxine in the Treatment of Hypothyroidism: A Randomized, Double-Blind, Crossover Study. *The Journal of Clinical Endocrinology & Metabolism, 98*(5), 1982-1990. doi:10.1210/jc.2012-4107

General References:

- Howdeshell, K. L. (2002). A Model of the Development of the Brain as a Construct of the Thyroid System. *Environmental Health Perspectives, 110*(S3), 337-348. doi:10.1289/ehp.02110s3337

- Turyk, M. E., Anderson, H. A., & Persky, V. W. (2007). Relationships of Thyroid Hormones with Polychlorinated Biphenyls, Dioxins, Furans, and DDE in Adults. *Environmental Health Perspectives, 115*(8), 1197-1203. doi:10.1289/ehp.10179

- Zimmermann, M. B., & Köhrle, J. (2002). The Impact of Iron and Selenium Deficiencies on Iodine and Thyroid Metabolism: Biochemistry and Relevance to Public Health. *Thyroid, 12*(10), 867-878. doi:10.1089/105072502761016494

- Kralik, A., Eder, K., & Kirchgessner, M. (1996). Influence of Zinc and Selenium Deficiency on Parameters Relating to Thyroid Hormone Metabolism. *Hormone and Metabolic Research, 28*(05), 223-226. doi:10.1055/s-2007-979169

- Hammouda, F., Messaoudi, I., Hani, J. E., Baati, T., Saïd, K., & Kerkeni, A. (2008). Reversal of Cadmium-Induced Thyroid Dysfunction by Selenium, Zinc, or Their Combination in Rat. *Biological Trace Element Research, 126*(1-3), 194-203. doi:10.1007/s12011-008-8194-8

- Smyth, P. P., & Duntas, L. H. (2005). Iodine Uptake and Loss - Can Frequent Strenuous Exercise Induce Iodine Deficiency? *Hormone and Metabolic Research,37*(9), 555-558. doi:10.1055/s-2005-870423

- Sang, Z., Wang, P. P., Yao, Z., Shen, J., Halfyard, B., Tan, L., . . . Zhang, W. (2011). Exploration of the safe upper level of iodine intake in euthyroid Chinese adults: a randomized double-blind trial. *American Journal of Clinical Nutrition, 95*(2), 367-373. doi:10.3945/ajcn.111.028001

- Laurberg, P. (2006). The Danish investigation on iodine intake and thyroid disease, DanThyr: status and perspectives. *European Journal of Endocrinology,155*(2), 219-228. doi:10.1530/eje.1.02210

- Contempré, B., Duale, N. L., Dumont, J. E., Ngo, B., Diplock, A. T., & Vanderpas, J. (1992). Effect of selenium supplementation on thyroid hormone metabolism in an iodine and selenium deficient population. *Clinical Endocrinology, 36*(6), 579-583. doi:10.1111/j.1365-2265.1992.tb02268.x

- Stepien, T., Krupinski, R., Sopinski, J., Kuzdak, K., Komorowski, J., Lawnicka, H., & Stepien, H. (2010). Decreased 1-25 Dihydroxyvitamin D3 Concentration in Peripheral Blood Serum of Patients with Thyroid Cancer. *Archives of Medical Research, 41*(3), 190-194. doi:10.1016/j.arcmed.2010.04.004

- Baisier, W. V., Hertoghe, J., & Eeckhaut, W. (2000). Thyroid Insufficiency. Is TSH Measurement the Only Diagnostic Tool? *Journal of Nutritional & Environmental Medicine, 10*(2), 105-113. doi:10.1080/13590840050043521

- Canaris, G. J., Manowitz, N. R., Mayor, G., & Ridgway, E. C. (2000). The Colorado Thyroid Disease Prevalence Study. *Archives of Internal Medicine, 160*(4), 526. doi:10.1001/archinte.160.4.526

- Takashima, N., Niwa, Y., Mannami, T., Tomoike, H., & Iwai, N. (2007). Characterization of Subclinical Thyroid Dysfunction From Cardiovascular and Metabolic Viewpoints. *Circulation Journal, 71*(2), 191-195. doi:10.1253/circj.71.191

- Tuzcu, A., Bahceci, M., Gokalp, D., Tuzun, Y., & Gunes, K. (2005). Subclinical Hypothyroidism may be Associated with Elevated High-sensitive C-Reactive Protein (Low Grade Inflammation) and Fasting Hyperinsulinemia. *Endocrine Journal, 52*(1), 89-94. doi:10.1507/endocrj.52.89

- Chueire, V. B., Romaldini, J. H., & Ward, L. S. (2007). Subclinical hypothyroidism increases the risk for depression in the elderly. *Archives of Gerontology and Geriatrics, 44*(1), 21-28. doi:10.1016/j.archger.2006.02.001

- Alevizaki, M., Mantzou, E., Cimponeriu, A. T., Alevizaki, C. C., & Koutras, D. A. (2005). TSH may not be a good marker for adequate thyroid hormone replacement therapy. *Wiener klinische Wochenschrift, 117*(18), 636-640. doi:10.1007/s00508-005-0421-0

- Pavia, M. A., Paier, B., Noli, M. I., Hagmuller, K., & Zaninovich, A. A. (1997). Evidence suggesting that cadmium induces a non-thyroidal illness syndrome in the rat. *Journal of Endocrinology, 154*(1), 113-117. doi:10.1677/joe.0.1540113

- Puri, H. S. (2003). Rasayana: Ayurvedic Herbs for Longevity and Rejuvenation: Volume 2 of Traditional Herbal Medicines for Modern Times. *The Journal of Alternative and Complementary Medicine, 9*(2), 331-332. doi:10.1089/10755530360623446

- Hoang, T. D., Olsen, C. H., Mai, V. Q., Clyde, P. W., & Shakir, M. K. (2013). Desiccated Thyroid Extract Compared With Levothyroxine in the Treatment of Hypothyroidism: A Randomized, Double-Blind, Crossover Study. *The Journal of Clinical Endocrinology & Metabolism, 98*(5), 1982-1990. doi:10.1210/jc.2012-4107

Chapter 36: Sex Hormones—Happy or Cranky?

In-text citations:

1. DUTCH Test: The Most Informative Hormone Test. (n.d.). Retrieved March 02, 2017, from http://articles.mercola.com/sites/articles/archive/2016/05/08/dutch-hormone-test.aspx

2. Schneider, A. P., Zainer, C. M., Kubat, C. K., Mullen, N. K., & Windisch, A. K. (2014, August). The breast cancer epidemic: 10 facts. Retrieved September 10, 2017, from https://www.ncbi.nlm.nih.gov/pmc/articles/PMC4135458/

3. Rocca, W. A., Bower, J. H., Maraganore, D. M., Ahlskog, J. E., Grossardt, B. R., Andrade, M. D., & Melton, L. J. (2007). Increased risk of parkinsonism in women who underwent oophorectomy before menopause. Neurology, 70(3), 200-209. doi:10.1212/01.wnl.0000280573.30975.6a

4. Parker, W. H., Broder, M. S., Chang, E., Feskanich, D., Farquhar, C., Liu, Z., . . . Manson, J. E. (2009). Ovarian Conservation at the Time of Hysterectomy and Long-Term Health Outcomes in the Nurses' Health Study. Obstetrics & Gynecology, 113(5), 1027-1037. doi:10.1097/aog.0b013e3181a11c64

5. Moorman, P. G., Myers, E. R., Schildkraut, J. M., Iversen, E. S., Wang, F., & Warren, N. (2011). Effect of Hysterectomy With Ovarian Preservation on Ovarian Function. Obstetrics & Gynecology, 118(6), 1271-1279. doi:10.1097/aog.0b013e318236fd12

General References:

- Vanderhaeghe, L. (2011). Fitzhenry and Whiteside.

- Moorman, P. G., Myers, E. R., Schildkraut, J. M., Iversen, E. S., Wang, F., & Warren, N. (2011). Effect of Hysterectomy With Ovarian Preservation on Ovarian Function. *Obstetrics & Gynecology,118*(6), 1271-1279. doi:10.1097/aog.0b013e318236fd12

- Xenoestrogens: Plastic's Dirty Secret. (n.d.). Retrieved March 02, 2017, from http://besynchro.com/blogs/blog/12492461-xenoestrogens-plastics-dirty-secret

- 25% Of The Body's Cholesterol Is In The Brain, Keeping You Alzheimer's-Free. (2015, October 05). Retrieved March 02, 2017, from http://www.healthy-holistic-living.com/fat-and-cholesterol-affect-the-brain.html

- Stress and Body Shape: Stress-Induced Cortisol Secretion Is... : Psychosomatic Medicine. (n.d.). Retrieved March 02, 2017, from http://journals.lww.com/psychosomaticmedicine/Abstract/2000/09000/Stress_and_Body_Shape__Stress_Induced_Cortisol.5.aspx

- Epsom Salt - The Magnesium-Rich, Detoxifying Pain Reliever. (2015, September 21). Retrieved March 02, 2017, from https://draxe.com/epsom-salt/

- Michnovicz, J. J., & Bradlow, H. L. (1990). Induction of Estradiol Metabolism by Dietary Indole-3-carbinol in Humans. *JNCI Journal of the National Cancer Institute,82*(11), 947-949. doi:10.1093/jnci/82.11.947

- The world's top new source on natural health. (n.d.). Retrieved March 02, 2017, from http://www.naturalnews.com/027227_cancer_breast_estrogen.html&sa=D&ust=1488504795406000&usg=AFQjCNH2xiRnbBGhc4Bce2uj29UEw-gNAw

- Kirschner, M. A., Samojlik, E., Drejka, M., Szmal, E., Schneider, G., & Ertel, N. (1990). Androgen-Estrogen Metabolism in Women with Upper BodyVersusLower Body Obesity.* *The Journal of Clinical Endocrinology & Metabolism, 70*(2), 473-479. doi:10.1210/jcem-70-2-473

- Fogle, R. H., Stanczyk, F. Z., Zhang, X., & Paulson, R. J. (2007). Ovarian Androgen Production in Postmenopausal Women. *Obstetrical & Gynecological Survey,62*(12), 791-793. doi:10.1097/01.ogx.0000292008.97616.c7

- Melton, L. J., Khosla, S., Malkasian, G. D., Achenbach, S. J., Oberg, A. L., & Riggs, B. L. (2003). Fracture Risk After Bilateral Oophorectomy in Elderly Women. *Journal of Bone and Mineral Research, 18*(5), 900-905. doi:10.1359/jbmr.2003.18.5.900

- Rocca, W. A., Grossardt, B. R., Geda, Y. E., Gostout, B. S., Bower, J. H., Maraganore, D. M., . . . Melton, L. J. (2008). Long-term risk of depressive and anxiety symptoms after early bilateral oophorectomy. *Menopause, 15*(6), 1050-1059. doi:10.1097/gme.0b013e318174f155

- Parker, W. H., Broder, M. S., Berek, J. S., Liu, Z., Shoupe, D., & Farquhar, J. S. (2005). Ovarian Conservation at the Time of Hysterectomy for Benign Disease. *Obstetrics & Gynecology, 106*(5, Part 1), 1107. doi:10.1097/01.aog.0000186258.37099.a2

- Farquhar, C. M., Sadler, L., Harvey, S. A., & Stewart, A. W. (2005). The association of hysterectomy and menopause: a prospective cohort study. BJOG: *An International Journal of Obstetrics and Gynaecology, 112*(7), 956-962. doi:10.1111/j.1471-0528.2005.00696.x

- Pinkerton, J. V., & Santoro, N. (2015). Compounded bioidentical hormone therapy. *Menopause, 22*(9), 926-936. doi:10.1097/gme.0000000000000420
- Zoeller, R. T., Brown, T. R., Doan, L. L., Gore, A. C., Skakkebaek, N. E., Soto, A. M., . . . Saal, F. S. (2012). Endocrine-Disrupting Chemicals and Public Health Protection: A Statement of Principles from The Endocrine Society. *Endocrinology, 153*(9), 4097-4110. doi:10.1210/en.2012-1422
- Michnovicz, J. J., & Bradlow, H. L. (1990). Induction of Estradiol Metabolism by Dietary Indole-3-carbinol in Humans. *JNCI Journal of the National Cancer Institute, 82*(11), 947-949. doi:10.1093/jnci/82.11.947

Chapter 37: Blood Sugar—How Is It Impacting Your Weight and Your Health?

In-text citations:

1. Walton, A. G. (2012, August 30). How Much Sugar Are Americans Eating? [Infographic]. Retrieved March 02, 2017, from https://www.forbes.com/sites/alicegwalton/2012/08/30/how-much-sugar-are-americans-eating-infographic/#66c51b384ee7

2. What Happens in Your Body When You Eat Too Much Sugar? (n.d.). Retrieved September 10, 2017, from http://articles.mercola.com/sugar-side-effects.aspx

3. The 5 Worst Artificial Sweeteners. (2015, July 01). Retrieved March 02, 2017, from https://draxe.com/artificial-sweeteners/

4. Monte, S. M., & Wands, J. R. (2008, November). Alzheimer's Disease Is Type 3 Diabetes–Evidence Reviewed. Retrieved September 10, 2017, from https://www.ncbi.nlm.nih.gov/pmc/articles/PMC2769828/

5. Kodl, C. T., & Seaquist, E. R. (2008, June). Cognitive Dysfunction and Diabetes Mellitus. Retrieved September 10, 2017, from https://www.ncbi.nlm.nih.gov/pmc/articles/PMC2528851/

6. What Is Metabolic Syndrome? (2016, June 22). Retrieved September 10, 2017, from https://www.nhlbi.nih.gov/health/health-topics/topics/ms

General References:

- Leptin and Leptin Resistance: Everything You Need to Know. (2016, August 18). Retrieved March 02, 2017, from https://authoritynutrition.com/leptin-101/
- Stöppler, M. M. (n.d.). Insulin Resistance Symptoms, Signs, Test, Diet, and Food List. Retrieved March 02, 2017, from http://www.medicinenet.com/insulin_resistance/article.htm
- Hyman, M. (2014). *The blood sugar solution: the ultra healthy program for losing weight, preventing disease, and feeling great now!* New York, NY: Little, Brown and Company.
- Stress and Diabetes. (n.d.). Retrieved March 02, 2017, from http://www.webmd.com/diabetes/features/stress-diabetes
- Mozaffarian, D., Cao, H., King, I. B., Lemaitre, R. N., Song, X., Siscovick, D. S., & Hotamisligil, G. S. (2010). Trans -Palmitoleic Acid, Metabolic Risk Factors, and New-Onset Diabetes in U.S. Adults. *Annals of Internal Medicine, 153*(12), 790. doi:10.7326/0003-4819-153-12-201012210-00005
- Hyperglycemia and hypoglycemia in type 2 diabetes. (2014, June 04). Retrieved March 02, 2017, from https://www.ncbi.nlm.nih.gov/pubmedhealth/PMH0072694/
- Neuhouser, M. L., Schwarz, Y., Wang, C., Breymeyer, K., Coronado, G., Wang, C., . . . Lampe, J. W. (2011). A Low-Glycemic Load Diet Reduces Serum C-Reactive Protein and Modestly Increases Adiponectin in Overweight and Obese Adults. *Journal of Nutrition, 142*(2), 369-374. doi:10.3945/jn.111.149807
- Schenk, S., Saberi, M., & Olefsky, J. M. (2008). Insulin sensitivity: modulation by nutrients and inflammation. *Journal of Clinical Investigation, 118*(9), 2992-3002. doi:10.1172/jci34260
- Andreasen, A. S., Larsen, N., Pedersen-Skovsgaard, T., Berg, R. M., Møller, K., Svendsen, K. D., . . . Pedersen, B. K. (2010). Effects of Lactobacillus acidophilus NCFM on insulin sensitivity and the systemic inflammatory response in human subjects. *British Journal of Nutrition, 104*(12), 1831-1838. doi:10.1017/s0007114510002874
- Zhang, H., Wei, J., Xue, R., Wu, J., Zhao, W., Wang, Z., . . . Jiang, J. (2010). Berberine lowers blood glucose in type 2 diabetes mellitus patients through increasing insulin receptor expression. *Metabolism, 59*(2), 285-292. doi:10.1016/j.metabol.2009.07.029
- Suez, J., Korem, T., Zeevi, D., Zilberman-Schapira, G., Thaiss, C. A., Maza, O., . . . Elinav, E. (2015). Artificial Sweeteners Induce Glucose Intolerance by Altering the Gut Microbiota. *Obstetrical & Gynecological Survey, 70*(1), 31-32. doi:10.1097/01.ogx.0000460711.58331.94
- Simental-Mendía, L. E., Sahebkar, A., Rodríguez-Morán, M., & Guerrero-Romero, F. (2016). A systematic review and meta-analysis of randomized controlled trials on the effects of magnesium supplementation on insulin sensitivity and glucose control. *Pharmacological Research, 111*, 272-282. doi:10.1016/j.phrs.2016.06.019

SECTION 8: GET YOUR GUT AND IMMUNE SYSTEM PERFORMING OPTIMALLY

Chapter 38: Your Gut—Understanding How It Works and What Could Go Wrong

In-text citations:

1. Mayer et al. (2014). Gut Microbes and the Brain. J. *Neuroscience. 34*(46): 15490-15496

2. Figure 2f from: Irimia R, Gottschling M (2016) Taxonomic revision of Rochefortia Sw. (Ehretiaceae, Boraginales). Biodiversity Data Journal 4: e7720. https://doi.org/10.3897/BDJ.4.e7720. (n.d.). doi:10.3897/bdj.4.e7720.figure2f

3. Survey shows 74 percent of Americans living with GI discomfort. (n.d.). Retrieved January 09, 2018, from http://www.foxnews.com/health/2013/11/22/survey-shows-74-percent-americans-experience-gi-discomfort.html

4. Plummer, D. (n.d.). *The Human Microbiome: A Key Driver in Lifelong Health & Disease.*

5. Julie-Ann Amos on June 30. (2012, June 30). Acid Reflux (GERD) Statistics and Facts. Retrieved September 10, 2017, from http://www.healthline.com/health/gerd/statistics

6. Vighi, G., Marcucci, F., Sensi, L., Cara, G. D., & Frati, F. (2008, September). Allergy and the gastrointestinal system. Retrieved September 10, 2017, from https://www.ncbi.nlm.nih.gov/pmc/articles/PMC2515351/

General References:

- Do You Have SIBO? Here is ALL You Need to Know! (2015, June 30). Retrieved March 02, 2017, from https://draxe.com/sibo-symptoms/
- Hanaway, P. (2014). Diversity: From Diet to Flora to Life. *Global Advances in Health and Medicine, 3*(3), 6-8. doi:10.7453/gahmj.2014.022
- Khanna, S., & Tosh, P. K. (2014). A Clinician's Primer on the Role of the Microbiome in Human Health and Disease. *Mayo Clinic Proceedings, 89*(1), 107-114. doi:10.1016/j.mayocp.2013.10.011
- Kumamoto, C. A. (2011). Inflammation and gastrointestinal Candida colonization. *Current Opinion in Microbiology, 14*(4), 386-391. doi:10.1016/j.mib.2011.07.015
- Turnbaugh, P. J., Hamady, M., Yatsunenko, T., Cantarel, B. L., Duncan, A., Ley, R. E., . . . Gordon, J. I. (2008). A core gut microbiome in obese and lean twins. *Nature, 457*(7228), 480-484. doi:10.1038/nature07540

- Konkel, L. (2013). *The Environment Within: Exploring the Role of the Gut Microbiome in Health and Disease. Environmental Health Perspectives, 121*(9). doi:10.1289/ehp.121-a276

- Pimentel, M., Chow, E. J., & Lin, H. C. (2000). Eradication of small intestinal bacterial overgrowth reduces symptoms of irritable bowel syndrome. *The American Journal of Gastroenterology, 95*(12), 3503-3506. doi:10.1111/j.1572-0241.2000.03368.x

- Halmos, E. P., Power, V. A., Shepherd, S. J., Gibson, P. R., & Muir, J. G. (2014). A Diet Low in FODMAPs Reduces Symptoms of Irritable Bowel Syndrome. *Gastroenterology, 146*(1). doi:10.1053/j.gastro.2013.09.046

- Marcason, W. (2012). What Is the FODMAP Diet? *Journal of the Academy of Nutrition and Dietetics, 112*(10), 1696. doi:10.1016/j.jand.2012.08.005

- Pedersen, N. (2014). Ehealth monitoring in irritable bowel syndrome patients treated with low fermentable oligo-, di-, mono-saccharides and polyols diet. *World Journal of Gastroenterology, 20*(21), 6680. doi:10.3748/wjg.v20.i21.6680

- Abraham, B. P., & Kane, S. (2012). Fecal Markers: Calprotectin and Lactoferrin. *Gastroenterology Clinics of North America, 41*(2), 483-495. doi:10.1016/j.gtc.2012.01.007

- Fecal calprotectin: a biomarker for intestinal inflammation. (2015). Inflammation and Cell Signaling. doi:10.14800/ics.563

- Devaraj, S., Hemarajata, P., & Versalovic, J. (2013). The Human Gut Microbiome and Body Metabolism: Implications for Obesity and Diabetes. *Clinical Chemistry,59*(4), 617-628. doi:10.1373/clinchem.2012.187617

- Duncan, S. H., & Flint, H. J. (2013). Probiotics and prebiotics and health in aging populations. *Maturitas, 75*(1), 44-50. doi:10.1016/j.maturitas.2013.02.004

- Mattson, M. P., Duan, W., Wan, R., & Guo, Z. (2004). Prophylactic activation of neuroprotective stress response pathways by dietary and behavioral manipulations. *Neurotherapeutics, 1*(1), 111-116. doi:10.1007/bf03206571

- Herbal therapy is equivalent to rifaximin for the treatment of small intestinal bacterial overgrowth. (n.d.). Retrieved March 02, 2017, from https://www.ncbi.nlm.nih.gov/pubmed/24891990

Chapter 39: The Immune System—Is Yours Strong Enough?

General References:

- Fasano, A. (2011). Leaky Gut and Autoimmune Diseases. *Clinical Reviews in Allergy & Immunology,42*(1), 71-78. doi:10.1007/s12016-011-8291-x

- Bubbs, M. (2015). *The Paleo Project: the 21st century guide to looking leaner, getting stronger and living longer.* Victoria, BC: Friesen Press.

- Mercola, J. (2016). *Effortless healing: 9 simple ways to sidestep illness, shed excess weight, and help your body fix itself.* New York: Harmony Book.

- Antibiotics & The Immune system. (n.d.). Retrieved March 02, 2017, from http://immunedisorders.homestead.com/antibiotics.html

- Forsgren, A., & Riesbeck, K. (2010). Antibiotics and the immune system. *Antibiotic and Chemotherapy,*104-109. doi:10.1016/b978-0-7020-4064-1.00007-5

- Food allergies and sensitivities. (2002). *Nutrition & Food Science,32*(3). doi:10.1108/nfs.2002.01732cab.014

- Flu Shot/Flu Vaccine Side Effects & Dangers - FREE Report! (n.d.). Retrieved March 02, 2017, from http://www.mercola.com/downloads/bonus/beat-the-flu-without-a-shot/report.htm

- The Health Dangers of Triclosan in Personal Care Products. (n.d.). Retrieved March 02, 2017, from http://articles.mercola.com/sites/articles/archive/2012/08/29/triclosan-in-personal-care-products.aspx#!

- Sleep and the Immune System: Implications for Health and Mortality. (2011). Sleep & Safety,52-59. doi:10.2174/978160805271410052

- Mälzer, J. N., Schulz, A. R., & Thiel, A. (2016). Environmental Influences on the Immune System: The Aging Immune System. *Environmental Influences on the Immune System,*55-76. doi:10.1007/978-3-7091-1890-0_3

- Dawson, M. (1978). THE ROLE OF the human APPENDIX IN IMMUNITY TO INFECTIONS. *Journal of Pharmacy and Pharmacology,30*(S1). doi:10.1111/j.2042-7158.1978.tb10797.x

- Sigthorsson, G., Tibble, J., Hayllar, J., Menzies, I., Macpherson, A., Moots, R., . . . Bjarnason, I. (1998). Intestinal permeability and inflammation in patients on NSAIDs. *Gut,43*(4), 506-511. doi:10.1136/gut.43.4.506

- Harel, M. (2006). Predicting and Preventing Autoimmunity, Myth or Reality? *Annals of the New York Academy of Sciences, 1069*(1), 322-345. doi:10.1196/annals.1351.031

- Diaz-Sanchez, D. (2000). Pollution and the immune response: atopic diseases - are we too dirty or too clean? *Immunology, 101*(1), 11-18. doi:10.1046/j.1365-2567.2000.00108.x

- Prasad, A. S. (2009). Zinc: role in immunity, oxidative stress and chronic inflammation. *Current Opinion in Clinical Nutrition and Metabolic Care, 12*(6), 646-652. doi:10.1097/mco.0b013e3283312956

Chapter 40: Inflammation—What Does It Mean for Your Health?

In-text citations:

1. Block, G., Jensen, C., Dalvi, T., Norkus, E., Hudes, M., Crawford, P., . . . Harmatz, P. (2009). Vitamin C treatment reduces elevated C-reactive protein. *Free Radical Biology and Medicine,46*(1), 70-77. doi:10.1016/j.freeradbiomed.2008.09.030

2. Nonsteroidal Anti-inflammatory Drug (NSAID) Toxicity. (2017, August 30). Retrieved September 10, 2017, from http://emedicine.medscape.com/article/816117-overview

General References:

- Griffin, R. M. (n.d.). Pain Relief: How NSAIDs Work. Retrieved March 02, 2017, from http://www.webmd.com/arthritis/features/pain-relief-how-nsaids-work#2

- Ciaccia, L. (2011, March). Fundamentals of Inflammation. Retrieved March 02, 2017, from https://www.ncbi.nlm.nih.gov/pmc/articles/PMC3064252/

- Nordqvist, C. (n.d.). Inflammation: Causes, Symptoms and Treatment. Retrieved March 02, 2017, from http://www.medicalnewstoday.com/articles/248423.php

- Pischon, T. (2003). Habitual Dietary Intake of n-3 and n-6 Fatty Acids in Relation to Inflammatory Markers Among US Men and Women. *Circulation, 108*(2), 155-160. doi:10.1161/01.cir.0000079224.46084.c2

- Aggarwal, B. B., & Sung, B. (2009). Pharmacological basis for the role of curcumin in chronic diseases: an age-old spice with modern targets. *Trends in Pharmacological Sciences, 30*(2), 85-94. doi:10.1016/j.tips.2008.11.002

- Moussaieff, A., Shohami, E., Kashman, Y., Fride, E., Schmitz, M. L., Renner, F., . . . Mechoulam, R. (2007). Incensole Acetate, a Novel Anti-Inflammatory Compound Isolated from Boswellia Resin, Inhibits Nuclear Factor- B Activation. *Molecular Pharmacology, 72*(6), 1657-1664. doi:10.1124/mol.107.038810

- Dahmen, U., Gu, Y., Dirsch, O., Fan, L., Li, J., Shen, K., & Broelsch, C. (2001). Boswellic acid, a potent antiinflammatory drug, inhibits rejection to the same extent as high dose steroids. *Transplantation Proceedings, 33*(1-2), 539-541. doi:10.1016/s0041-1345(00)02131-x

- Kane, S. (2000). Use of Bromelain for Mild Ulcerative Colitis. *Annals of Internal Medicine, 132*(8), 680. doi:10.7326/0003-4819-132-8-200004180-00026

- Huang, T. H., Tran, V. H., Duke, R. K., Tan, S., Chrubasik, S., Roufogalis, B. D., & Duke, C. C. (2006). Harpagoside suppresses lipopolysaccharide-induced iNOS and COX-2 expression through inhibition of NF-KappaB activation. *Journal of Ethnopharmacology, 104*(1-2), 149-155. doi:10.1016/j.jep.2005.08.055
- Mncwangi, N., Chen, W., Vermaak, I., Viljoen, A. M., & Gericke, N. (2012). Devil's Claw—A review of the ethnobotany, phytochemistry and biological activity of Harpagophytum procumbens. *Journal of Ethnopharmacology, 143*(3), 755-771. doi:10.1016/j.jep.2012.08.013
- Jeong, H. W., Hsu, K. C., Lee, J., Ham, M., Huh, J. Y., Shin, H. J., . . . Kim, J. B. (2009). Berberine suppresses proinflammatory responses through AMPK activation in macrophages. AJP: *Endocrinology and Metabolism, 296*(4). doi:10.1152/ajpendo.90599.2008

Chapter 41: Food Sensitivities—Is Your Body Angry with What You Are Eating?

In-text citations:

1. Skip the skim milk and go full fat. (2016, January 05). Retrieved September 10, 2017, from http://www.buzznutrition.com/skip-the-skim-milk-and-go-full-fat/
2. Meats, U. W. (n.d.). Dairy: Food of the Gods? |USWM. Retrieved September 10, 2017, from http://blog.grasslandbeef.com/dairy-food-of-the-gods
3. Institute of Medicine (US) Committee to Review Dietary Reference Intakes for Vitamin D and Calcium. (1970, January 01). Overview of Calcium. Retrieved September 10, 2017, from https://www.ncbi.nlm.nih.gov/books/NBK56060/
4. Milk Allergy. (n.d.). Retrieved September 10, 2017, from https://www.foodallergy.org/common-allergens/milk
5. Gundry, S. R., & Buehl, O. B. (2017). *The plant paradox: the hidden dangers in "healthy" foods that cause disease and weight gain.* New York, NY: Harper Wave, an imprint of HarperCollins .
6. Processing Milk. (n.d.). Retrieved September 10, 2017, from http://www.mercola.com/article/milk/no-milk.aspx
7. Why Dairy Is Scary. (2016, July 18). Retrieved September 10, 2017, from https://www.theodysseyonline.com/got
8. D. (2017, August 01). Dr. Mark Hyman: Are You Still Consuming Dairy? Retrieved September 10, 2017, from https://www.ecowatch.com/mark-hyman-dairy-2467918213.html
9. Calcium and Cancer Prevention. (n.d.). Retrieved September 10, 2017, from https://www.cancer.gov/about-cancer/causes-prevention/risk/diet/calcium-fact-sheet
10. Dairy: 6 Reasons You Should Avoid It at all Costs. (2017, January 03). Retrieved March 02, 2017, from http://drhyman.com/blog/2010/06/24/dairy-6-reasons-you-should-avoid-it-at-all-costs-2/
11. Sales and Trends. (n.d.). Retrieved September 10, 2017, from http://www.soyfoods.org/soy-products/sales-and-trends
12. About GE Foods. (n.d.). Retrieved December 23, 2017, from https://www.centerforfoodsafety.org/issues/311/ge-foods/about-ge-foods

General References:.

- Davis, D., About Dr. DavisCardiologist Dr. William Davis is a New YorkTimes #1 Best Selling author and the Medical Director of the Wheat Belly Lifestyle Institute and the Cureality.com program. Nothing here should be construed as medical advice, but only topics for further discussion with your doctor. I practice cardiology in Milwaukee, Wisconsin., B., S., Epps, P., D., . . . J. (2012, February 14). Wheat is NOT "genetically-modified." Retrieved March 02, 2017, from http://www.wheatbellyblog.com/2012/02/wheat-is-not-genetically-modified/
- Winters, C. (n.d.). The Best Way to Boost Your Immune System. Retrieved March 02, 2017, from http://www.consumerreports.org/conditions-treatments/best-ways-to-boost-your-immune-system/
- Why You Need to Avoid Low Fat Milk and Cheese. (n.d.). Retrieved March 02, 2017, from http://articles.mercola.com/sites/articles/archive/2011/05/21/why-you-need-to-avoid-low-fat-milk-and-cheese.aspx
- Whole Milk vs Skim Milk: Full Fat Is Better for Your Health. (n.d.). Retrieved March 02, 2017, from http://time.com/4279538/low-fat-milk-vs-whole-milk/
- The relationship between high-fat dairy consumption and obesity, cardiovascular, and metabolic disease. (n.d.). Retrieved March 02, 2017, from https://www.ncbi.nlm.nih.gov/pubmed/22810464
- Is Soy Bad For You, or Good? The Shocking Truth. (2016, August 18). Retrieved March 02, 2017, from https://authoritynutrition.com/is-soy-bad-for-you-or-good/
- Punder, K. D., & Pruimboom, L. (2013). The Dietary Intake of Wheat and other Cereal Grains and Their Role in Inflammation. *Nutrients, 5*(3), 771-787. doi:10.3390/nu5030771
- Atkinson, W. (2004). Food elimination based on IgG antibodies in irritable bowel syndrome: a randomised controlled trial. *Gut, 53*(10), 1459-1464. doi:10.1136/gut.2003.037697
- Guo, H., Jiang, T., Wang, J., Chang, Y., Guo, H., & Zhang, W. (2012). The Value of Eliminating Foods According to Food-Specific Immunoglobulin G Antibodies in Irritable Bowel Syndrome with Diarrhoea. *Journal of International Medical Research, 40*(1), 204-210. doi:10.1177/147323001204000121
- Sapone, A., Lammers, K. M., Casolaro, V., Cammarota, M., Giuliano, M. T., Rosa, M. D., . . . Fasano, A. (2011). Divergence of gut permeability and mucosal immune gene expression in two gluten-associated conditions: celiac disease and gluten sensitivity. *BMC Medicine, 9*(1). doi:10.1186/1741-7015-9-23
- Peters, S. L., Biesiekierski, J. R., Yelland, G. W., Muir, J. G., & Gibson, P. R. (2014). Randomised clinical trial: gluten may cause depression in subjects with non-coeliac gluten sensitivity - an exploratory clinical study. *Alimentary Pharmacology & Therapeutics, 39*(10), 1104-1112. doi:10.1111/apt.12730
- Untersmayr, E. (2005). Anti-ulcer drugs promote IgE formation toward dietary antigens in adult patients. *The FASEB Journal.* doi:10.1096/fj.04-3170fje
- Sapone, A., Bai, J. C., Ciacci, C., Dolinsek, J., Green, P. H., Hadjivassiliou, M., . . . Fasano, A. (2012). Spectrum of gluten-related disorders: consensus on new nomenclature and classification. *BMC Medicine, 10*(1). doi:10.1186/1741-7015-10-13
- Kurzer, M. S. (2002, March). Hormonal effects of soy in premenopausal women and men. Retrieved September 10, 2017, from https://www.ncbi.nlm.nih.gov/pubmed/11880595
- Fasano, A., Sapone, A., Zevallos, V., & Schuppan, D. (2015). Nonceliac Gluten Sensitivity. *Gastroenterology, 148*(6), 1195-1204. doi:10.1053/j.gastro.2014.12.049
- Khamsi, R. (2014). The Trouble with Gluten. *Scientific American, 310*(2), 30-32. doi:10.1038/scientificamerican0214-30
- Fasano, A. (2015). A Clinical Conversation: Celiac Disease and Gluten-Related Disorders: Integrative Clinical Approaches. *Alternative and Complementary Therapies, 21*(1), 18-21. doi:10.1089/act.2015.21109
- Fasano, A. (2009). Surprises from Celiac Disease. *Scientific American, 301*(2), 54-61. doi:10.1038/scientificamerican0809-54
- Sapone, A., Lammers, K. M., Casolaro, V., Cammarota, M., Giuliano, M. T., Rosa, M. D., . . . Fasano, A. (2011). Divergence of gut permeability and mucosal immune gene expression in two gluten-associated conditions: celiac disease and gluten sensitivity. *BMC Medicine, 9*(1). doi:10.1186/1741-7015-9-23
- Junker, Y., Zeissig, S., Kim, S., Barisani, D., Wieser, H., Leffler, D. A., . . . Schuppan, D. (2012). Wheat amylase trypsin inhibitors drive intestinal inflammation via activation of toll-like receptor 4. *The Journal of Experimental Medicine, 209*(13), 2395-2408. doi:10.1084/jem.20102660

Chapter 42: Histamine Intolerance—Could It Be Contributing to Your Allergies?

General References:

- Histamine Intolerance causes|symptoms|treatment Histamine Intolerance info. (n.d.). Retrieved March 02, 2017, from http://www.histamine-intolerance. info/
- Histamine intolerance investigated by Dr Janice Joneja. (n.d.). Retrieved March 02, 2017, from http://www.foodsmatter.com/allergy_intolerance/histamine/ articles/histamine_joneja.html
- The Food List. (n.d.). Retrieved March 02, 2017, from http://www.histamineintolerance.org.uk/about/the-food-diary/the-food-list/

SECTION 9: GET YOUR BRAIN TURNED ON TO ITS FULL POWER

Chapter 43: Brain 101—How Does Your Brain Work?

In-text citations:

1. Wallis, L. (2013, September 23). Is 25 the new cut-off point for adulthood? Retrieved September 10, 2017, from http://www.bbc.com/news/ magazine-24173194

General References:

- Medina, J. (2008). *Brain rules: 12 principles for surviving and thriving at work, home, and school.* Seattle, WA: Pear Press.
- Why SPECT. (n.d.). Retrieved March 05, 2017, from http://www.amenclinics.com/why-spect/
- Freudenrich, P. C., & Boyd, R. (2001, June 06). How Your Brain Works. Retrieved March 05, 2017, from http://science.howstuffworks.com/life/inside-the-mind/human-brain/brain7.htm
- Dear Mark: How Much Glucose Does Your Brain Really Need? (2014, June 19). Retrieved March 05, 2017, from http://www.marksdailyapple.com/how-much-glucose-does-your-brain-really-need/
- "Brain Structures and their Functions." *Serendip Studio.* N.p., n.d. Web. 06 Mar. 2017.
- Braverman, Eric R. *Edge effect.* New York, NY: Sterling Publishing Co., Inc., 2004. Print.
- "Your Gut May Hold the Key to Better Brain Health." *Mercola.com.* N.p., n.d. Web. 06 Mar. 2017.
- "2. The 4 Pillars of Brain Maintenance." *SharpBrains.* N.p., 08 Apr. 2010. Web. 06 Mar. 2017.
- Amen, Daniel G. *Change your brain, change your life: the breakthrough program for conquering anxiety, depression, obsessiveness, lack of focus, anger, and memory problems.* New York: Harmony , 2015. Print.
- Mendelsohn, A. R., & Larrick, J. W. (2013). Sleep Facilitates Clearance of Metabolites from the Brain: Glymphatic Function in Aging and Neurodegenerative Diseases. *Rejuvenation Research, 16*(6), 518-523. doi:10.1089/rej.2013.1530
- Exercise, Yoga, and Meditation for Depressive and Anxiety ... (n.d.). Retrieved April 2, 2017, from https://www.aafp.org/afp/2010/0415/p981.pdf

Chapter 44: Neurotransmitters—Nutritional Support for Optimal Brain-Body Communication

In-text citations:

1. C, U. (2013). Capsule Endoscopy: A New Era of Gastrointestinal Endoscopy. *Endoscopy of GI Tract.* doi:10.5772/52732

General References:

- Amen, Daniel G. *Change your brain, change your life: the breakthrough program for conquering anxiety, depression, obsessiveness, lack of focus, anger, and memory problems.* New York: Harmony , 2015. Print.
- Adnan, Amna. "Neurotransmitters and its types." *Neurotransmitters and its types.* N.p., n.d. Web. 06 Mar. 2017.
- Braverman, Eric R. *Edge effect.* New York, NY: Sterling Publishing Co., Inc., 2004. Print.
- Ratey, John J., and Eric Hagerman. *Spark: the revolutionary new science of exercise and the brain.* New York: Little, Brown, 2013. Print.
- Hansell, James, and Lisa Damour. *Abnormal psychology.* Chichester: John Wiley, 2008. Print.
- "No one knows a prescription drug's side effects like the person taking it." RxISK. N.p., n.d. Web. 06 Mar. 2017.
- "Science, Psychiatry and Social Justice." *Mad In America.* N.p., n.d. Web. 06 Mar. 2017.
- "Welcome to benzo.org.uk : Main Page." *Welcome to benzo.org.uk : Main Page.* N.p., n.d. Web. 06 Mar. 2017.
- "Benzodiazepines: How They Work & How to Withdraw, Prof C H Ashton DM, FRCP, 2002." *Benzodiazepines: How They Work & How to Withdraw, Prof C H Ashton DM, FRCP, 2002.* N.p., n.d. Web. 06 Mar. 2017.
- "Stressed By His Short Allele." *Brain Blogger Stressed By His Short Allele Comments.* N.p., n.d. Web. 06 Mar. 2017.
- "THE BRAIN FROM TOP TO BOTTOM." *THE BRAIN FROM TOP TO BOTTOM.* N.p., n.d. Web. 06 Mar. 2017.
- Clouse, Rhiannon. "The Effects of Dopamine on the Brain." *LIVESTRONG.COM.* Leaf Group, 08 Oct. 2015. Web. 06 Mar. 2017.
- Gotlib, Ian H., Jutta Joormann, Kelly L. Minor, and Joachim Hallmayer. "HPA Axis Reactivity: A Mechanism Underlying the Associations Among 5-HTTLPR, Stress, and Depression." *Biological Psychiatry*63.9 (2008): 847-51. Web.
- "You can and should feel on top of the world!" *Antianxiety Food Solution Improve Mood End Cravings Trudy Scott.* N.p., n.d. Web. 06 Mar. 2017.
- Comer, R. J. (2015). *Abnormal psychology.* New York, NY: Worth , a Macmillan Higher Education imprint.
- Purves, Dale. "Neurotransmitters." *Neuroscience. 2nd edition.* U.S. National Library of Medicine, 01 Jan. 1970. Web. 06 Mar. 2017.
- 1Ratey, J. J., & Hagerman, E. (2013). *Spark: the revolutionary new science of exercise and the brain.* New York: Little, Brown.

Chapter 45: The Nervous System—Is Yours Turned On?

In-text citations:

1. Stephenson, R. W., & Price, G. R. (1999). *Chiropractic textbook.* Davenport, IA: Palmer College of Chiropractic.
2. The 33 Chiropractic Principles. (2009, April 16). Retrieved January 09, 2018, from https://pureandpowerful.com/welcome/the-33-chiropractic-principles/
3. T. F. O. T. E. S. O. C. T. N. A. S. Electrophysiology. (1996). Heart Rate Variability : Standards of Measurement, Physiological Interpretation, and Clinical Use. *Circulation, 93*(5), 1043-1065. doi:10.1161/01.cir.93.5.1043

General References:

- *National Institutes of Health.* U.S. Department of Health and Human Services, n.d. Web. 06 Mar. 2017.
- Gray, Henry, and Carmine D. Clemente. *Anatomy of the human body.* Philadelphia: Lea & Febiger, 1985. Print.
- Bitenieks, Madars. *Chiropractic Leadership Alliance.* N.p., n.d. Web. 06 Mar. 2017.
- Bitenieks, Madars. "The COREscore: Simplified, Powerful reporting." *Chiropractic Leadership Alliance.* N.p., 05 July 2012. Web. 06 Mar. 2017.
- "Nervous System." *InnerBody.* N.p., n.d. Web. 06 Mar. 2017.

Chapter 46: Sharpening Your Brain—How to Mitigate Cognitive Decline

In-text citations:

1. Macrowe. "How to Keep a Sharp Mind and Good Attitude." *WikiHow.* WikiHow, 06 Mar. 2017. Web. 06 Mar. 2017.

General References:

- "Mint Scent Boosts the Brain, Improves Problem Solving and Memory." *Natural Society.* N.p., 07 May 2014. Web. 06 Mar. 2017.
- Nixon, Robin. "10 Ways to Keep Your Mind Sharp." *LiveScience.* Purch, 18 Feb. 2011. Web. 06 Mar. 2017.
- Publications, Harvard Health. "6 simple steps to keep your mind sharp at any age." *Harvard Health.* N.p., n.d. Web. 06 Mar. 2017.
- Medina, John. *Brain rules: 12 principles for surviving and thriving at work, home, and school.* Seattle, WA: Pear Press, 2008. Print.

Chapter 47: Epigenetics—You Are What You Think

In-text citations:

1. Twins become more different as they age. (n.d.). Retrieved September 10, 2017, from https://phys.org/news/2005-07-twins-age.html
2. Feinberg, C. (2014, March 03). The Mindfulness Chronicles. Retrieved September 10, 2017, from http://harvardmagazine.com/2010/09/the-mindfulness-chronicles

General References:

- Dispenza, Joe. *You are the placebo: making your mind matter.* Carlsbad, CA: Hay House, Inc., 2015. Print.
- Lipton, Bruce H. *The Biology of Beliefs.* Burgrain: Koha-Verl., 2012. Print.
- Weinhold, Bob. "Epigenetics: The Science of Change." *Environmental Health Perspectives.* National Institute of Environmental Health Sciences, Mar. 2006. Web. 06 Mar. 2017.
- 07.24.07, Posted. "Epigenetics." *PBS.* Public Broadcasting Service, n.d. Web. 06 Mar. 2017.
- "Epigenetics: DNA Isn't Everything." *ScienceDaily.* ScienceDaily, n.d. Web. 06 Mar. 2017.
- Weissenbach, J. "Human Genome Project: Past, Present, Future." *The Human Genome*(2002): 1-9. Web.
- Friedman, Lauren F. "A radical experiment tried to make old people young again - and the results were astonishing." *Business Insider.* Business Insider, 06 Apr. 2015. Web. 06 Mar. 2017.
- "An Overview of the Human Genome Project." *National Human Genome Research Institute (NHGRI).* N.p., n.d. Web. 06 Mar. 2017.

Chapter 48: Aging—Slowing the Process

In-text citations:

1. And, C. C. (2009, September 01). CARSTEN CARLBERG. Retrieved September 10, 2017, from http://ar.iiarjournals.org/content/29/9/3485.long
2. (n.d.). Retrieved January 09, 2018, from https://www.sciencedaily.com/releases/2010/08/100823172327.htm

General References:

- Uribarri, J., Cai, W., Sandu, O., Peppa, M., Goldberg, T., & Vlassara, H. (2005). Diet-Derived Advanced Glycation End Products Are Major Contributors to the Body's AGE Pool and Induce Inflammation in Healthy Subjects. *Annals of the New York Academy of Sciences, 1043*(1), 461-466. doi:10.1196/annals.1333.052
- Richie, J. P., Nichenametla, S., Neidig, W., Calcagnotto, A., Haley, J. S., Schell, T. D., & Muscat, J. E. (2014). Randomized controlled trial of oral glutathione supplementation on body stores of glutathione. *European Journal of Nutrition,54*(2), 251-263. doi:10.1007/s00394-014-0706-z

SECTION 10: GET REST, RECHARGE AND BE MORE ZEN

Chapter 49: Sleep—More Than Just Beauty Rest

In-text citations:

1. (2005, November 16). Retrieved September 11, 2017, from http://www.statcan.gc.ca/daily-quotidien/051116/dq051116a-eng.htm
2. (n.d.). Retrieved September 11, 2017, from https://web.stanford.edu/~dement/sleeppoll.html
3. Brain may flush out toxins during sleep. (2015, September 17). Retrieved September 11, 2017, from https://www.nih.gov/news-events/news-releases/brain-may-flush-out-toxins-during-sleep
4. Sleep. (2016, April 13). Retrieved September 11, 2017, from https://www.hsph.harvard.edu/obesity-prevention-source/obesity-causes/sleep-and-obesity/

General References:

- Lopresti, A. L., Hood, S. D., & Drummond, P. D. (2013). A review of lifestyle factors that contribute to important pathways associated with major depression: Diet, sleep and exercise. *Journal of Affective Disorders, 148*(1), 12-27. doi:10.1016/j.jad.2013.01.014
- Reid, K. J., Baron, K. G., Lu, B., Naylor, E., Wolfe, L., & Zee, P. C. (2010). Aerobic exercise improves self-reported sleep and quality of life in older adults with insomnia. *Sleep Medicine, 11*(9), 934-940. doi:10.1016/j.sleep.2010.04.014
- Medina, John. *Brain rules: 12 principles for surviving and thriving at work, home, and school.* Seattle, WA: Pear Press, 2008. Print.
- "Sleep Problems Solution – Tips on How to Sleep Better." *Mercola.com.* N.p., n.d. Web. 06 Mar. 2017.
- "Lack of Sleep Affects Hormone Levels 9/3/00 cortisol, growth hormone, adrenal gland, sleep, pineal." *Mercola.com.* N.p., n.d. Web. 06 Mar. 2017.
- "Want to Prevent Cancer? Make Sure You Sleep Well 10/22/03." *Mercola.com.* N.p., n.d. Web. 06 Mar. 2017.

- "The Effect of Short Sleep Duration on Coronary Heart Disease Risk is Greatest Among Those with Sleep Disturbance: A Prospective Study from the Whitehall II Cohort." *Sleep*(2010): n. pag. Web.
- Stevens, R. G. "Epidemiology of Uriniary Melatonin in Women and Its Relation to Other Hormones and Night Work." *Cancer Epidemiology Biomarkers & Prevention*14.2 (2005): 551. Web.
- Kim, Jee Hyun, and Hyang Woon Lee. "Melatonin and Human Sleep." *Journal of Korean Sleep Research Society*2.1 (2005): 10-15. Web.
- Hirshkowitz, Max, Constance A. Moore, and Gisele Minhoto. "The basics of sleep." *Understanding sleep: The evaluation and treatment of sleep disorders.*(n.d.): 11-34. Web.
- Vgontzas, A. N., E. Zoumakis, E. O. Bixler, H.-M. Lin, H. Follett, A. Kales, and G. P. Chrousos. "Adverse Effects of Modest Sleep Restriction on Sleepiness, Performance, and Inflammatory Cytokines." *The Journal of Clinical Endocrinology & Metabolism*89.5 (2004): 2119-126. Web.
- Bianchi, Matt T. "Sleep Deprivation and Neurological Diseases." *Sleep Deprivation and Disease*(2013): 47-63. Web.
- "10 Things to Hate About Sleep Loss." *WebMD.* WebMD, n.d. Web. 06 Mar. 2017.

Chapter 50: Meditation—You Don't Have to Be a Monk

General References:

- Smith, J. C. (2004). Alterations In Brain And Immune Function Produced By Mindfulness Meditation: Three Caveats. *Psychosomatic Medicine,66*(1), 148-149. doi:10.1097/00006842-200401000-00022
- "76 Scientific Benefits of Meditation." *Live and Dare.* N.p., 22 Jan. 2017. Web. 06 Mar. 2017.
- Delmonte, M. M. (1984). Electrocortical Activity and Related Phenomena Associated with Meditation Practice: A Literature Review. *International Journal of Neuroscience,24*(3-4), 217-231. doi:10.3109/00207458409089810
- Maclean, C. R., Walton, K. G., Wenneberg, S. R., Levitsky, D. K., Mandarino, J. P., Waziri, R., . . . Schneider, R. H. (1997). Effects of the transcendental meditation program on adaptive mechanisms: Changes in hormone levels and responses to stress after 4 months of practice. *Psychoneuroendocrinology,22*(4), 277-295. doi:10.1016/s0306-4530(97)00003-6
- Newberg, A., & Iversen, J. (2003). The neural basis of the complex mental task of meditation: neurotransmitter and neurochemical considerations. *Medical Hypotheses,61*(2), 282-291. doi:10.1016/s0306-9877(03)00175-0
- Brown, KW & Ryan (2003)., RM. The Benefits of Being Present: Mindfulness and Its Role in Psychological Well-Being. *Journal of Personality and Social Psychology;* 84(4); 822-848.
- "23 Types of Meditation - Find The Best Techniques For You." *Live and Dare.* N.p., 22 Jan. 2017. Web. 06 Mar. 2017.
- "Meditation and Wellbeing." *Masculinity, Meditation and Mental Health*(n.d.): n. pag. Web.
- Aujla, Rupy, Rupy Aujla Says, Farzanah Says, and The Reluctant Salonniere Says. "IFM 2016 Top 5 Lifestyle Tips." *The Doctors Kitchen.* N.p., 26 May 2016. Web. 06 Mar. 2017.
- "Top Five Benefits of Meditation." *STRENGTH SENSEI.* N.p., 15 Dec. 2016. Web. 06 Mar. 2017.

Chapter 51: De-Stressing—Explore the Tapping Technique

In-text citations:

1. "Emotional Freedom Technique (EFT) - Emotional Health." *Mercola.com.* N.p., n.d. Web. 06 Mar. 2017.
2. The Gary Craig Official EFT™ Training Centers. (n.d.). Retrieved September 11, 2017, from https://www.emofree.com/eft-tutorial/tapping-basics/what-is-eft.html

General References:

- "Emotional Freedom Techniques (EFT) Helps Relieve Stress & Anxiety." *Mercola.com.* N.p., n.d. Web. 06 Mar. 2017.
- "EFT: Tap Away Your Pain with This Extraordinary Healing Tool." *Mercola.com.* N.p., n.d. Web. 06 Mar. 2017.
- "The Home of Gold Standard EFT™(Emotional Freedom Techniques)." *What is EFT? - Theory, Science and Uses | PART I For Everyone: The EFT Tapping Basics | Official EFT Tutorial.* N.p., n.d. Web. 06 Mar. 2017.
- "What is EFT?" *What is EFT - Emotional Freedom Techniques.* N.p., n.d. Web. 06 Mar. 2017.

Chapter 52: Electromagnetic Field—What You Don't See Can Still Hurt You!

In-text citations:

1. Cellular Phones. (n.d.). Retrieved September 11, 2017, from https://www.cancer.org/cancer/cancer-causes/radiation-exposure/cellular-phones.html
2. EMF GOOD VS. BAD – MagnoPro. (n.d.). Retrieved September 11, 2017, from http://www.electromeds.com/magnopro/emf-good-vs-bad/
3. The Effects of Electromagnetic Fields:. (n.d.). Retrieved September 12, 2017, from http://www.weness.org/emfs/effects-electromagnetic-fields.html
4. Electromagnetic fields and public health: mobile phones. (n.d.). Retrieved September 12, 2017, from http://www.who.int/mediacentre/factsheets/fs193/en/
5. Bilton, N. (2015, March 18). The Health Concerns in Wearable Tech. Retrieved September 12, 2017, from https://www.nytimes.com/2015/03/19/style/could-wearable-computers-be-as-harmful-as-cigarettes.html
6. Research on Wireless Health Effects. (n.d.). Retrieved September 12, 2017, from https://ehtrust.org/science/research-on-wireless-health-effects/
7. Zhang, Y., Li, Z., Gao, Y., & Zhang, C. (2015, March). Effects of fetal microwave radiation exposure on offspring behavior in mice. Retrieved September 12, 2017, from https://www.ncbi.nlm.nih.gov/pmc/articles/PMC4380045/
8. The WORST Place to Store Your Cell Phone | EMF Dangers. (n.d.). Retrieved September 12, 2017, from http://articles.mercola.com/sites/articles/archive/2012/06/16/emf-safety-tips.aspx
9. BREAKING: Massive government study concludes cell phone radiation causes brain cancer. (n.d.). Retrieved September 12, 2017, from http://www.naturalnews.com/054165_cell_phone_radiation_brain_tumors_government_study.html

General References:

- "EMFs from Cell Phones and WiFi Are Making People Sick." *Mercola.com.* N.p., n.d. Web. 06 Mar. 2017.
- Wyde, Michael, Mark Cesta, Chad Blystone, Susan Elmore, Paul Foster, Michelle Hooth, Grace Kissling, David Malarkey, Robert Sills, Matthew Stout, Nigel Walker, Kristine Witt, Mary Wolfe, and John Bucher. "Report of Partial findings from the National Toxicology Program Carcinogenesis Studies of Cell Phone Radiofrequency Radiation in Hsd: Sprague Dawley® SD rats (Whole Body Exposure)." *BioRxiv.* Cold Spring Harbor Labs Journals, 01 Jan. 2016. Web. 06 Mar. 2017.
- Maron, Dina Fine. "Major Cell Phone Radiation Study Reignites Cancer Questions." *Scientific American.* N.p., 27 May 2016. Web. 06 Mar. 2017.

- *Hedron Life Source.* N.p., n.d. Web. 06 Mar. 2017.
- "Graham-Stetzer Microsurge Meter (to measure Dirty Electricity)." *EMF Solutions.* N.p., n.d. Web. 06 Mar. 2017.
- "The Top Five Sources of EMF Exposure." *Mercola.com.* N.p., n.d. Web. 06 Mar. 2017.
- "What Is EMF?" *Electromagnetic Field (EMF) Safety from Safe Space Protection.* N.p., n.d. Web. 06 Mar. 2017.
- "Exposure effects of RF-EMF on the cerebral microcirculation in rats." *SciVee*(n.d.): n. pag. Web.

Chapter 53: Earthing—Recharging with Nature

General References:

- Mercola, Joseph. *Effortless healing: 9 simple ways to sidestep illness, shed excess weight, and help your body fix itself.* New York: Harmony Book, 2016. Print.
- "Earthing.com." *Earthing.* N.p., n.d. Web. 06 Mar. 2017.
- "All about Grounding/Earthing Technology for Health & EMF Protection." *Groundology.* N.p., n.d. Web. 06 Mar. 2017.
- "The Health Effects of Grounding." *Mercola.com.* N.p., n.d. Web. 06 Mar. 2017.

SECTION 11: GET IN CONTROL–YOU AND YOUR WELLNESS TEAM

Chapter 54: It's Your Health—Who Is in Charge?

General References:

- Dweck, Carol S. *Mindset.* London: Robinson, an imprint of Constable & Robinson Ltd, 2017. Print.
- Miller, John G. *QBQ!: the question behind the question.* Denver, CO: Denver Press, 2001. Print.

Chapter 55: Know Your Numbers—Understanding Your Test Results to Take Control of Your Health

In-text citations:

1. Nakanga, W., Crampin, A., & Nyirenda, M. (2016, March). Should haemoglobin A1C be used for diagnosis of diabetes mellitus in Malawi? Retrieved September 12, 2017, from https://www.ncbi.nlm.nih.gov/pmc/articles/PMC4864390/
2. Fascinating Facts You Never Knew About the Human Brain. (n.d.). Retrieved December 18, 2017, from https://articles.mercola.com/sites/articles/archive/2009/01/22/fascinating-facts-you-never-knew-about-the-human-brain.aspx
3. Mastering Blood Chemistry (2006) Datis Kharazian
4. Ordovas, J. M., & Mooser, V. (2004, April). Nutrigenomics and nutrigenetics. Retrieved January 09, 2018, from https://www.ncbi.nlm.nih.gov/pubmed/15017352
5. MELISA – MELISA testing. (n.d.). Retrieved January 09, 2018, from http://www.melisa.org/

General References:

- "D-Spot." *Rocky Mountain Analytical.* N.p., 01 Feb. 2017. Web. 08 Mar. 2017.
- Chaudhary, A. K. (2015). Study on Diastolic Dysfunction in Newly Diagnosed Type 2 Diabetes Mellitus and its Correlation with Glycosylated Haemoglobin (HbA1C). *Journal Of Clinical And Diagnostic Research.* doi:10.7860/jcdr/2015/13348.6376
- Mayo Clinic Staff Print. "Complete blood count (CBC)." *Mayo Clinic.* N.p., 18 Oct. 2016. Web. 08 Mar. 2017.
- "Liver Panel." *Lab Tests Online: Empower Your Health. Understand Your Tests. A public resource on clinical laboratory testing.*N.p., n.d. Web. 08 Mar. 2017.
- "Cholesterol." *Lab Tests Online: Empower Your Health. Understand Your Tests. A public resource on clinical laboratory testing.*N.p., n.d. Web. 08 Mar. 2017.
- "Renal Function Panel | Blood test for Kidney Function." *Request A Test.* N.p., n.d. Web. 08 Mar. 2017.
- "Glucose Tests." *Lab Tests Online: Empower Your Health. Understand Your Tests. A public resource on clinical laboratory testing.*N.p., n.d. Web. 08 Mar. 2017.

Chapter 56: Your Wellness Team—You Don't Have to Do It Alone

General References:

- "Benefits of Physiotherapy." *Benefits of Physiotherapy | Physiotherapy Association of British Columbia.* N.p., n.d. Web. 08 Mar. 2017.
- Dentistry, The Center For Natural. "What is Holistic Dentistry?" *Natural Dentistry in Encinitas, CA | Cosmetic Dentistry, Holistic Dentistry, Restorative Dentistry, & More! | The Center for Natural Dentistry.* The Center For Natural Dentistry, 09 Oct. 2009. Web. 08 Mar. 2017.

Chapter 57: Accountability—Who Is Helping You Grow?

General references:

- *Built to Last Successful Habits of Visionary Companies.* N.p.: Paw Prints, 2011. Print.
- Rubin, Gretchen. *Better than before.* New York: Crown Publishers, 2015. Print.
- "True North Groups Reviews." *Bill George Headshot.* N.p., n.d. Web. 08 Mar. 2017.
- "True North Groups Stories." *Bill George Headshot.* N.p., n.d. Web. 08 Mar. 2017.

SECTION 12: GET ON PURPOSE–DESIGNING THE LIFE YOU WANT

Chapter 58: Life Purpose—Are You Living Yours?

General References:

- Csikszentmihalyi, Mihaly. *Flow: the psychology of optimal experience.* New York: Harper Perennial Modern Classics, 2009. Print.
- Pink, Daniel H. *Drive.* N.p.: n.p., 2009. Print.
- Seligman, Martin. *Authentic happiness.* S.l.: Nicholas Brealey Pub, 2017. Print.
- *Abraham Maslow: the hierarchy of needs.* Corby: Institute of Management Foundation, 1998. Print.
- Burchard, Brendon. *The motivation manifesto: 9 declarations to claim your personal power.* London: Simon & Schuster, 2014. Print.

Chapter 59: Strengths Finder—How to Find and Develop Yours

General References:

- Wright, David E. *Discover your inner strength: cutting edge growth strategies from the industry's leading experts.* Sevierville, TN: Insight Publishing, 2009. Print.
- Gallup, Inc. "Clifton StrengthsFinder." *Clifton StrengthsFinder.* N.p., n.d. Web. 08 Mar. 2017.
- Rath, Tom. *Strengths finder 2.0.* New York: Gallup, 2007. Print.
- Seligman, Martin E. P., and Jane Gillham. *The science of optimism & hope: research essays in honor of Martin E.P. Seligman.* Philadelphia: Templeton Foundation Press, 2000. Print.
- Payne, Mark. *Pareto principle.* Place of publication not identified: Publishamerica, 2012. Print.
- Polly, Shannon, Kathryn Britton, and Senia Maymin. *Character strengths matter: how to live a full life.* Charleston, SC?: Positive Psychology News, LLC, 2015. Print.

Chapter 60: 10x Your Life—Are You Thinking Big Enough?

General References:

- Cardone, Grant. *The 10x rule: the only difference between success and failure.* Hoboken, NJ: Wiley, 2011. Print.

Chapter 61: Philosophy—We All Need It

General References:

- Rand, Ayn, Lloyd James, and Leonard Peikoff. *Philosophy: who needs it.* Ashland, OR: Blackstone Audio, 2006. Print.
- Gentempo, P. (2014, December 14). *Unleashing The Power of Philosophy* [TEDx Talk].